Decision Making in Health and Medicine

Integrating Evidence and Values

Second Edition

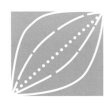

Decision Making in Health and Medicine

Integrating Evidence and Values

Second Edition

M.G. Myriam Hunink
Milton C. Weinstein

Eve Wittenberg
Michael F. Drummond
Joseph S. Pliskin
John B. Wong
Paul P. Glasziou

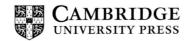

CAMBRIDGE
UNIVERSITY PRESS

CAMBRIDGE
UNIVERSITY PRESS

University Printing House, Cambridge CB2 8BS, United Kingdom

Cambridge University Press is part of the University of Cambridge.

It furthers the University's mission by disseminating knowledge in the pursuit of education, learning and research at the highest international levels of excellence.

www.cambridge.org
Information on this title: www.cambridge.org/9781107690479

Second Edition © M. G. Myriam Hunink, Milton C. Weinstein, et al. (the authors) 2014

First Edition © M. G. Myriam Hunink, Paul P. Glasziou, et al. (the authors) 2001

Second Edition first published 2014

First Edition first published 2001

Printed in Spain by Grafos SA, Arte sobre papel

A catalog record for this publication is available from the British Library

Library of Congress Cataloging in Publication data
Hunink, M. G. Myriam, author.
Decision making in health and medicine : integrating evidence and values / M.G. Myriam Hunink,
Milton C. Weinstein, Eve Wittenberg, Michael F. Drummond, Joseph S. Pliskin, John B. Wong,
Paul P. Glasziou. – Second edition.
    p. ; cm.
Preceded by Decision making in health and medicine : integrating evidence and values / M.G. Myriam
Hunink ... [et al.]. 2001.
Includes bibliographical references and index.
ISBN 978-1-107-69047-9 (Paperback)
I. Title.
[DNLM: 1. Decision Making.   2. Delivery of Health Care.   3. Decision Support
Techniques.   4. Evidence-Based Medicine.   5. Uncertainty.   W 84.1]
R723.5
610–dc23   2014000260

ISBN 978-1-107-69047-9 Paperback

Additional resources for this publication are available at www.cambridge.org/9781107690479

Cambridge University Press has no responsibility for the persistence or accuracy
of URLs for external or third-party internet websites referred to in this publication,
and does not guarantee that any content on such websites is, or will remain,
accurate or appropriate.

....

In memoriam
Howard S. Frazier
Jane C. Weeks

Contents

Additional resources can be found at www.cambridge.org/9781107690479

Foreword

Suppose we are sitting in a room, and I tell you that if you walk out a certain door, you will die instantly. However, if you remain in your chair for another five minutes, you can leave when you like with no ill effects. If you believe me, and you value your life, you will stay put, at least for five minutes.

This situation poses an easy choice. It requires little thought and no analysis, and the best option is transparently clear. A number of attributes make this an easy case: First, the choice is stark, with only two extreme outcomes, live or die. Second, the consequences are certain-live if you stay, die if you leave. Third, the outcomes are immediate, with no time delay. Fourth, there are no financial costs involved, and if anything the preferred choice (staying in your chair) is easier than getting up and leaving. And finally, you are making this choice for yourself; you are the one who decides and who will experience the outcomes.

Unfortunately, real-life situations related to medicine and health are murkier and more complicated. The choices are much more varied than "stay or go" and may involve a range of possible tests and treatments, as well as watchful waiting. The attainable outcomes include many possible states of ill-health, ranging from minor inconvenience to severe pain and disability, as well as death. The intermediate and ultimate results are rife with uncertainty, and the various states of illness may play out over a long time period. Typically, both a doctor and a patient are involved in decision-making, and, in some cases, perhaps family members and others as well. The doctor generally knows more about what may happen, and the patient understands more about their own preferences, and both information and values bear on the best decision. Layer on top of all this the emotionality and urgency that occasionally attends to health and medical care. And then try to contemplate questions of cost and choices that can affect the health of an entire population.

This book presents a systematic approach to identifying, organizing, and considering these many complexities in health and medical care. In a sense, all of the tools described in these pages are designed to convert the complex and uncertain realities of health and medicine into the decision-equivalent of the simple "stay or go" question posed above. For example, probability analysis converts the array of uncertain, intermediate, and ultimate states into an overall expectation of what will or will not happen (as if they were simply certain to live or certain to die). Utility assessment allows a decision maker to rank the value of all possible outcomes on a scale (between life and death) that is quantitatively meaningful for decisions. Discounting allows one to set equivalents for outcomes that play out at different times (as if the outcomes were all to occur now). Modeling enables one to take account of complex interactions and the iterative quality of many disease processes over time (as if they were clear-cut and instantaneous). Tools such as balance sheets and decision diagrams enable one to take account of the problem as a whole and to focus at different times on specific parts without losing sight of the whole, something the unaided human mind cannot possibly accomplish. And cost-effectiveness analysis enables one to consider systematically the most efficient means of achieving one's aims, when costs matter. And today, costs frequently matter.

The Institute of Medicine (IOM) has long been a champion of patient-centered care. It is one of the six core attributes of quality defined by the IOM and arguably the most fundamental aim. If we are truly centered on the needs of patients, and on the health needs of people more generally, the goals of safe, effective, timely, efficient, and equitable care naturally follow as part of attaining higher-quality care. The tools and techniques outlined in this text will not make an uncaring physician more compassionate, nor an indifferent caregiver more centered on the needs of the patient. However, for doctors who are compassionate and caring, these tools will strengthen their ability to reach decisions with patients that truly serve the patient's interests in health and medicine.

President, Institute of Medicine   **Harvey V. Fineberg, M.D., Ph.D.**
June 2014

Foreword to the first edition (2001)

> ... high Arbiter *Chance* governs all.
>
> John Milton, *Paradise Lost*, book II, lines 909–10

When the predecessor to this book was being prepared in the late 1970s (Weinstein et al., 1980), medical decision making seemed to have become more complicated than ever before. The number of diagnostic and therapeutic options dwarfed those of an earlier generation, and the costs of care were growing relentlessly. Increasing numbers of patients expected to play an active role in decisions that affected their lives, and many physicians were acclimating themselves to a less authoritarian doctor–patient relationship. The tools of decision analysis permitted the clinician and patient to break down the complexity of a medical situation into its constituent parts, to identify and assess the pertinent uncertainties and values, and to reassemble the pieces into a logical guide to action.

Today, a generation later, the dilemma of medical decision making seems even more problematic. This is not merely the result of scientific and technologic advances – ingenious new devices, pharmaceuticals, surgical possibilities, and other interventions. The environment of decision making has itself become confounded by government agencies and service delivery systems playing a more direct (and directive) role in decision making. Today, not only are the costs of care a prime concern, so, too, is the quality of care. Patients no longer need rely mainly on their physicians to gain access to medical information – the internet has given millions a direct line to abundant information, though of variable accuracy and pertinence. In light of progress in mapping the human genome, clinicians may soon face profound ethical questions that only a generation ago were the stuff of science fiction.

These dynamic changes in medicine, in science, and in the health-care environment make this new book more valuable than ever. This volume conveys both fundamental and sophisticated methods that can render complex health-care situations more comprehensible. It would be a mistake, however, to think that the methods described in this volume apply only to the exceptional case, to the rare clinical encounter. The task of integrating scientific knowledge, clinical evidence, and value judgments into coherent decisions remains the daily task of medical care.

Much of what counts for differences in outcome related to medicine comes not from failure to access experimental and expensive technology. It comes rather from the failure to deploy relatively inexpensive and proven technology to all those who need it: vaccine against pneumonia for those at risk, beta-blockers in the period following myocardial infarction, appropriate screening for cancer, and much more. The challenge for quality improvement is not the extraordinary case and exceptional decision so much as the challenge to implement systematically the preventive, diagnostic, and therapeutic measures for all who would benefit at reasonable cost. The lessons in this book can reinforce the case for sounder everyday decisions in medicine and health care.

Regardless of how far science and health care advance, the element of chance will remain a fixture in medical encounters. A refined understanding of causation and prognosis will alter how much we know about the likelihood of certain consequences, but uncertainty will persist. Much of medical learning can be interpreted as an effort to reduce the range of uncertainty in medical care. The ideas and methods provided in this volume teach how to make informed decisions in the face of the uncertainty which inevitably remains.

The methods in this book to aid decision makers are simply tools. They are tools for the willing clinician. They are tools for the worried patient. They are tools for the concerned policy maker and payer. They will not make a hazardous situation safe, nor will they make a lazy or incompetent clinician into a superior caregiver. If the methods do not eliminate controversy, they can clarify the reasons for differences of opinion. In dealing with the realities and uncertainties of life and illness, they will enable the thoughtful clinician, the honest patient, and the open-minded policy maker to reach more reasoned conclusions.

Provost, Harvard University   **Harvey V. Fineberg**

REFERENCE

Weinstein MC, Fineberg HV, Elstein AS, et al. *Clinical Decision Analysis.* Philadelphia, USA: WB Saunders; 1980. ISBN 0-7216-9166-8.

Preface

How often do you find yourself struggling with a decision, be it a medical decision, a policy decision, or a personal one? In clinical medicine and health-care policy, making decisions has become a very complicated process: we have to make trade-offs between risks, benefits, costs, and preferences. We have to take into account the rapidly increasing evidence – some good, some poor – presented in scientific publications, on the worldwide web, and by the media. We have to integrate the best available evidence with the values relevant to patient and society; and we have to reconcile our intuitive notions with rational analysis.

In this book we explain and illustrate tools for integrating quantitative evidence-based data and subjective outcome values in making clinical and health-policy decisions. The book is intended for all those involved in clinical medicine or health-care policy who would like to apply the concepts from decision analysis to improve their decision making process. The audience we have in mind includes (post-)graduate students and health-care professionals interested in medical decision making, clinical decision analysis, clinical epidemiology, evidence-based medicine, technology assessment in health care, and health-care policy. The main part of the book is written with graduate students as audience in mind. Some chapters cover advanced material and as such we would recommend reserving this material for advanced courses in decision modeling (the second half of Chapters 4 and 7, and the entire Chapters 10, 11, and 12).

The authors' backgrounds ensure that this is a multidisciplinary text. Together we represent general practice, internal medicine, radiology, mathematics, decision sciences, psychology of decision making, health economics, health-care policy and management. The examples in the book are taken from both clinical practice and from health policy.

There is a previous version of this book (Weinstein et al., 1980), but the name of the book has changed, the content is 80% different, the publisher has changed, and the list of authors has changed. The main message is, however, the same! And the main message is the same: decisions in clinical medicine and health care in general can benefit from a proactive approach to decision making in which evidence and values are integrated into one framework. In addition, substantial changes have been made compared with the first edition of this book (Hunink et al., 2001): Chapters 11 and 13 are totally new, all existing chapters have been thoroughly revised to present current insights, examples throughout the book have been updated to be clinically relevant in today's practice, figures have been improved (especially in Chapter 6) and more figures have been added, and the supplementary material has been expanded and revised.

The book comes with a website. The book itself can, however, be read without immediate access to the website, that is, in a comfortable chair or on a couch! The website supplies additional materials: assignments and their solutions, examples of the decision models in the book programmed using decision analytical software, supplementary materials for the chapters including some useful spreadsheets and model templates, and the references. Access to the teachers' website, which contains additional useful material, is available on request.

We hope you enjoy reading. Good (but calculated) luck with your decision making!

M.G. Myriam Hunink
on behalf of all the authors

REFERENCE

Hunink MGM, Glasziou PP, Siegel JE, Weeks JC, Pliskin JS, Elstein AS, Weinstein MC. *Decision Making in Health and Medicine: Integrating Evidence and Values*. Cambridge: Cambridge University Press, Cambridge; 2001. ISBN 978-0521770293.

Weinstein MC, Fineberg HV, Elstein AS, et al. *Clinical Decision Analysis*. Philadelphia, USA: WB Saunders; 1980. ISBN 0-7216-9166-8.

Acknowledgments

A book never gets prepared by the authors only. Numerous people helped to make this book come into being. We would like to thank those who reviewed the manuscript, edited, revised, and helped prepare the exercises, solutions, references, and supplementary material. For the second edition this included: Marieke Langhout, Ursula Rochau, Isha Argawal, Bart Ferket, Bob van Kempen, Steffen Petersen, Jane Weeks, Ewout Steyerberg, and Bas Groot Koerkamp.

We would especially like to acknowledge the contributions of the authors of the previous version and the authors of the first edition of the book who were not directly involved this time: Harvey V. Fineberg, Howard S. Frazier, Duncan Neuhauser, Raymond R. Neutra, Barbara J. McNeil, Joanna E. Siegel, Jane C. Weeks, and Arthur S. Elstein. Also, we would like to thank the reviewers of the first edition.

Writing a book consists not only of putting text on paper, making illustrations, and having the chapters proofread, but also the thoughts, ideas, and intellectual input from many, too numerous to list and often difficult to identify, have played a role in getting this book together. We are grateful for the intellectual input from our colleagues, students, and postgraduates at the University of Queensland, Bond University, Ben Gurion University, University of York, Erasmus University Medical Center Rotterdam, Netherlands Institute of Health Sciences, Tufts University Medical School, Harvard School of Public Health, and members of the Society for Medical Decision Making.

Last, but certainly not least, we would like to thank our families for being supportive and giving us the opportunity to spend time working on the book during many evenings and weekends.

Abbreviations

ACP	American College of Physicians
ASR	age–sex–race
CABG	coronary artery bypass grafting
CAD	coronary artery disease
CDC	Centers for Disease Control and Prevention
CEA	carotid endarterectomy
CEA	cost-effectiveness analysis
CE25	certainty equivalent 25
CE50	certainty equivalent 50
CE ratio	cost-effectiveness ratio
CI	confidence interval
CPI	Consumer Price Index
CRC	colorectal cancer
CT	computed tomography
CTA	computed tomography angiography
CVD	cardiovascular disease
DALY	disability-adjusted life year
DRG	diagnostic-related group
DVT	deep venous thrombosis
EBCT	electron beam computed tomography
EKG	electrocardiogram
EQ-5D	EuroQol with five dimensions
EU	expected utility
EVCI	expected value of clinical information
EVPI	expected value of perfect information
EVPPI	expected value of partial perfect information
EVSI	expected value of sample information
FNR	false-negative ratio
FOBT	fecal occult blood test

FPR	false-positive ratio
HBV	hepatitis B virus
HDL	high-density lipoprotein
HIV	human immunodeficiency virus
HMO	health maintenance organization
HRR	hazard rate ratio
HUI	Health Utilities Index
IV	intravenous
LE	life expectancy
LR	likelihood ratio
MeSH	Medical Subject Headings
MI	myocardial infarction ('heart attack')
MISCAN	Microsimulation of Screening for Cancer
MRI	magnetic resonance imaging
MRA	magnetic resonance angiography
NHB	net health benefit
NMB	net monetary benefit
OME	otitis media with effusions ('glue ear')
OR	odds ratio
ORS	oral rehydration solution
PAD	peripheral artery disease
PAT	paroxysmal atrial tachycardia
PE	pulmonary embolism
PTA	percutaneous transluminal angiography
PV	present value
QALE	quality-adjusted life expectancy
QALY	quality-adjusted life year
QWB	Quality of Well-Being scale
RCT	randomized controlled trial
ROC	receiver operating characteristic
RR	relative risk
RRR	relative risk reduction
RRTO	risk–risk trade-off
RS	rating scale
SF-36	36-Item Short Form
SG	standard gamble
SIP	Sickness Impact Profile
TNR	true-negative ratio
TPR	true-positive ratio
VAS	visual analog scale
V/Q scan	ventilation–perfusion scan
WTP	willingness to pay

About the authors

M.G. Myriam Hunink, B.Sc., M.D., Ph.D. trained and practiced as an interventional and cardiovascular radiologist. Currently she directs the Assessment of Radiological Technology (ART) program and the division of Clinical Epidemiology at the Erasmus MC and dedicates herself to research and teaching. She is Professor of Clinical Epidemiology and Radiology at the Erasmus University Medical Center, Rotterdam, the Netherlands and Adjunct Professor of Health Decision Sciences at Harvard School of Public Health, Harvard University, Boston. She is a past president of the Society for Medical Decision Making and a recipient of their Distinguished Service award. Her main research interests are comparative effectiveness research and health technology assessment studies of diagnostic and prognostic imaging tests (biomarkers) and image-guided therapies, in particular for cardiovascular disease. Other research interests include integrated diagnostics, computerized decision support for evidence-based use of imaging tests, and (imaging to measure) the effectiveness of lifestyle interventions. Her vision is to optimize medical decisions by combining the best available quantitative evidence on risks and benefits from diverse sources and integrating patient values, preferences, quality of life, and costs.

Milton C. Weinstein, A.B./A.M., M.P.P., Ph.D. is the Henry J. Kaiser Professor of Health Policy and Management at the Harvard School of Public Health and Professor of Medicine at the Harvard Medical School. At the Harvard School of Public Health he is Academic Director of the Center for Health Decision Science, and Director of the Program on Economic Evaluation of Medical Technology. He is best known for his research on cost-effectiveness of medical practices and for developing methods of economic evaluation and decision analysis in health care. He is a co-developer of the CEPAC (Cost-Effectiveness of Preventing AIDS Complications) computer simulation model, and has conducted studies on prevention and treatment of HIV infections. He was the co-developer of the Coronary Heart Disease Policy Model, which has been used to evaluate the cost-effectiveness of cardiovascular prevention and treatment. He consults with industry and government and is a Principal Consultant with Optuminsight. He is an elected member of the Institute of Medicine of the National Academy of Sciences, a past president and recipient of the Career Achievement Award of the Society for Medical Decision Making, and the Avedis Donabedian Lifetime Achievement Award from the International Society for Pharmacoeconomics and Outcomes Research.

Eve Wittenberg, M.P.P., Ph.D. is a Senior Research Scientist at the Center for Health Decision Science at the Harvard School of Public Health. Her interests include the conceptualization and measurement of well-being and values across individuals and health conditions, and the application of this information to clinical decision making and policy. She has estimated economic utilities for conditions ranging from cancer to intimate partner violence, and has a special focus on health issues for vulnerable and under-studied populations. Her recent work includes studies of choice-based methods to inform preference research and design of interventions, as well as measurement approaches to capture family spillover effects of illness. She teaches in the decision science curriculum at the Harvard School of Public Health and advises students in health policy.

Michael F. Drummond, B.Sc., M.Com., D.Phil. is Professor of Health Economics and former Director of the Centre for Health Economics at the University of York, UK. His particular field of interest is in the economic evaluation of health care treatments and programmes. He has undertaken evaluations in a wide range of medical fields including care of the elderly, neonatal intensive care, immunization programs, services for people with AIDS, eye health care and pharmaceuticals. He has acted as a consultant to the World Health Organization and was Project Leader of a European Union Project on the Methodology of Economic Appraisal of Health Technology. He has been President of the International Society of Technology Assessment in Health Care, and the International Society for Pharmacoeconomics and Outcomes Research. He was previously a member of the Guidelines Review Panels of the National Institute for Health and Clinical Excellence (NICE) in the UK, is a Principal Consultant for Optuminsight, and editor-in-chief of Value in Health. He has been awarded two honorary degrees, from City University, London (2008) and Erasmus University, Rotterdam (2012). In 2010 he was made a member of the Institute of Medicine of the National Academies in the USA and in 2012 he was the recipient of The John Eisenberg Award, in recognition of exemplary leadership in the practical application of medical decision-making research, by the Society for Medical Decision Making.

Joseph S. Pliskin, B.Sc., S.M., Ph.D. is the Sidney Liswood Professor of Health Care Management at Ben Gurion University of the Negev, Beer-Sheva, Israel. He was chairman of the Department of Health Systems Management and is a member of the Department of Industrial Engineering and Management. He is also an Adjunct Professor in the Department of Health Policy and Management at the Harvard School of Public Health, Boston, USA. His research interests focus on clinical decision making, operations management in health care organizations, cost–benefit and cost-effectiveness analysis in health and medicine, technology assessment, utility theory, and decision analysis. He has published extensively on issues relating to end-stage renal disease, heart disease, Down syndrome, technology assessment, and methodological issues in decision analysis. In 2004 he received the Career Achievement Award of the Society for Medical Decision Making and in 2012 he was the recipient of a Harvard School of Public Health teaching award.

John B. Wong, B.S., M.D. is a general internist, Chief of the Division of Clinical Decision Making at Tufts Medical Center, Director of Comparative Effectiveness Research at Tufts Clinical Translational Science Institute, and Professor of Medicine at the Tufts University School of Medicine. He is a past president of the Society for Medical Decision Making and a recipient of their Distinguished Service award. He has been an invited member of the ISPOR-SMDM Modeling Good Research Practices Task Force and of guideline committees for the American Association for the Study of Liver Disease, European League Against Rheumatism, the AMA Physician Consortium for Performance Improvement Work Groups on Coronary Artery Disease, Hypertension, Heart Failure, Cardiac Imaging, and Hepatitis C, and the Technical Panel for the ACCF Appropriate Use Criteria for Diagnostic Catheterization and Multi-modality Imaging. His research focuses on the application of decision analysis to help patients, physicians, and policymakers choose among alternative tests, treatments, or policies, thereby promoting rational evidence-based efficient and effective patient-centered care. As a content editor at the Informed Medical Decisions Foundation, he has helped develop award winning decision aid programs for testing, treatment, and management of heart disease to facilitate shared decision making.

Paul P. Glasziou, F.R.A.C.G.P., Ph.D. is Professor of Evidence-based Medicine and Director, Centre for Research in Evidence-based Practice, Bond University, Australia. He was a general practitioner at the Inala Community Health Centre, and at Beaumont St, Oxford. He teaches evidence-based practice to medical students and other health care workers. He holds honorary positions as Professor at the University of Oxford, and Professor at the University of Sydney. Dr Glasziou was the co-editor of the BMJ's *Journal of Evidence-Based Medicine*, and Director of the Centre for Evidence-based Medicine, University of Oxford. His research interests focus on identifying and removing the barriers to using high-quality research in everyday clinical practice.

Elements of decision making in health care

And take the case of a man who is ill. I call two physicians: they differ in opinion. I am not to lie down and die between them: I must do something.

Samuel Johnson

1.1 Introduction

How are decisions made in practice, and can we improve the process? Decisions in health care can be particularly awkward, involving a complex web of diagnostic and therapeutic uncertainties, patient preferences and values, and costs. It is not surprising that there is often considerable disagreement about the best course of action. One of the authors of this book tells the following story (1):

> Being a cardiovascular radiologist, I regularly attend the vascular rounds at the University Hospital. It's an interesting conference: the Professor of Vascular Surgery really loves academic discussions and each case gets a lot of attention. The conference goes on for hours. The clinical fellows complain, of course, and it sure keeps me from my regular work. But it's one of the few conferences that I attend where there is a real discussion of the risks, benefits, and costs of the management options. Even patient preferences are sometimes (albeit rarely) considered.
>
> And yet, I find there is something disturbing about the conference. The discussions always seem to go along the same lines. Doctor R. advocates treatment X because he recently read a paper that reported wonderful results; Doctor S. counters that treatment X has a substantial risk associated with it, as was shown in another paper published last year in the world's highest-ranking journal in the field; and Doctor T. says that given the current limited health-care budget maybe we should consider a less expensive alternative or no treatment at all. They talk around in circles for ten to 15 minutes, each doctor reiterating his or her opinion. The professor, realizing that his fellows are getting irritated, finally stops the discussion. Practical chores are waiting; there are patients to be cared for. And so the professor concludes: 'All right. We will offer the patient treatment X.' About 30% of those involved in the decision-making process nod their heads in agreement; another 30% start bringing up objections which get stifled quickly by the fellows who *really* do not want an encore, and the remaining 40% are either too tired or too flabbergasted to respond, or are more concerned about another objective, namely their job security.

The authors of this book are all familiar with conferences like this. We suspect our readers also recognize the scenario and that they too have wondered, 'Isn't there a better way to make clinical decisions? Isn't there a better way for health professionals, policy makers, patients, and the general public to communicate with each other and talk things out when the going gets tough?'

This book addresses these questions. The methods we present can be helpful to all decision makers in the health-care arena – patients; physicians, nurses, other providers of clinical services; public health and hospital administrators; health-care payers in both the private and public sectors; and clinical and public health researchers whose job it is to offer wise and reasoned counsel.

Health-care decisions have become complex. As recently as a century ago, a physician had only a narrow range of possible diagnoses, a handful of simple tests, and a few, mostly ineffective, treatments to choose from. For example, the first edition of the justly famous *Merck Manual* (1899) ran to 192 pages. Since then our understanding of disease processes and our ability to control them have vastly increased, but so too has the complexity of health-care decisions. The 1999 centennial edition of the *Merck Manual* runs to 2833 pages (2). Currently our health-care technologies are expanding even further and faster, as is our knowledge about them, making modern electronic media indispensable in providing up-to-date information. Websites and mobile applications summarizing the evidence have proliferated over the last decade. All this knowledge needs to be integrated in a logical and wise fashion in order to optimize the decisions we make.

While new treatments have improved the outcome for many conditions, and even eliminated some diseases such as smallpox, many treatments are 'halfway' technologies that improve a condition but do not cure. For example, in cancer, there are many new, useful but sometimes taxing treatments that improve the prognosis without curing. Along with this increase in management options, we now contemplate treatment in a broader range of diseases, from mild hypertension to major disfigurement. This combination of a broad range of illnesses and imperfect treatment options increases our potential to help, but it also increases costs and makes decision making more complex and difficult. In this chapter, we outline a systematic approach to describing and analyzing decision problems. This approach, decision analysis, is intended to improve the quality of decisions and of communication between physicians, patients, and other health-care professionals. Decision analysis is designed to deal with choice under uncertainty and so it is naturally suited to both clinical and public health settings. We believe that decision analysis is a valuable tool for physicians and others concerned with health-care decision making, both for decisions affecting individual patients and for health policy decisions affecting populations of patients. The ability of physicians collectively to command a vast array of powerful and expensive diagnostic and therapeutic interventions carries with it a social responsibility to use these resources wisely. Decision analysis is a systematic, explicit, quantitative way of making decisions in health care that can, we believe, lead to both enhanced communication about clinical controversies and better decisions. At a minimum, the methods we expound can illuminate what we disagree about and where better data or clearer goals are needed. At best, they may assure us that the decisions we make are the logical consequences of the evidence and values that were the inputs to the decision. That is no small achievement.

1.2 Decision making and uncertainty

Unlike most daily decisions, many health-care decisions have substantial consequences and involve important uncertainties and trade-offs. The uncertainties may be about the diagnosis, the accuracy of available diagnostic tests, the natural history of the disease, the effects of treatment in an individual patient or the effects of an intervention in a group or population as a whole. With such complex decisions, it can be difficult to comprehend all options 'in our heads,' let alone to compare them. We need to have some visual or written aids. Hence a major purpose of decision analysis is to assist in comprehension of the problem and to give us insight into what variables or features of the problem should have a major impact on our decision. It does this by allowing and encouraging the decision maker to divide the logical structure of a decision problem into its components so that they can be analyzed individually and then to recombine them systematically so as to suggest a decision. Here are two representative situations that can be addressed with this approach:

EXAMPLE 1   As a member of the State Committee for common childhood diseases, you have been asked to help formulate a policy on the management of chronic otitis media with effusions (also known as 'glue ear'). Glue ear is the most common cause of hearing problems in childhood and can lead to delayed language development. Many treatment choices exist, including grommets (pressure-equalizing tympanostomy tubes), analgesics, antibiotics, vaccinations (pneumococcal and influenza) and hearing aids (3). However, since glue ear usually resolves spontaneously, you might also choose to do nothing, at least initially. Given these various treatment options, should your committee recommend monitoring for hearing loss, treatment with grommet insertion, or the use of hearing aids? For example, tympanometry, which measures the eardrum's ability to move, can be used as a monitoring tool, though an audiogram is needed to confirm the degree of any hearing loss. How do you proceed with formulating a recommendation? How can you systematically approach such a decision?

EXAMPLE 2   A 70-year-old man with severe three-vessel coronary artery disease is being evaluated for coronary artery bypass grafting (CABG). An ultrasound demonstrates a
90% asymptomatic stenosis (a narrowing) of one of the carotid arteries leading to
the brain. The decision faced by the team of physicians is whether to:
(a) perform coronary artery bypass surgery, without further diagnostic workup or
     treatment of the carotid artery stenosis;
(b) perform a carotid CT angiography to confirm the diagnosis and then a carotid
     endarterectomy (i.e., surgery to clear the obstruction in the carotid artery) prior
     to coronary artery bypass surgery;
(c) perform carotid CT angiography and if the diagnosis is confirmed then perform
     carotid endarterectomy during the same procedure as the bypass surgery.

Medical decisions must be made, and they are often made under conditions of
uncertainty. Uncertainty about the current state of the patient may arise from
erroneous observation or inaccurate recording of clinical findings or misin-
terpretation of the data by the clinician. For example, was the carotid artery
stenosis really asymptomatic? Did the patient ever have a transient ischemic
attack (temporary symptoms due to loss of blood flow to a region of the brain)
that went unnoticed or that he interpreted as something else?

Uncertainty may also arise due to ambiguity of the data or variations in
interpretation of the information. For example, if you repeated the ultrasound
examination, would you get the same result? Uncertainty exists too about the
correspondence between clinical information and the presence or absence of
disease. The ultrasound is not perfect: how accurately does it indicate the
presence or absence of a carotid artery stenosis? Some patients with a stenosis
may be falsely classified as not having the disease, and some patients without a
stenosis may be falsely classified as having the disease. Does our patient really
have a carotid artery stenosis?

Finally, the effects of treatment are uncertain. In Example 1, there is
essentially no diagnostic uncertainty, but there is uncertainty about the
outcomes of treatment and about whether a trial of watchful waiting might
allow the glue ear to clear up without medical or surgical intervention and
without harm to the child. An important uncertainty, therefore, is the natural
history of the disease. In Example 2, there would be uncertainty about the
outcome of treatment, even if the diagnosis is certain and the treatment is well
established. The rate of treatment failure may be known, but in whom it will
fail is unpredictable at the time the treatment is initiated. For our 70-year-old
patient we cannot predict whether performing a carotid endarterectomy will
really protect him from a stroke during the CABG.

To deal with the uncertainties associated with the decision problem you need to find the best available evidence to support or refute your assumptions, and you need a framework for combining all of these uncertainties into a coherent choice. In a decision analysis process we first make the problem and its objectives explicit; then we list the alternative actions and how these alter subsequent events with their probabilities, values, and trade-offs; and finally we synthesize the balance of benefits and harms of each alternative. We shall refer to this as the PROACTIVE approach (problem – reframe – objectives – alternatives – consequences and chances – trade-offs – integrate – value – explore and evaluate) to health-care decision making. This has three major steps, each with three substeps. (The steps are a modification of the PrOacTive approach suggested by Hammond et al. in their book *Smart Choices* (4)). Though we present this as a linear process, you should be aware that often iteration through some steps will be required, and that sometimes the solution will be apparent before all steps are complete.

1.3 Step 1 – PROactive: the problem and objectives

You should begin by making sure you are addressing the right problem. This first requires that you make explicit what the possible consequences are that you are seeking to avoid or achieve. This may not be straightforward, as there are often different ways of viewing the problem and there may be competing objectives. Exploring these dimensions before analyzing the alternative actions is important to steer the analysis in the right direction. After the initial attempt at defining the *problem*, you should *reframe* the problem from other perspectives, and finally, identify the fundamental *objectives* that you are hoping to attain.

1.3.1 P: Define the problem

What are your principal concerns? A good way to clarify management problems is to begin by asking, 'What would happen if you took no immediate action?' This simple question seeks to uncover the outcomes that you might wish to avoid or achieve. Carefully answering this question should lead to a description of the possible sequences of events in the natural history of the condition. You may need to follow up by asking 'and what then?' several times. For example, a common cause of a very rapid heart beat is paroxysmal supraventricular tachy-cardia or PSVT (episodes of rapid heart beat initiated by the conducting system in the upper heart chambers). A patient with PSVT will typically experience a sudden onset of rapid heart beat (around 200 beats/min), which ceases suddenly after minutes to hours. It is usually accompanied by some anxiety, since patients worry that there is something very wrong with their heart, but it usually causes no

Table 1.1 Consequence table for the wait-and-see option for the problem of otitis media with effusion (glue ear)(6)

Consequences	Wait-and-see option
Hearing	Slow improvement over months to years
Behavior	Poor hearing may lead to disruptive behavior
Language development	Delayed articulation and comprehension (with possible long-term consequences)
Acute middle-ear infections	Recurrent episodes
Long-term complications	Possible conductive problems

other physical discomfort. If a patient presents after such an episode, you may analyze the problem by asking: 'What would happen if you took no immediate action?' A recent study in a cohort of nearly five million eligible patients demonstrated a statistically significant two-fold increase in the incidence of stroke in patients with PSVT compared to those without PSVT (5), demonstrating that the natural history potentially has dire consequences.

Other problems we will consider as illustrative examples in later chapters include management of needlestick injuries, smallpox vaccination, suspected pulmonary embolism, fatigue and iron deficiency anemia, imaging test for chest pain, testing for the BrCa1 gene for breast cancer, and atrial fibrillation. Each of these problems has a complex sequence of uncertain but potentially serious consequences. Visual aids that help describe the problem include decision trees, state-transition diagrams, influence diagrams, and survival plots. These descriptions are necessarily schematic: just as a map is useful to describe a territory, these visual aids help chart the possible course of events. They are helpful in describing and communicating the consequences and hence help navigate the decision-making process. The most straightforward tool to begin with is a *consequence table*, i.e., a tabulation of the principal concerns. Table 1.1 shows this for the management options for glue ear.

DEFINITION   A *consequence table* tabulates the consequences of a choice and considers all relevant perspectives and important dimensions.

1.3.2 R: Reframe from multiple perspectives

Does the problem look different from different perspectives? You should understand how the problem you are dealing with appears to others. In the clinical setting this requires that you broaden, at least temporarily, your focus from a disease framework to one that includes the concerns for the patient. In the context of public health this requires broadening your perspective to include the aggregate limits on resources, as well as the individual perspectives of the patient, the provider, the payer, and the public policy maker.

How does the problem of glue ear appear from different perspectives? You might consider different disciplinary perspectives. For example, biologically, glue ear is a problem of microbes, immune responses, and anatomical dysfunctions. From a psychological perspective, it is one of difficulties in language development. From a sociological perspective, it might be seen to be a problem of classroom behavior and family interactions. A public health practitioner may want to focus attention on adequate vaccination schemes to avoid infections. The child, the parents, the teacher, the primary care physician, the pediatrician, the public health practitioner, and the health-care insurance company will all view the problem differently and have overlapping objectives but with different emphases.

1.3.3 O: Focus on the objective

The main objective of health care is to avert or diminish the consequences of a disease. Sometimes this means prevention or cure; sometimes it may be slowing the disease's progress or preventing the disease's complications; sometimes it may be only the alleviation of symptoms or dysfunction. In our first example, only time will 'cure' the age-related anatomical problem with the Eustachian tube that leads to glue ear, but meanwhile you may alleviate the major problem – deafness – by removing fluid from the middle ear, or you may simply use a hearing aid.

If you framed and reframed the problem appropriately, the pivotal concerns and objectives should have become apparent. However, before proceeding to develop and evaluate options, you should check that you have a clear idea of the objectives. What elements are of most concern to the patient or population? What are the short-term and long-term objectives and concerns, and how do these vary between patients? Sometimes these objectives are straightforward. For example, the objective of immunization decisions is to reduce morbidity and mortality from infectious diseases. However, often there are multiple competing objectives. For example, in managing patients with advanced cancer there may be competing objectives of comfort, function, and length of life, and these may be different for patient and caregivers. If there are trade-offs between the objectives, it is obviously important to understand what the objectives are.

When listing the objectives, you should clearly distinguish between *means objectives* and *fundamental objectives*. A means objective is an intermediate goal but which is only a stepping stone to what we truly value. In our second example, the coronary artery bypass surgery is not a goal in itself, but a means of achieving the fundamental objectives of improved quality of life (less angina, i.e., chest pain) and avoidance of early mortality.

The nature of objectives may be clarified by repeatedly asking 'because?' or 'why?' In our first example, you might consider that insertion of a tympanostomy tube (grommet) will achieve the objective of resolving the glue ear, which may appear to be an objective. Why do you want the glue ear to resolve? Because that will lead to normal hearing. And why do you want normal hearing? Normal hearing will improve quality of life and it is important for proper language development. Why do you want proper language development? Because it improves quality of life. And why do we want to improve quality of life? That is something we intrinsically value, and hence it is a fundamental objective. Thus resolving the glue ear and obtaining normal hearing and proper language development are means objectives, whereas a good quality of life is a fundamental objective.

Understanding the fundamental objectives can help us generate options that achieve such objectives through different means. For example, focusing on quality of life instead of the fluid in the middle ear suggests that analgesics and a hearing aid may be good treatments to consider. Similarly, with the coronary artery bypass graft, you may need to step back and reconsider other options to manage the angina, such as stent placement or optimal medical therapy. Committing too early to a means objective rather than the fundamental objective can unnecessarily narrow our view of the possible options.

1.4 Step 2 – proACTive: the alternatives, consequences, and trade-offs

1.4.1 A: Consider all relevant alternatives

To be able to choose the best alternative in a particular circumstance, you need to know the range of reasonable alternatives. This list may be very long, so it is helpful to have a generic list. All alternatives may be placed in one of three categories: (i) a wait-and-see, watchful waiting, or a 'do-nothing' policy; (ii) initiate an intervention, e.g., treatment now; or (iii) obtain more information before deciding, such as ordering a diagnostic test or doing a population survey. These alternatives are illustrated in the decision tree of Figure 1.1.

The initial line is labeled with the population or problem you are considering (such as glue ear or coronary artery disease). The square represents a

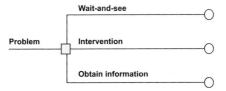

Figure 1.1   Generic decision tree for the initial decision node.

decision node at which just one of the several alternative actions, represented by the subsequent lines, must be chosen. At the decision node, the decision maker is in control. From each alternative action, there will usually be a subsequent chance node (the circles), with branches representing the possible outcomes of each option. The probabilities of events and the ultimate outcomes will depend on the alternative chosen. Let us look in more detail at each of the three generic alternative decisions.

DEFINITION   A *decision tree* is a visual representation of all the possible options and the consequences that may follow each option.

1.4.1.1 Wait-and-see, watchful waiting, or do-nothing policy

A wait-and-see, watchful waiting, or do-nothing policy may take several forms. You may decide to do nothing about the condition. For example, this might be a reasonable choice for benign skin lesions or other variants of 'normal.' However, usually you will have a contingent policy that requires action depending on the disease course over time. The contingencies may be classified as either *monitoring*, where a regular check is made, or *triggering*, where you wait for a change in the type or severity of symptoms.

With monitoring, a check is made at fixed times to see whether the condition has improved, remained the same, or become worse. Action is then based on this progression. For example, you may decide not to treat patients with mild hypertension until their blood pressure increases or they develop other risk factors; the criterion for action is the condition becoming worse. For the glue ear case, you may decide that action is required if no improvement is seen at two months; the criterion is either no change in the condition or a worsening. If a condition is unchanged, why should its persistence indicate a need for action? Imagine that there are two types of the condition: those that spontaneously resolve and those that never resolve. Waiting will allow us to differentiate these. Effectively this is a test-of-time. In reality, the groups will not be so distinct, and the test-of-time will be imperfect. So there will be a trade-off: delay may reduce the benefits for the persistent case but avoid the harm of unnecessary treatment for those who would resolve spontaneously.

With triggering, the patient is advised to return if particular events occur. In family practice this method is known as safety netting – a patient is instructed in the criteria required to catch a potentially ominous change. Clearly, wait-and-see is a strategy rather than a single action. Thus a *strategy* is in fact a sequence of choices contingent on the observed events at chance nodes. In some cases it may be useful to consider several different wait-and-see strategies.

1.4.1.2 Intervention

The next step is to list the active intervention alternatives, refraining from any evaluation of their merit at this point so that the full range of options can be considered. In the glue ear example, intervention would be treatment which may be aimed at cure, at arresting the progress of the disease, at preventing complications, or at alleviating the symptoms. As described earlier, glue ear may be managed by attempting to resolve the effusion (cure), or by prescribing analgesics and use of a hearing aid, which would alleviate the principal symptoms of pain and hearing loss and the consequences.

Where do you get the list of alternatives? Websites, mobile applications, discussions with colleagues and experts, textbooks, and literature searches all contribute. An important component is a search of controlled trials, since these are often the source of the best-quality evidence on the benefits and risks of interventions. The Cochrane Library is a good place to start: it contains systematic reviews of randomized controlled trials (RCTs) and references to RCTs. A search of the Cochrane Library for 'otitis media with effusion' (performed in Sept 2013) provided 12 systematic reviews and 532 RCTs that include: (i) antibiotics, such as ceftibuten, cefixime, amoxicillin, and cotrimoxazole; (ii) oral corticosteroids, such as betamethasone, prednisolone, and prednisone; (iii) intranasal corticosteroids such as beclomethasone; (iv) nonsteroidal anti-inflammatory drugs, such as naproxen and tranilast; (v) tympanostomy tubes (ventilation tubes/grommets) with two major different types; (vi) adenoidectomy; (vii) mucolytics such as carboxymethylcysteine and bromhexine; (viii) autoinflation (mechanical maneuvers which force air up the Eustachian tube); (ix) decongestants and antihistamines; and (x) hearing aids. Some of these options, such as antihistamines, are clearly ineffective. Others, such as mucolytics, autoinflation, and nonsteroidal anti-inflammatory drugs, are of doubtful or uncertain value. The remaining treatments show a range of effectiveness and harms, which need to be compared.

Figure 1.2 shows the start of a decision tree for our second example. In this example, the do-nothing option is to refrain from treating the carotid artery

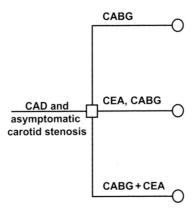

Figure 1.2

Decision tree fragment for Example 2: asymptomatic 90% carotid artery stenosis in a male planned for coronary artery bypass grafting (CABG) for severe three-vessel coronary artery disease (CAD). The options are: perform CABG only; perform carotid endarterectomy (CEA) and then CABG (CEA, CABG); or perform CABG and CEA in a combined procedure (CABG + CEA).

stenosis and proceed directly to CABG. There are at least two alternative treatment options: to either do a combined procedure, or to do the carotid endarterectomy first and then proceed to CABG. Note that this decision tree does not include an 'obtain more information' strategy.

1.4.1.3 Obtain information

If you are uncertain about the prognosis or diagnosis, further information, such as from a diagnostic test, may help in selecting the best intervention. In clinical medicine, diagnostic tests are frequently performed to determine the diagnosis in a patient presenting with symptoms. In public health, performing a diagnostic test usually implies screening to detect disease at a pre-clinical stage or to identify individuals at high risk of developing disease who may be worth targeting for primary prevention. Obtaining more information may also imply determining the prevalence of disease, doing a population survey, or measuring the level of a toxin. Useful information for making a clinical diagnosis may include symptoms, signs, laboratory tests, or imaging tests. Most tests will, however, produce some false-positive and false-negative results. In Chapters 5, 6, and 7, we will look in detail at interpreting such imperfect tests.

Even if the diagnosis is clear, testing may still be helpful to plan treatment, to determine the responsiveness to treatment, or to clarify the prognosis. For example, deciding that CABG should be performed for a patient with angina will require angiography to decide which coronary arteries need to be bypassed and where to place the anastomoses. With glue ear, the test-of-time helps by identifying those who are likely to have a sustained problem. Some tests specifically help to identify those most likely to respond. In women with breast cancer, for example, the presence of estrogen receptors identifies cancers more likely to respond to hormonal treatments such as tamoxifen.

1.4.2 C: Model the consequences and estimate the chances

You need to think through the sequence of consequences of each decision option and the chances of each event. Both short-term and long-term consequences should be considered. For each consequence you need to find the best available evidence to support your arguments. Having listed the alternatives, you next need to consider the consequences of each. This was partly accomplished when you outlined the natural history in Step 1, since natural history outlines the consequences of the do-nothing option. In Chapter 2 we will detail the types of probabilities you will encounter in decision making. These include the risks and benefits of interventions (Chapters 3, 8) and the accuracy and interpretation of diagnostic test information (Chapters 5, 6, and 7). Depending on the type of decision, the relevant outcomes may be identified based on the patient's values and preferences (Chapter 4) and/or the resource costs (Chapter 9).

Each alternative will lead to a different distribution of outcomes which need to be quantified. The relevant outcomes depend on the particular problem at hand. It may be the number of days of illness avoided or deaths prevented by a vaccine for influenza; or the chances of permanent hearing loss if glue ear is untreated; or the chances of five- or ten-year stroke-free survival for the 70-year-old man with coronary artery disease and asymptomatic carotid artery stenosis. Some of the consequences may be better described in diagrams than words. For example, the possible consequences following the combined CABG and carotid endarterectomy operation for our patient in Example 2 might be described as in Figure 1.3, which shows one representation of the *chance tree*.

The round circles (chance nodes) are used to indicate time points at which there are two or more possible consequences. Several sequences of chance nodes may be needed to describe a problem. For Example 2, choosing to do the combined CABG and carotid endarterectomy might result in one of three possible outcomes. Which of the three occurs is beyond our control. However, the likelihood of each can be indicated by the probabilities shown below the branches emanating from the chance node. We will return to the simple mathematics of probability in Chapter 2; for now, note that the probabilities are all between 0 and 1 (or between 0% and 100%, if expressed as percentages), and the sum of the probabilities of all of the branches from a single chance node adds up to 1 (that is, 100%). This reflects the fact that one, and

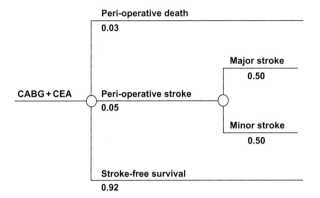

Figure 1.3   Chance tree for combined coronary artery bypass grafting (CABG) and carotid
endarterectomy (CEA) (Example 2).

only one, of the possibilities at each chance node may occur. From each chance arm, there may either be a further division into possible outcomes, such as the major or minor stroke shown in Figure 1.3, or further decisions to be made. The decision tree thus assists in structuring the sequence of choices and outcomes over time.

DEFINITION   A *chance tree* is a visual representation of a series of random discrete linked events. It visualizes the chance that each event can occur.

Sometimes consequences are simple. For example, in patients who have had ventricular fibrillation (a fatal arrhythmia unless resuscitation is given), the main concern is sudden death from a recurrence. Decisions about appropriate drugs or implantable defibrillators will focus around this obviously important outcome. Many disease conditions, however, involve multiple consequences. For these, comparison of the benefits and harms across different options is assisted by a balance sheet.

DEFINITION   A *balance sheet* tabulates the consequences of different options and considers all relevant perspectives and important dimensions.

Table 1.2 provides an example of a balance sheet for some of the alternatives for managing glue ear. Usually, the first alternative will be a wait-and-see strategy and the balance sheet will then incorporate the consequence table from Step 1 (Table 1.1). The subsequent columns will show the consequences of each alternative. Note that the probabilities of uncertain outcomes are also included, e.g., the spontaneous resolution rate and the complication rates.

Table 1.2 Balance sheet for some options for managing glue ear

	Alternatives		
	Monitor (wait-and-see)	**Grommet insertion (short-term tube)**	**Hearing aid**
Potential treatment benefits			
Improve hearing and behavior	Slow improvement of months to years (resolution at 1, 3, and 6 months is 60%, 74%, and 88%)	Rapid improvement with grommet until it falls out in 8 months (range 6–12 months)	Immediately improved
Language development	Delayed (possibly permanent)	'Normal'	'Normal'
Acute middle-ear infections	1–2 episodes per year	Reduced by 0.5 episodes per year	1–2 episodes per year
Long-term complications of glue ear	Uncertain: possible conductive problems	Uncertain effects	Uncertain: possible conductive problems
Potential treatment harms and costs			
Long-term complications of treatment	None	Tympanosclerosis (scarred drum): 40%; retraction: 18%; grommet lost into middle ear[a]: 0.4%; perforation[a]: 0.4%; chronic: 5%	None
Restrictions	None	(Some) swimming restrictions while grommet in place	Need to wear hearing aid
Short-term complications	None	Ear discharge: Brief: 40%	Child may lose hearing aid
Cost	Low	$2400	$600–1500

[a] These complications will require further surgery to retrieve the grommet or patch the perforation.

The balance sheet can be assembled by either describing the outcomes with each alternative, or by describing the relative effects of each alternative (relative to the wait-and-see strategy). Both methods are reasonable, and often one will be more convenient than the other. However, only one method should be used within a single table to insure consistent interpretation of the information presented.

The table will also describe the potential harms and resource use (or costs) of treatment alternatives. These harms and costs will include: (i) the direct burden or discomfort from the intervention; (ii) the complications and adverse effects of the intervention; and (iii) the cost to the health-care system, patients, and their families, including management of any complications. The direct burden may vary considerably. This burden might also include changes in the patient's self-perception. For example, the burden of a diagnosis of hypertension includes not just the taking of a daily medication but also the change in self-perception which has been shown to result in increased sick days taken and poorer career progress. The complications can range from minor dose-related side effects to major surgical complications or drug reactions. Finally, the burden to the health-care system is the cost of the intervention, including personnel, materials, overheads, and costs to patients and families (see Chapter 9).

1.4.3 T: Identify and estimate the trade-offs

In decision analysis it is essential to identify the relevant trade-offs and to capture these in the model. Common trade-offs in medical decisions are the immediate risk of a procedure vs. improved long-term prognosis, quality of life vs. length of life, and health gained vs. costs.

If you are only concerned with a single adverse consequence, such as mortality, then the issue is simply a question of which alternative offers the lowest (expected) probability of that consequence or the highest probability of survival. If there are several disparate consequences, however, the choice of alternative might depend on how we value them. For example, how important is quality of life in relationship to length of life.

With the alternatives for managing glue ear, the inconvenience and perhaps embarrassment of wearing a hearing aid must be weighed against the small probability of complications from grommet insertion. Such trade-offs require clarification of the values involved. In some problems values can be clarified by trying out one of the alternatives. For example, a child with glue ear might borrow a hearing aid to test practicality and satisfaction with the results. Information about the experience of others may also be helpful in deciding whether an alternative is worth trying. In a study of 48 English children with glue ear, 71% reported complete satisfaction with a hearing aid and experienced improved speech and hearing.

Many decisions do not allow such a trial period. A common dilemma is a treatment that offers relief of symptoms but at a small risk of serious adverse consequences. Example 2 is a vivid illustration of this issue. There is a measurable risk of peri-operative mortality to be balanced against the better quality of life and longevity to be gained with successful surgery. Other examples include: total hip replacement for severe arthritis, a procedure which relieves pain and can restore mobility but has a small risk of peri-operative mortality or major complications; non-steroidal anti-inflammatory drugs, which provide relief for several conditions but with a very small risk of stomach bleeding; and a blood transfusion which may relieve symptoms of anemia but has a small risk of a transfusion reaction or blood-borne infection. Because of the processes for drug and device approval in place in most of the industrialized world, the benefits are likely to outweigh the adverse consequences for most commonly used treatments. However, the balance will depend on the individual's disease severity and prognosis as well as on the magnitude of the potential harms and the strength of each individual's outcome preferences. For example, women with the BrCa1 gene are at increased risk of breast cancer, and this risk may be decreased by undergoing bilateral mastectomy, which may affect quality of life. Clearly this is an individual decision and women may have very different values and attitudes towards the risks and outcomes of each choice. Methods for quantifying preferences and values are discussed in Chapter 4. Resource constraints limit the ability of health care to meet all the needs of patients and society and the method of cost-effectiveness analysis is the topic of Chapter 9.

1.5 Step 3 – proactIVE: integration and exploration

Once the probabilities and values of each outcome have been identified, it is time to figure out which option is best. To do this we may need to calculate the expected value – that is, the average value gained from choosing a particular alternative. The option with the highest expected value will generally be chosen, provided we have captured the major decision elements in the analysis. However, you should also explore how sensitive the decision is to the exact probabilities and values chosen. Let us look at these three subcomponents.

1.5.1 I: Integrate the evidence and values

After explicitly formulating the problem, the options, and the associated risks, benefits, and values, it sometimes becomes obvious which option is optimal. Further analysis is unnecessary. But this is not always the case. If there are multiple dimensions, a useful next step is to focus on the important differences between options. To do this with the balance sheet you might first rank the issues in order of importance. The rearranged table on glue ear – with only the two relevant treatment options – is shown in Table 1.3, with the rankings done separately within the benefits and harms. Next, those rows for which the consequences are fairly even may be struck out. These consequences can be ignored, as they are not altered by the available choices. For the treatment of

Table 1.3 Balance sheet with reduction of items to consider by striking out those consequences that are fairly even across the options

	Alternatives	
	Grommet insertion (short-term tube)	Hearing aid
Potential treatment benefits		
Language development	~~Normal~~	~~Normal~~
Improve hearing and behavior	Rapid improvement with grommet until it falls out in 8 months (range 6–12 months)	Immediately improved
Long-term complications of glue ear	~~Uncertain effects~~	~~Uncertain: possible conductive problems~~
Acute middle-ear infections	Reduced by 0.5 episodes per year	1–2 episodes per year
Potential treatment harms and costs		
Long-term complications of treatment	Tympanosclerosis (scarred drum): 40%; retraction: 18%; grommet lost into middle ear[a]: 0.4%; perforation[a]: 0.4%	None
Restrictions	~~(Some) swimming restrictions while grommet in place~~	~~Need to wear hearing aid~~
Short-term complications	Ear discharge: brief: 40%; chronic: 5%	None
Cost	$2400	$600–1500

[a] These complications will require further surgery to retrieve the grommet or patch the perforation.

glue ear, the simplified table suggests that grommet insertion has more complications and slightly greater expense than a hearing aid but reduces the number of acute middle-ear infections.

The balance sheet can help tease out the different dimensions of a problem. However, for some dimensions the sequence of events is complex and will be better represented by a chance tree. If we combine the chance trees for all the options we have a decision tree. With the decision tree we perform a formal calculation of the expected probability of each outcome for each option. In addition, in problems that involve both outcome values and probabilities, the decision tree helps us calculate the expected value of each option.

The process of calculating expected values is described further in Chapter 3. Furthermore, we may want to take quality of life into account, and calculate the expected quality-adjusted life years, which will be described in Chapter 4. Sometimes we will want to consider two different dimensions of the outcomes simultaneously and separately calculate the expected value for each. For example, in Chapter 9 we will incorporate costs, separately calculating expected benefits and expected economic costs, allowing us to calculate the cost per unit of benefit gained.

DEFINITION	The *expected value* of an option is the sum of the values of all the consequences of that option, each value weighed by the probability that the consequence will occur.

1.5.2 V: Optimize the expected value

You have now evaluated each alternative, but which should you choose? Decision analysis employs an explicit principle for making choices: maximize expected utility. The complex and sometimes conflicting information about outcomes, harms, and benefits represented in our list are combined and integrated by a multiplication-and-addition procedure: the probability of each outcome is multiplied by its value, and for each alternative, these products are added. You obtain an expected value for each alternative, and these expectations are the basis for recommending one.

In theory, you should prefer the alternative with the best net expected value, that is, the one that appears to give the best overall utility, taking into account both the chances and value of each consequence. If the outcome values have been expressed as desirable values, we would want to maximize the expected value. If the outcome values have been expressed as undesirable values, we would want to minimize the expected value. Other decision goals are defensible, especially if you think that some especially important objectives or features of the problem have not been included in the analysis. For example, in some situations, some decision makers prefer to minimize the chance of the worst outcome (a mini-max strategy). This 'fear-of-flying' strategy focuses on avoiding a single catastrophic outcome without regard to its probability. It would rule out total hip replacement for hip arthritis because of the small risk of operative mortality, and would eschew medication for anything but life-threatening illnesses because of the small risk of an adverse reaction that was worse than the illness being treated. Precedent, authority, habit, religious considerations, or local consensus may also play a part in making a decision. We think that the approach we have described, which leads to the maximum net expected value, should generally be preferred because it balances considerations of the harms and benefits of all outcomes, weighed by the probability that they will occur.

1.5.3 E: Explore the assumptions and evaluate uncertainty

The approach we have described uses numbers to talk about both the probabilities and the values of treatment outcomes. Clearly some of these numbers will be well established in the clinical literature, while others may be very 'soft.' You may not be sure they are really right. You may be uncertain about whether some probabilities retrieved from the literature apply to our patient, or, if you have to estimate some key probabilities, you may be uncertain about the accuracy of our estimates or concerned about various cognitive biases that have been shown to affect probability estimates (which are discussed in Chapter 13). If you have consulted patients to elicit their values and preferences, you may be uncertain about the stability of the numbers obtained from these inquiries, especially if the patients have been asked to evaluate health states they have not yet experienced (see Chapter 4). What if some or all of these numbers were different? Would our decision change? How much change in any of these numbers will change the recommended decision? Or is the recommendation insensitive to any plausible change in either the probabilities or the utilities?

To understand the effects of these uncertainties on our decision, you should perform a 'what-if' analysis, also known as a *sensitivity analysis*. By varying the uncertain variables over the range of values considered plausible, you can calculate what the effect of that uncertainty is on the decision. If the decision is not sensitive to a plausible change in a parameter value, then the precise value of that parameter is irrelevant. If the decision does change, this warrants further study to find out more precisely what the value is. In Example 2, a sensitivity analysis for age and peri-operative risk in a published decision analysis (7) could enable a decision maker to apply the results to her particular case, or to gain confidence that her decision was best. A quantitative, formal sensitivity analysis permits us to gain insight into what particular variables really drive a decision. If the key variables causing changes are probabilities, we say the decision is 'probability-driven.' More research may be needed to get better or more updated evidence. If the decision hinges on values and preferences, it is said to be 'utility-driven.' These uncertainties cannot be resolved by better evidence, because they are not about the facts but about values and preferences. But they can be ameliorated by value clarification: whose values are at issue? How clear are the decision makers about what they really want? Do they understand the trade-offs that may be involved? Many recently developed decision aids for patients aim to assist in clarifying the patient's values and understanding of the treatment options.

1.6 Using the results

What is the end product of this decision process? You might consider that 'the decision' is the major outcome. However, the insight gained will be useful for other similar decisions. So you should explicitly consider how to capture this insight for future use.

So, how can you apply the results of an analysis to other patients or target populations? Future patients may differ in many ways, so it is not usually the decision that is reapplied but rather the analysis process. Elements of the problem that, if different, are likely to change the decision are the critical factors in applying the decision analysis more broadly. Probabilities, such as the likelihood of having a disease, the likelihoods of observing various test results given the presence or absence of a disease, and the responses to treatments, are among the most important factors. Also important, and often more important, are the values attached to the various dimensions of outcome, such as survival, functional status, and symptoms. Consideration of these factors is assisted by sensitivity and threshold analysis, which we shall cover in several chapters, particularly 3, 6, and 12. Here we shall look briefly at how the results of an analysis might be summarized as a guideline for future decisions.

1.6.1 Guidelines for specific clinical decisions

A clinically useful decision guide (or aid) should meet two requirements. First, it should give the clinician information about how outcomes of a recommended practice are likely to vary with different patient characteristics. Second, the outcomes should be presented in a way that permits incorporating patients' preferences. For example, a summary showing how quality-adjusted life years (see Chapter 4) vary with predictors is helpful for decision making at the level of public health, but it is insufficient at the bedside, as it does not allow each patient's unique values to be incorporated. In constructing a decision guide that will fulfill these two requirements and take account of individual prognosis and values, a decision analyst needs to be mindful of the practicalities and constraints of using a guide in clinical practice: the more it provides for tailoring to an individual patient, the more time it will take to use it, and so it may be less used as its complexity increases. On the other hand, insufficient flexibility also threatens its acceptability in clinical practice.

Decision guides have several formats. These vary in the degree to which they satisfy our two requirements. The most common guide is the section on management in clinical textbooks. These will generally describe some of the alternatives and heuristics for making a choice, along the lines of: 'unless the patient is allergic to penicillin, the first-line treatment should be . . ..' However, these texts are usually not written with the requirements outlined and rarely meet them. There are two other major formats for decision guides: clinical algorithms and balance sheets.

1.6.2 Clinical algorithms

A clinical algorithm consists of a structured sequence of questions and recommended actions based on the answers to those questions. They are also called clinical protocols, clinical pathways, or flow charts. The questions will divide patients into subgroups based on features such as disease severity, allergies, other diseases, etc., which will then lead to a sequence of actions such as investigation or treatment. These algorithms are usually represented as a tree of questions and actions, as illustrated in Figure 1.4.

If we were to develop a decision tree, then prune away the suboptimal alternatives at each decision node and leave out the probability and value estimates, the result would be a clinical algorithm. Thus, decision analysis can be used to develop a clinical algorithm, but not all clinical algorithms are developed using decision analysis. Indeed, most are not.

Algorithms may be developed in different ways, using the opinions and recommendations of individual experts, or of a hospital guideline committee, or of a national consensus group. The development process may be informal or formal, using methods such as the PROACTIVE approach. Clinical algorithms are particularly useful to assist rapid and consistent decision making

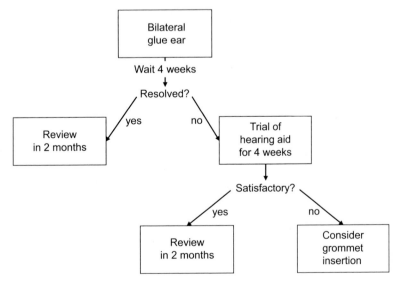

Figure 1.4   A possible clinical algorithm for the management of glue ear (Example 1).

when patient preferences are not crucial. For example, clinical algorithms are common and helpful for the management of cardiac arrests, treatment of anaphylaxis, or preparation for bowel surgery.

A drawback of simply pruning away the non-optimal alternatives is that we cannot readily adapt the steps to different circumstances and patient values. Thus clinical algorithms do not usually satisfy either of our requirements, and therefore have a price in flexibility. An algorithm is usually devised for a well-defined set of circumstances, and it is difficult to broaden it to cover others, even if they are plausibly related to the base condition. For example, if an urgent magnetic resonance imaging scan is recommended, what do you do when the local machine is unavailable for 24 hours and the nearest alternative is 300 km away? Without an estimate of the consequences of following or disregarding a recommendation, we have no guide to action. Thus, not specifying the outcomes used to construct the algorithm limits its applicability. This limitation is most relevant for a decision in which patient values are crucial, such as the choice of contraception, or treatments for prostate and breast cancer. These decisions have no single 'right' choice but depend on the patient's view of the consequences. Algorithms can neglect patients' preferences, however, and still be useful, even in these instances. We return to these issues in Chapter 4.

1.6.3 Balance sheets

An alternative format for a decision guide is the balance sheet. Whether this is in the form of a table (such as Table 1.2) or a graph, the aim is to present quantitative estimates of the consequences of the different reasonable alternatives. It may or may not make a specific recommendation, but it does present the data needed for an informed choice. Hence, we should be able to see the consequences of deviation from the recommended alternative.

1.6.4 Patient-oriented decision aids

For value-sensitive decisions, informing patients adequately may take considerable time that is not available in practice. To break free of this constraint, several investigators have developed patient decision aids that use paper, video, or interactive computer-guided information that describe the problem, the alternatives, and the consequences (8). The informed patient and clinician can then meet to make a final decision. Many of these patient-oriented decision aids are based on the principles expounded in the following chapters, but they generally avoid making a formal recommendation based on expected-utility maximization. Instead, they concentrate on explaining the harms and benefits of each alternative treatment, and leave the decision up to the patients and their clinicians.

1.7 Why are these tools helpful?

What do the tools we have discussed add to decision making in health care? Surely patients, physicians, and public policy makers think in terms of risks and benefits when making medical decisions? The tools enable us to lay out our assumptions, the evidence, and our goals explicitly and systematically, and they help us overcome some well-documented cognitive limitations. A major problem in making decisions without some kind of aid, even one as simple as a consequence table, is that our capacity to deal with complex problems is limited (9, 10). We tend to think we can manage more information at once than is really possible (11, 12). We are inclined to hone in on one particular piece of the problem, and it is difficult to consider the other parts in a balanced way at the same time. We focus first on one aspect, then move on to another, and so on. By the time we have reviewed the entire set of choices, we may have forgotten what was said (or thought) at the beginning. Even if we remember all of the steps in our deliberations, it is difficult to fit all of the pieces together into a coherent package. We run the risk of going round in circles and getting stuck in our thinking and our discussions. We may focus on optimizing one tiny piece and forget to think about whether optimizing that piece serves our global goal, or we may respond to minor variations in the formulation of the problem, features that should not affect our decision (13–15). Or we may be influenced by the sheer number of available alternatives (16). Visual aids and other logical thinking tools help us take a broad perspective. They help us to think through the problem from all angles, to identify conflicting objectives and trade-offs, and to think and communicate in a systematic logical way. It is like 'going to the balcony' and getting a general overview of what's happening.

1.7.1 But are they practical?

How practical are these tools and this sequence of steps? Not all steps will be required for every decision. Sometimes the first few steps will resolve the decision problem. Sometimes knowing the natural history, reassuring the patient, and instructing them when to return will be sufficient. Many other decisions can be resolved by finding the evidence about the effects of different alternatives and clearly describing the consequences – the optimal choice may then be obvious. For many decisions, however, more steps are needed because of the complex trade-off between the consequences.

To complete all nine steps usually takes far more time than is available for the typical patient–physician encounter. Hence, we suggest that for 'once-only' decisions, it is advisable to check the evidence and draw a rough consequence table, even if there is not enough time to draw a complete decision tree. If the decision is one that you or your colleagues will face repeatedly, then spending the time to do all the steps and develop a decision guide for future cases may improve decisions, help with patient education and communication, and reduce future decision-making time. With the growth of clinical guidelines, it is worth understanding the steps and asking whether the guidelines you employ have used a similar process and presentation, or whether they can be supplemented or replaced using the techniques described in this book. Finally, when it comes to public health policy-making, decision modeling, taking into account both effectiveness and costs, is invariably required in order to optimize the use of available health-care resources.

The basic concepts and tools of decision analysis are useful in many situations and are valuable in day-to-day practice even when a formal decision analysis cannot be fully performed. We hope that these fundamental concepts become part of your entire approach to clinical reasoning and health-care decision making. We have tried to show how these tools grow out of a formal theory of decision making, even if they do not invoke it explicitly or employ all of the steps involved in a complete decision analysis.

1.8 Summary

We have outlined a systematic rational approach to decision making in health care. The process itself helps health-care decision makers to gain an overview of the issues and think beyond the perspective most of us are most inclined to take. Table 1.4 presents these steps, summarized with a convenient mnemonic – PROACTIVE.

Decision analysis may appear to be a serial process, i.e., the steps are followed consecutively. This is because we can only describe it sequentially. In reality the process is far more a recursive circular process with feedback loops. For example, we structure the problem and consider all the possible options. Subsequently, as we search the literature for evidence, we may find other diagnostic or treatment options that we had not yet considered, or we realize that the way we structured the problem does not accurately reflect the best available evidence. We then have to go back and adjust our initial formulation of the problem and expand the list of options. Analogously, after completing the analysis we may find ourselves confronted with varying cases and conditions that force us to adjust our assumptions and estimates. A conflict between the plan we had in mind before the analysis and that

Table 1.4 Summary of the PROACTIVE approach to decision making: the steps, considerations, tools, and corresponding chapter (Ch) numbers.

	Step	Considerations	Tools
Step 1 PRO			
Problem	Define the problem	What will happen if I do nothing? Is there a problem?	"Go to the balcony" (Ch 1) Visualize with a consequence table or sketch (Ch 1)
Reframe	Reframe from multiple perspectives	Consider the perspective of the patient, physician, department, hospital, payer, and society	Communicate with those involved in the decision (Ch 1, 13) Step to their side, understand their perspective (Ch 1, 13)
Objective	Focus on the objective	Consider diagnostic uncertainty, medical effectiveness, psychosocial, micro- and macroeconomics, political, ethical, and philosophical aspects	Ask those involved: "Why? What is the goal?" (Ch 1) Distinguish means objectives from fundamental objectives (Ch 1)
Step 2 ACT			
Alternatives	Consider all relevant alternatives	Wait-and-see, intervention, obtain information	Logical and lateral thinking
		Different combinations, sequences, and positivity criterion of diagnostic tests	Expand the options: brainstorm first, decide later
Consequences and Chances	Model the consequences and estimate the chances	Model disease and events Estimate the corresponding probabilities	Balance sheet (Ch 1, 2) Find the evidence (Ch 8) Meta-analysis (Ch 8) Bayesian probability revision (Ch 5) Decision tree (Ch 3, 6) Markov cohort model (Ch 10) Microsimulation model (Ch 12)
Trade-offs	Identify and estimate value trade-offs	Immediate risk vs. long-term risk Quality of life vs. length of life Health outcome vs. costs	Balance sheet (Ch 1, 2) Meta-analysis (Ch 8) Utility assessment (Ch 4) Cost analysis (Ch 9)

Table 1.4 (*cont.*)

	Step	Considerations	Tools
Step 3 IVE			
Integrate	Integrate the evidence and values	Qualitatively Quantitatively	Reduce data in balance sheet (Ch 1) Average out: calculate expected value (Ch 1, 3) Fold back: apply decision criterion to choose (Ch 3)
Value	Optimize expected value	Maximize desirable outcomes Minimize undesirable outcomes	Multiattribute outcomes (Ch 3, 4, 9)
Explore and Evaluate	Explore assumptions	Evaluate heterogeneity Evaluate parameter uncertainty Evaluate model structure uncertainty	Microsimulation (Ch 12) One-way, two-way, three-way sensitivity analysis (Ch 3, 12) Probabilistic sensitivity analysis (Ch 12)

recommended by the model may cause us to consider whether important variables have been omitted from our analysis or if our thinking has been inconsistent. Thus, the analytic process helps us continually to reflect on the important trade-offs and issues involved in the decision problem.

Time is needed for a fully fledged decision analysis involving all of these steps. Consequently, a complete decision model is generally developed only for commonly recurring problems that necessitate and justify detailed analysis. A detailed analysis is necessary if there are competing diagnostic or treatment strategies, where consensus has not been established, and where there is considerable uncertainty. In these circumstances, decision analyses can help formulate a clinical guideline or health policy statement for health-care practice or at least clarify the issues at the heart of the controversy.

1.9 Overview of the book

In Chapter 2, we expand on managing uncertainty by developing fundamental rules of probability and the concept of expected value. We show how to calculate the expected value of simple monetary lotteries, as a preparation for calculating expected value in more complex clinical situations, involving life expectancy, quality of life, and health states between perfect health and death.

Chapter 3 discusses the proactive approach to a clinical problem and explains the use of decision trees to determine the best treatment under diagnostic uncertainty. Maximization of expected utility is employed as the criterion for decision making under uncertainty.

Chapter 4 outlines utility assessment. It discusses different methods that are employed to quantify outcome values, for both individual clinical decision making and for health policy or population-based decisions.

Chapter 5 develops Bayes' theorem, the basic tool of decision analysis for revising opinion with imperfect information. The theorem is widely used in clinical diagnosis, to revise diagnostic opinion with physical findings, tests, or laboratory studies that we know are not 100% accurate. We begin with an analysis of tests with dichotomous results (positive and negative).

Chapter 6 revisits decision trees, this time adding Bayes' theorem. We shall explore a family of decision problems with three options – do not treat, treat without further testing, and test-and-treat – and show how to determine in which region you are operating.

Chapter 7 deepens the analysis of tests, moving from dichotomous test results to tests with multiple results and combining results from multiple tests. The material covered in the second half of this chapter is fairly advanced and can be skipped without loss of the general flow of the text of the book.

In Chapter 8, we will discuss techniques for rapidly identifying the best available relevant data and how to manage the limitations of such data.

Chapter 9 discusses the problems of societal decision making with limited financial resources. It introduces cost-effectiveness analysis and cost–utility analysis and shows how to apply decision analytic principles to select among health-care programs using a cost-effectiveness criterion.

Chapter 10 introduces an additional complexity, showing how to model clinical situations in which patients move from one health state to another over time and when events can occur at any uncertain point in the future. Decision trees do not handle these situations conveniently, but state-transition models do, and we shall discuss these models in some detail.

Chapter 11 considers methods for estimating variable values that are the inputs of the decision model. This can be done either directly from (literature) data or indirectly using the decision model through calibration methods. This chapter also discusses validation methods that are used to check whether the decision model produces outputs that are accurate. This chapter covers advanced material and would not be recommended for an introductory course.

Chapter 12 discusses methods to explore and evaluate heterogeneity and uncertainty. Several sophisticated approaches are explained, including micro-simulation, probabilistic sensitivity analysis, and value of information analysis.

This chapter covers advanced material and would not be recommended for an introductory course.

Chapter 13 addresses the psychological aspects relevant to judgment and decision making. These issues are relevant to diagnostic errors, decision making in clinical practice and health policy, obtaining expert opinion, and implementing the results of decision models.

We hope you will conclude that you made the right decision in picking up this book – enjoy it!

REFERENCES

1. Hunink MG. In search of tools to aid logical thinking and communicating about medical decision making. *Med Decis Making.* 2001;21(4):267–77.
2. Beers MH, Berkow R, eds. *The Merck Manual Of Diagnosis And Therapy.* 17th edn. Whitehouse Station, NJ: Merck & Co; 1999.
3. Lieberthal AS, Carroll AE, Chonmaitree T, et al. The diagnosis and management of acute otitis media. *Pediatrics.* 2013 February 25, 2013.
4. Hammond JS, Keeney RL, Raiffa H. *Smart Choices: A Practical Guide to Making Better Decisions.* Boston: Harvard Business School Press; 1999.
5. Kamel H, Elkind MSV, Bhave PD, et al. Paroxysmal supraventricular tachycardia and the risk of ischemic stroke. *Stroke.* 2013;44(6):1550–4.
6. Rosenfeld RM, Bluestone CD. *Evidence-based Otitis Media.* Hamilton, Ontario: B.C. Decker; 1999.
7. Cronenwett JL, Birkmeyer JD, Nackman GB, et al. Cost-effectiveness of carotid endarterectomy in asymptomatic patients. *J Vasc Surg.* 1997;25(2):298–309; discussion 10–11.
8. O'Connor AM, Bennett CL, Stacey D, et al. Decision aids for people facing health treatment or screening decisions. *Cochrane Database Syst Rev.* 2009(3):CD001431.
9. Newell A, Simon HA. *Human Problem Solving.* Englewood Cliffs, NJ: Prenticehall; 1972.
10. Redelmeier DA, Rozin P, Kahneman D. Understanding patients' decisions. Cognitive and emotional perspectives. *JAMA.* 1993;270(1):72–6.
11. Dawson NV, Arkes HR. Systematic errors in medical decision making: judgment limitations. *J Gen Intern Med.* 1987;2(3):183–7.
12. Miller GA. The magical number seven, plus or minus two: some limits on our capacity for processing information. *Psychol Rev.* 1956;63:81–97.
13. Kahneman D. *Thinking, Fast and Slow.* New York: Farrar, Straus and Giroux; 2011.
14. Tversky A, Kahneman D. Judgment under uncertainty: Heuristics and biases. *Science.* 1974;185:1124–31.
15. Tversky A, Kahneman D. The framing of decisions and the psychology of choice. *Science.* 1981;211(4481):453–8.
16. Redelmeier DA, Shafir E. Medical decision making in situations that offer multiple alternatives. *JAMA.* 1995;273(4):302–5.

Managing uncertainty

Much of medical training consists of learning to cope with pervasive uncertainty and with the limits of medical knowledge. Making serious clinical decisions on the basis of conflicting, incomplete, and untimely data is routine.

J.D. McCue

2.1 Introduction

Much of clinical medicine and health care involves uncertainties: some reducible, but some irreducible despite our best efforts and tests. Better decisions will be made if we are open and honest about these uncertainties, and develop skills in estimating, communicating, and working with such uncertainties. What types of uncertainty exist? Consider the following example.

EXAMPLE	**Needlestick injury:**

It has been a hard week. It is time to go home when you are called to yet another heroin overdose: a young woman has been found unconscious outside your clinic. After giving intravenous (IV) naloxone (which reverses the effects of heroin), you are accidentally jabbed by the needle. After her recovery, despite your reassurances, the young woman flees for fear of the police. As the mêlée settles, the dread of human immunodeficiency virus (HIV) infection begins to develop. You talk to the senior doctor about what you should do. She is very sympathetic, and begins to tell you about the risks and management. The good news is that, even if the patient was HIV-positive, a needlestick injury *rarely* leads to HIV infection (about 3 per 1000). And if she was HIV-positive then a basic two-drug regime of antivirals such as zidovudine (AZT) plus lamivudine are *likely* to be able to prevent most infections (perhaps 80%).

Unfortunately, the HIV status of the young woman who had overdosed is unknown. Since she was not a patient of your clinic, you are uncertain about whether she is infected, but think that it is *possible* since she is an IV drug user. The Centers for Disease Control and Prevention (CDC) guidelines (1) suggest: 'If the exposure source is *unknown*, use of post-exposure prophylaxis should be decided on a case-by-case basis. Consider the severity of exposure and the epidemiologic likelihood of HIV.' What do you do?

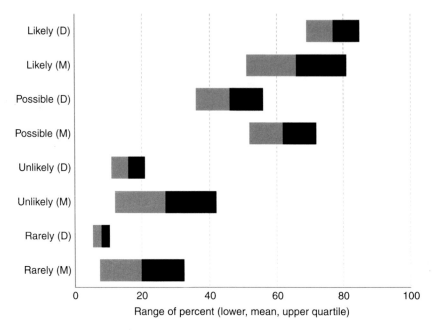

Figure 2.1   Median, interquartile range (box), and range (whiskers), for percentages assigned to expressions by 100 mothers (M) and 50 doctors and medical students (D). Reproduced from Shaw, N.J. and Dear, P.R. (1990). How do parents of babies interpret qualitative expressions of probability? *Arch. Dis. Child.*, **65**, 520–3, with permission of the BMJ Publishing Group.

The example illustrates several types of uncertainty: we are uncertain of the HIV status of the heroin user, of the chance of HIV transmission, and of the effectiveness of prophylactic treatment. Regardless of these uncertainties, we must make a choice. Even doing nothing is a choice; inaction should not be an evasion of decision making but a deliberate choice, which should be made only if it is better than the alternatives. In health care we are often reluctant 'gamblers,' who must place our stakes as wisely as possible in the face of multiple and irreducible uncertainties. To enable us to choose wisely we must make these uncertainties explicit.

When communicating and reasoning about uncertainties, verbal expressions create problems. For example, what do the words 'rarely,' 'likely,' and 'possible' mean to you? Do they mean the same thing to a co-worker or patient? Unfortunately, several surveys demonstrate wide variation in the interpretation of such verbal expressions. This makes them a poor vehicle for communication about uncertainty, risk, and probability. For example, Figure 2.1 shows an assessment of these words by 100 mothers of infants and 50 doctors and medical students (2).

To some extent we can predict people's differences in meaning for probabilistic terms. For example, patients with previous experience of an adverse event tend to ascribe its 'likely' occurrence a higher probability than those who have not experienced it (3). This is in line with a general tendency to give a higher probability to events that are more 'available' to us, that is, that we have seen more frequently or more recently or that are especially memorable. Similarly, patients' interpretations of 'rare' were higher if the event was more severe. However, such differences are not sufficiently predictable to enable repair of our faulty risk communication. We may know what we mean by a particular risk expression but we do not know what other people mean by the same expression. This can have undesirable consequences for important decisions involving uncertainty. Being explicit has practical advantages: doctors' agreement about decisions to treat hypothetical cases was improved when given numerical rather than verbal expressions of probability (4).

Patients generally express a desire for risk communication, and most prefer this to be quantitative. For example, of the mothers interviewed for the data in Figure 2.1, 53% wanted numerical statements of risk; 37% wanted a verbal expression; and 10% had no preference (2). Despite this, doctors have been reluctant to communicate risk either quantitatively or qualitatively. Given the inevitability of uncertainties in many health-care decisions, we believe that both health-care workers and patients would be best served by learning how to express uncertainty numerically. If it is difficult to give a single figure, using a range still provides a clearer statement than a verbal expression. This approach requires that health-care workers develop skills in understanding, assessing, and manipulating information about probabilities.

Some physicians may question the use of probabilities for an individual patient and wonder whether any probability estimates, such as the probability that the patient has a particular disease or the likelihood that the patient will survive an illness, can possibly be valid and meaningful for a given individual. After all, one might argue that this patient either has the disease or does not and will either recover or not. There is no probability involved. Furthermore, the argument continues, since each patient is unique, probability estimates derived from experience with previous patients or from epidemiological studies cannot possibly apply to any individual case.

Decisions must be made in the present looking into the uncertain future, not looking back at the certain past. It is true that every patient is unique, either has the disease or does not, and will either recover or not. But in the situation we are discussing, both her underlying true state and future course of the illness (if any) are unknown and hence uncertain. What is important for a decision maker is the state of his or her beliefs and knowledge at the time of the decision and not what may then be – and perhaps may later emerge as – the truth.

The assignment of probabilities to the case of an individual patient may be viewed as a measure of the decision maker's ignorance about all of the special characteristics of that unique individual. We must be cognizant of what we know and do not know about each patient, but a refusal to quantify our ignorance will not lessen it. We argue that a physician should use probabilities to help decide on a strategy for an individual patient.

This chapter will begin by looking at the most common uncertainties in health care: diagnosis, prognosis, and the effects of treatment. We will express these uncertainties in probabilities and then discuss how these probabilities can be combined and manipulated. In the next chapter we will look at how, when either diagnosis or outcome is uncertain, explicit probabilities can be combined with a quantitative assessment of the outcomes to make better decisions.

2.2 Types of probability

Uncertainty may be expressed quantitatively in several different ways: as probabilities, proportions, frequencies, odds, percentages, and rates (Table 2.1). Probabilities, by definition, range in value from 0.0 to 1.0.

Table 2.1 Probability terms: definitions and relationships of various terms for probabilities

Term	Definition	Formula	Range
Probability	The chance of an event	p	0–1
Proportion	The relative frequency of a state	p	0–1
Prevalence	The proportion of a population with a specific disease	p	0–1
Percentage	Probability expressed as a frequency 'per 100'	$p \times 100$	0–100
Frequency	Probability expressed per sample (e.g., 1 per 1000)	p	0–denominator
Odds	The ratio of the probability of an event to its complement	$p/(1 - p)$	0–infinity
Probability measures involving time			
Incidence (or hazard) rate	The occurrence of new disease cases or events per unit of person-time	p/t	0–infinity
Cumulative incidence	The proportion of people who develop a new disease or have an event during a specified period of time	p	0–1
Risk	The probability that an individual develops a new disease or has an event during a specified period of time	p	0–1

A probability of 0 means that the event is impossible; a probability of 1.0 means that it is certain. A probability of 0.5 means the event is equally likely to occur as not to occur. Probabilities may also be expressed as percentages, where 0% corresponds to a probability of 0, and 100% corresponds to a probability of 1. A percentage expresses a probability as a frequency per 100, but other frequency expressions are common. For example, cancer incidence is often expressed as a frequency per 100 000. For consistency in this book, we will usually use probabilities rather than frequencies for working through problems. However, since many people find frequencies easier to interpret, you should generally express final results as frequencies, particularly when communicating with patients.

We shall not concern ourselves here with two types of distinctions that become crucial at a more advanced level. One such distinction concerns 'frequencies' and 'probabilities.' One school of thought, known as 'frequentist,' holds that the only meaningful sense in which probability can be discussed is in terms of empirical frequencies in a sample of observations. Another school of thought, known as 'subjectivist' or 'Bayesian,' holds that probability is fundamentally a degree of belief, and that, while frequency data may inform estimates of probability, they are not themselves probabilities. Chapter 8 describes an approach to probabilities and the data that inform their estimation, incorporating a healthy respect for empirical data while retaining the view that, in the end, decision makers must act on the probabilities they believe.

A second, more technical distinction, which we do not belabor here, but to which we return in Chapter 10 in the context of state-transition models, concerns rates and probabilities. Technically, a rate is an instantaneous change in the cumulative probability of an outcome per unit of time, rather than an average change. The formal definition of a rate requires calculus, as it is the first derivative of a cumulative probability with respect to time. Until we get to Chapter 10, we will rather loosely use the term 'rate' to apply to the probability of an event in a specified time interval.

There are several types of uncertainty in the needlestick example at the beginning of this chapter: the **diagnostic** uncertainty of whether the heroin user has an HIV infection; the **prognostic** uncertainty of how often the development of HIV (seroconversion) would occur after a needlestick injury from an HIV-infected patient; and the **treatment** uncertainty about the effectiveness of prophylactic treatment with antiviral drugs. These three uncertainties, all of which can be quantified using probabilities, will be examined in Sections 2.3, 2.4, and 2.5 respectively, looking at the measures of and data sources for each.

2.3 Diagnostic uncertainty

Diagnosis is a very uncertain art. Studies comparing clinicians' diagnoses show disagreement is very common (5). This is implicit in the differential diagnosis, which lists the possible causes of an individual illness. Skilled diagnosticians often generate a longer list, but also are better able to differentiate between the most and least likely causes. Good diagnosis depends on both knowing all the possibilities and accurately assessing their relative frequency. Diagnostic probabilities express our uncertainty about the list of differential diagnoses. For example, we might need to know the likelihood of different possible causes of sudden chest pain; or, in our needlestick example, we would like to know the chance that an IV drug user had a blood-borne infection such as HIV, hepatitis B, or hepatitis C.

2.3.1 The summation principle

There are some simple 'rules' that a differential diagnosis should follow. First, the differential diagnosis should include all possible single diseases and combinations of diseases and the sum of the probabilities of all possibilities must add up to 1 (the summation principle). Second, one and only one possibility must be true. This is a general requirement for the analysis of chance outcomes: they must be structured to be mutually exclusive (only one can occur) and collectively exhaustive (one must occur). For example, either a patient has HIV or not. The probabilities of these two possibilities add up to 1. In mathematical notation:

$$p(\text{HIV}) + p(\text{not HIV}) = 1 \qquad (2.1)$$

where $p(\text{HIV})$ is shorthand which is read as 'the probability of HIV.' Thus, with our needlestick example, if the probability of HIV is 0.25 then the complement, $p(\text{not HIV})$, must be $1 - 0.25 = 0.75$.

It is common to assume that only one diagnosis is causing a problem. This is usually true, as the likelihood of two illnesses with similar presentations occurring simultaneously is low. However, for longer-term illness this will not be true and among the elderly, multiple diseases are common. If multiple diseases are possible we need to be explicit about this. For example, if we were considering the chances of HIV and hepatitis B, then we would need to consider each alone, both, or neither, so that:

$$p(\text{HIV only}) + p(\text{hepatitis B only}) + p(\text{HIV and hepatitis B}) +$$
$$p(\text{neither}) = 1 \qquad (2.2)$$

More generally, the summation rule for n mutually exclusive possible diagnoses may be written as:

$$p(\text{possibility 1}) + p(\text{possibility 2}) + \ldots + p(\text{possibility n}) = 1 \qquad (2.3)$$

2.3.2 Conditional probabilities

Returning to our needlestick example, we need to assess the probability of HIV in the heroin user. We write this probability as $p(\text{HIV} \mid \text{IV drug use})$ which is read as 'the probability of HIV given IV drug use.' The symbol '|' is read as 'given' the particular group in whom we have estimated the probability.

If this conditional information makes no difference to the probability, then we say the two factors are (statistically, or probabilistically) independent. For example, if gender made no difference to our estimate of the probability of HIV, that is, $p(\text{HIV} \mid \text{female}) = p(\text{HIV} \mid \text{male}) = p(\text{HIV})$, then HIV status and gender are said to be independent (this will be formally defined in the section on combining probabilities at the end of this chapter).

DEFINITION   The probability that event E occurs, given that event F has occurred, is called the *conditional probability* of event E given event F. It is denoted by $p(E \mid F)$.

2.3.3 Sources of data

Where do diagnostic probabilities come from? We do not start with a blank slate: the patient's presenting problem, other symptoms and signs, his or her age, and gender all contribute to the likelihood of different possibilities. Estimates may come from (a combination of) personal experience, empirical data (the systematically collected experience of others), and our understanding of the different disease processes. The principal empirical information will be studies of consecutive patients with a particular presenting complaint. For example, if we wish to know the probabilities of different causes of headaches for patients in ambulatory care, then the ideal study will have collected a consecutive series of patients presenting with headache, then ascertained the cause through a standard protocol of tests and follow-up. However, our setting and the individual patient will usually differ in several ways from this study, so, while it may provide a useful starting point, some mental adjustment will be needed to particularize the results. Estimates based on personal experience are often called subjective probabilities, while those based on data are sometimes called objective, data-based, or frequency-based probabilities. For our purposes in this book, it is important to note that the rules for combining these probabilities are exactly the same, regardless of the source.

EXAMPLE (*cont.*) For our needlestick injury case, we need to know how likely an HIV infection is for an IV drug user. Clearly this will vary greatly in different locations. Ideally, we would like a recent serological survey of a representative sample of intravenous drug users in the local area. This is unlikely to be available. Our best data for US populations is probably from the CDC, which compiles data on HIV prevalence in many subgroups, including IV drug users. A systematic review (see Chapter 8) of prevalence studies (6) found a range of US prevalences among IV drug users from 0% in Milwaukee to 60% in New York. Clearly, the local data are relevant, and we should be more concerned in New York than in Milwaukee. For our example, we will use a large recent study from New York which found a prevalence of 14%.

2.4 Prognostic uncertainty

The television image of doctors suggests they are clairvoyant and can tell you that you have three months to live. Reality falls far short of this. For many conditions, the natural history is not well documented, and even when it is, the prediction is an average, which may not apply well to any single individual. For example, the average survival for a cancer may be two years, but the range of survival is wide and unpredictable, with some patients surviving only a few weeks and others many years. Prognostic uncertainty is uncertainty about future health states rather than current health states. For example, prognostic questions include the chance that someone who has survived a myocardial infarction (heart attack) will have another, or the long-term risk of liver failure in someone with hepatitis C. Thus prognosis involves probability over time. For example, cancer prognosis is often expressed as a five-year survival rate. There is nothing special about five years; we might also want to know the one-year and 20-year survival, though five-year survival gives a single convenient 'snapshot.'

Because of the time element, prognosis is often expressed through incidence and hazard rates, which measure the probability per unit time, e.g., percent per year. Since the rate may change, the most complete description of prognosis will usually be a survival curve, which shows the effects of risk over time, not simply at a defined interval.

2.4.1 'Survival' curves

Though the calculations can be difficult, the concept of a survival curve is straightforward: it plots the probability of being alive over a period of time. Figure 2.2 shows an example of a survival curve. It begins at time 0, with all

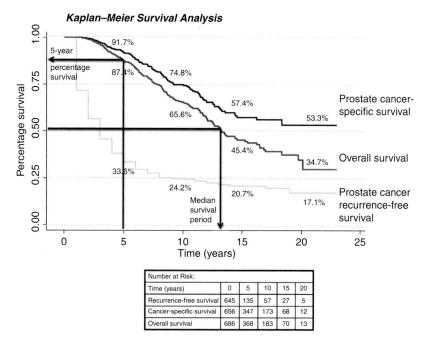

Figure 2.2   'Survival curve' indicating the five-year percentage survival and median survival period (7) (from: Pierorazio et al. Urology. 2010; 76(3): 715–21).

patients alive. As we follow the plot out over time, there is a progressive decrease in survival. As shown for the five-year point in the figure, the proportion alive (five-year survival), and its complement, the proportion dead (five-year mortality), can be read off by drawing a line from the survival curve and then to the vertical axis. 'Survival' curves are also useful to show the probability of other events over time: Figure 2.2 also shows the proportion of patients surviving and free of recurrence (lower line) – in which case the endpoint (or failure) is defined as either death or recurrence. Similarly, prostate cancer-specific survival has been plotted.

The overall survival can be summarized in several ways. First, from the graph we can read off the median survival – the point at which exactly 50% of patients have died and 50% are still alive – by drawing a line from the 0.50 on the vertical axis across to the survival curve and then down to the time (horizontal) axis. In this example, the median survival is about nine years. The expected value or mean (also called the life expectancy) is more difficult to calculate but corresponds to the area under the survival curve. We shall be returning frequently to the concept of life expectancy and its calculation, both in Chapter 4 on outcome values, and in Chapter 10, where we show how simple state-transition models can be used to generate estimates of life expectancy.

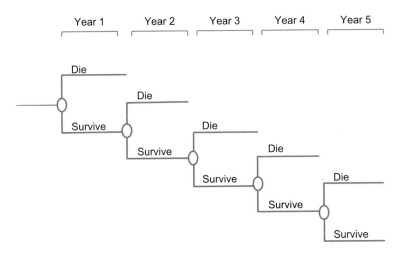

Year 1   Year 2   Year 3   Year 4   Year 5

Figure 2.3   Chance tree indicating the probability of dying in the first five years.

Survival curves can be constructed through published life tables, by apply-ing so-called product-limit (Kaplan–Meier) estimators to empirical data, or by estimating the parameters of survival functions statistically from data. For a detailed description of survival analysis we refer the reader to textbooks and articles on the subject (8).

2.4.2 Probability trees

In the most general sense, *prognosis* may be defined as the chance tree facing an individual, or population of individuals, given particular conditions. These conditions include *prognostic factors* (also called *risk factors*) and any health-care interventions that may be applied.

A survival curve is really a concise format for visually representing the chance tree of successive event rates (e.g., mortality rates) over time. For example, in Figure 2.2 the probability of dying during the first year can be calculated as the difference between the probability of being alive at year 0 (100%) and the probability of being alive at year 1 (approximately 91%), or about 0.09. This probability of dying in the first year could be represented as the first event in a sequence of chance nodes in a chance tree (Figure 2.3). The probabilities of dying in each successive year can be obtained similarly from the survival curve, taking care to divide each survival difference (between the nth year and the $(n-1)$th year) by the probability of being alive at year $n-1$. These annual probabilities of death would be represented as the remaining chance nodes in the chance tree that corresponds to the survival curve (Figure 2.3).

DEFINITION	An individual's *prognosis* is the chance tree describing future events, given a set of prognostic factors and interventions.

2.4.3 Prognostic factors

Everyone with the same disease does not have the same prognosis. Risk may be modified by many other factors, such as the stage of disease, and the patient's age and gender. Such prognostic factors enable us to refine our individual predictions. Again, when risk varies over time, the ideal description would be a survival curve for each particular subgroup. For example, for colorectal cancer the five-year survival is 92% for patients whose colorectal cancer is detected at an early stage, 64% if there is spread to nearby organs or lymph nodes, and only 7% if there is spread (metastasis) to distant parts of the body such as the liver or lungs. The term 'survival' is used to mean being event-free, however the event is defined. The duration of influenza, the time to cancer relapse, and the duration of pain in acute middle-ear infections have all been presented as 'survival' curves.

2.4.4 Sources of data

How can we obtain information on prognosis and prognostic factors? To understand the development of a disease over time, the ideal would be to have a large cohort of patients with all prognostic factors measured at the beginning of the disease, followed up to the end stage of the disease. This is usually referred to as an inception cohort. Such studies may be found through literature searches of MEDLINE, but finding the better-quality studies can be difficult. PubMed's Clinical Queries, which is part of the internet version of MEDLINE, provides filters that assist in identifying the better prognostic studies. There are some useful compilations and summaries of prognostic studies, such as that provided by *Best Evidence*, which contained all previous editions of the American College of Physicians' (ACP) *Journal Club* and *Evidence-based Medicine*. Among the most widely used inception cohorts for decision analysis is the Framingham Heart Study, which measured numerous risk factors for cardio-vascular disease every two years, and followed subjects for the occurrence of heart disease, stroke, and death at these intervals (9).

Such a study will describe the prognosis of patients given their particular treatments. If they had no specific treatment, the prognosis is known as the natural history. However, if they had specific treatment that modified the disease process, then the study provides evidence on the prognosis conditional

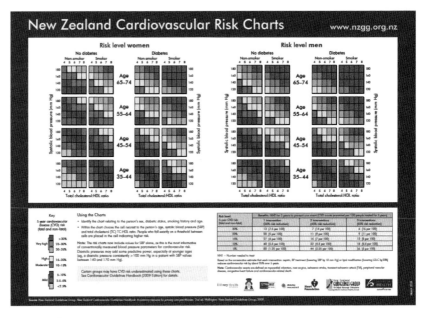

Figure 2.4   Guideline for managing cardiovascular risk from multiple risk factors. HDL: high-density lipoprotein cholesterol; CVD: cardiovascular disease; NNT: number-needed-to-treat. (Obtained from http://www.health.govt.nz/publication/new-zealand-cardiovascular-risk-charts; accessed Oct 15, 2013.)

on those treatments. Natural history is important, as it gives us the probabilities we need to estimate along the 'no-intervention' branch of a decision tree. By comparing it with the prognosis in the absence of the disease, the natural history also enables us to calculate the individual's potential benefit from treatment.

In general, the potential benefit will be greater in those with more severe disease and/or those who are at higher risk. Unfortunately, most treatments are neither perfect cures nor harmless. Most treatments provide symptomatic relief or a chance of cure, but usually with the risk of some adverse effects. This means that the net benefit a patient derives from treatment is usually less (sometimes considerably so) than the potential benefit.

DEFINITION   The *potential benefit* is the difference between the expected outcome based on an individual's prognosis if a harmless curative treatment is available and the expected outcome based on his or her current prognosis without specific treatment.

Integrating prognostic information as a function of patient characteristics is necessary when developing a guideline. For example, the guideline for managing cardiovascular risk shown in Figure 2.4 (10;11) provides explicit information on individual prognosis using six risk factors: gender, age, diabetes, smoking, blood pressure, and total cholesterol to high-density lipoprotein

(HDL) ratio. From these risk factors, the guide quantifies the five-year risk of a cardiovascular event (colored cells) and the benefit of treatment alternatives in terms of numbers needed to treat for five years to avoid one CVD event. The guide shows patients and clinicians by how much the risk of cardiovascular events is reduced through control of the risk factors that are manageable. We would suggest one additional step, to provide the 'harms' of the treatment alternatives, including the frequency of adverse events (for example, weight gain when people try to stop smoking, diabetes when using statins) and the effort involved in compliance and monitoring.

2.5 Treatment uncertainty

Few treatments have the dramatic impact of insulin for juvenile-onset diabetes or penicillin for pneumococcal pneumonia. The efficacy of such 'miracle' cures is clear: without treatment, the disease is usually progressive, while treatment cures almost all patients and has few or no adverse effects. However, usually the disease fluctuates or a proportion remits spontaneously; in either case the treatment effect is incomplete. For example, the vast majority of people with high blood pressure (hypertension) will not have a stroke (prognostic uncertainty); and lowering blood pressure will not prevent all strokes (treatment uncertainty). The effects of such imperfect treatments need to be weighed against their harms, such as mild adverse effects and the occasional severe or even fatal reaction, such as anaphylaxis. For those treatments that are not 'miracle' cures, we need an accurate assessment of their incremental benefit for comparison with possible harms.

How can we best assess treatment effects? The ideal study would compare two large similar groups of patients, one treated and the other not, observing how treatment influences the course of illness. This is the aim of controlled clinical trials. For several reasons, however, the results may need to be adapted for application to individual patients. First, any individual's prognosis, and hence the potential benefit, may be quite different from the average patient in the trial. Second, the individual's concomitant illnesses and risk factors may be different, modifying the potential benefit. Third, the effectiveness and cost of the intervention may differ by setting; for example, experienced surgeons may get better results than less experienced ones, or follow-up and monitoring may be more difficult in a rural setting.

2.5.1 Sources of data

Randomized controlled trials provide the best type of information on which to base an analysis. If there are several such trials, a systematic review of these is ideal (see Chapter 8). For controlled trials, there are two principal design problems: establishing two comparable groups and unbiased observation of the outcomes.

How can we establish comparable groups? Allowing the clinician and patient to choose either treatment is likely to lead to systematic differences. For example, older patients or smokers might prefer one of the treatments, and hence both these prognostic factors (determinants in epidemiological terminology) and the treatment would influence the outcome. These imbalanced prognostic factors are said to *confound* the treatment comparison.

DEFINITION	A *confounder* is a prognostic factor that is associated both with the exposure to an intervention (or with another determinant of outcome) and with the outcome (or disease) but is not an intermediate in the causal chain.

Statistical techniques can partly adjust for known prognostic factors but not for unknown prognostic factors. Randomization is the only secure method of obtaining balance between the treatment groups in both known and unknown prognostic factors. Since the first randomized trial of streptomycin for tuberculosis was published in 1948, over half a million randomized trials have been conducted.

How can we obtain unbiased observation of outcomes? As observers, we have a natural tendency to see what we want to see. The principal method of reducing observer bias is for the person assessing the outcome to be unaware of which treatment the patient was allocated to – known as *blinding*. Ideally, both patient and clinician will be unaware of the treatment allocation, known as a *double blind* trial. A common way to achieve this in pharmaceutical trials is using a placebo, which matches the active treatment for size, color, taste, and dosing schedule. If two pharmaceuticals are being compared, then either these need to match or each is provided with its own placebo (known as the double-dummy technique). Even when using a placebo is not feasible, one should ensure that the person assessing the outcome is unaware of the treatment allocation. For example, blinding in surgery, percutaneous interventions, and lifestyle programs is often extremely difficult but blind outcome assessment is still achievable for some outcomes.

Not all treatments can be, or need to be, subjected to a double-blind randomized controlled trial and, even when it is possible and necessary, it has not always been done. The aim is to use the best available evidence. Decisions, both individual treatment and policy decisions, need to be made even when 'perfect' evidence is lacking. To rank evidence from 'best' to 'worst,' several hierarchies of evidence for interventions have been proposed, but many do not distinguish between the different types of research needed for different types of uncertainty. Table 2.2

Table 2.2 Best sources of evidence for different types of uncertainty

Oxford Centre for Evidence-based Medicine (OCEBM) 2011 Levels of Evidence

Question	Step 1 (Level 1*)	Step 2 (Level 2*)	Step 3 (Level 3*)	Step 4 (Level 4*)	Step 5 (Level 5)
How common is the problem?	Local and current random sample surveys (or censuses)	Systematic review of surveys that allow matching to local circumstances**	Local non-random sample**	Case-series**	n/a
Is this diagnostic or monitoring test accurate? (Diagnosis)	Systematic review of cross-sectional studies with consistently applied reference standard and blinding	Individual cross-sectional studies with consistently applied reference standard and blinding	Non-consecutive studies, or studies without consistently applied reference standards**	Case-control studies, or 'poor' or non-independent reference standard**	Mechanism-based reasoning
What will happen if we do not add a therapy? (Prognosis)	Systematic review of inception cohort studies	Inception cohort studies	Cohort study or control arm of randomized trial*	Case-series or case-control studies, or poor-quality prognostic cohort study**	n/a
Does this intervention help? (Treatment benefits)	Systematic review of randomized trials or n-of-1 trials	Randomized trial or observational study with dramatic effect	Non-randomized controlled cohort/follow-up study**	Case-series, case-control, or historically controlled studies**	Mechanism-based reasoning
What are the COMMON harms? (Treatment harms)	Systematic review of randomized trials, systematic review of nested case-control studies, n-of-1	Individual randomized trial or (exceptionally) observational study with dramatic effect	Non-randomized controlled cohort/follow-up study (post-marketing surveillance)	Case-series, case-control, or historically controlled studies**	Mechanism-based reasoning

Table 2.2 (*cont.*)

Oxford Centre for Evidence-based Medicine (OCEBM) 2011 Levels of Evidence

Question	Step 1 (Level 1*)	Step 2 (Level 2*)	Step 3 (Level 3*)	Step 4 (Level 4*)	Step 5 (Level 5)
	trial with the patient you are raising the question about, or observational study with dramatic effect		provided there are sufficient numbers to rule out a common harm. (For long-term harms the duration of follow-up must be sufficient)**		
What are the RARE harms? (Treatment harms)	Systematic review of randomized trials or *n*-of-1 trial	Randomized trial or (exceptionally) observational study with dramatic effect			
Is this (early detection) test worthwhile? (Screening)	Systematic review of randomized trials	Randomized trial	Non-randomized controlled cohort/follow-up study**	Case-series, case-control, or historically controlled studies**	Mechanism-based reasoning

Data obtained from www.cebm.net, accessed June 5, 2013.

* Level may be graded down on the basis of study quality, imprecision, indirectness (study PICO does not match questions PICO), because of inconsistency between studies, or because the absolute-effect size is very small; level may be graded up if there is a large- or very large-effect size.

** As always, a systematic review is generally better than an individual study.

How to cite the Levels of Evidence table:

OCEBM Levels of Evidence Working Group.*** 'The Oxford 2011 Levels of Evidence.'.

Oxford Centre for Evidence-based Medicine. http://www.cebm.net/index.aspx?o=5653

*** *OCEBM Table of Evidence Working Group = Jeremy Howick, Iain Chalmers (James Lind Library), Paul Glasziou, Trish Greenhaigh, Carl Heneghan, Alessandro Liberati, Ivan Moschetti, Bob Phillips, Hazel Thornton, Olive Goddard, and Mary Hodgkinson.*

provides a summary of the types of research and resources you might look for (as a series of steps). Whatever evidence is found will need further appraisal (see Chapter 8): to grade the strength of the evidence, the system developed by the GRADE working group is the most complete (www.grade-workinggroup.org/).

A case-control study compares a group of individuals who have experienced an outcome of interest with a comparable group who have not, to determine the differences between their previous prognostic factors or other determinants of risk. A cohort study compares a group of individuals who have been exposed to an intervention or prognostic factor with a comparable group who have not, to determine the differences between their outcomes. The chief limitation of both of these study designs lies in insuring that the two groups are truly comparable in terms of all other prognostic factors. This can be accomplished to some degree by matching them according to known and measurable factors or by post-hoc statistical adjustment.

EXAMPLE (*cont.*) Unfortunately, the evidence on the effectiveness of antiviral drugs for needlestick injuries is limited. A case-control study of the use of zidovudine suggested that 81% of seroconversions to HIV could be prevented by prophylaxis. Less direct, but high-quality evidence comes from randomized trials of zidovudine and other antivirals to prevent vertical transmission of HIV, that is, transmission from mother to fetus. The first of these showed a 67% reduction. So we have some evidence of efficacy, but we do not precisely know how effective zidovudine alone is.

2.6 Combining probabilities

Many decision problems will involve more than one uncertainty. Decision analysis provides a means of weighing the competing benefits and harms for individuals or specific groups. We may need to combine the probabilities that represent diagnostic, prognostic, and treatment uncertainties. To combine these probabilities validly requires an understanding of a few important rules and ways of representing these probabilities in diagrams.

Recall the needlestick example, where there was both diagnostic uncertainty regarding the HIV status of the IV drug user, and prognostic uncertainty regarding the chance of developing HIV given a needlestick injury from an HIV-positive subject. Figure 2.5 shows the chance tree when no prophylactic treatment is given. In the bottom branch we have made explicit the assumption that, if the IV drug user was HIV-negative, then HIV cannot be transmitted to the health-care worker.

The overall probability of developing HIV is the sum of all the paths in the tree that result in HIV, that is: $(0.14 \times 0.005) + (0.86 \times 0) = 0.0007$. The final result could be more clearly presented in frequency terms: we can rewrite this probability and say that there is 1 chance in 1429 of developing HIV without prophylaxis ($1/0.0007 = 1429$).

Table 2.3 Observed distribution of human immunodeficiency virus (HIV) and hepatitis B virus (HBV) in 2202 intravenous drug users in Baltimore

	HBV +	HBV –	Total
HIV +	500 (23%)	40 (2%)	**540 (25%)**
HIV –	1360 (61%)	302 (14%)	**1662 (75%)**
Total	**1860 (84%)**	**342 (16%)**	2202

Data from (12). Numbers in parentheses are the percentages of the total population in each cell.

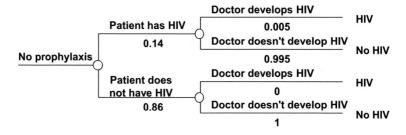

Figure 2.5   Chance tree for the needlestick example when no prophylaxis is given.

The chance tree here is quite simple, but the same process can be used to visualize far more complex sequences of probabilities, as we shall see in the chapters ahead.

2.6.1 Probability multiplication rules

To obtain the probability of HIV in the above example, we simply multiplied the two probabilities: diagnostic and prognostic. However, combining probabilities is sometimes less straightforward. Let us look at a second example that incorporates the possibility of other blood-borne infections. Specifically, let us consider the chance of an IV drug user having both HIV and hepatitis B virus (HBV) together. It is not sufficient to multiply the separate probabilities, since the two infections are likely to occur together, that is, they are not independent events. Examine the data in Table 2.3 from a 1988–89 serological study of consecutive IV drug users at a street outreach clinic in Baltimore (12). The table shows the observed joint distribution of HIV and HBV results: the cells of this 2 × 2 table show the numbers (and percentages) of those with both, either one, or neither infection. Keep in mind that the percentages in the cells of the table are calculated in relation to the total population (2202) in the study.

2.6.2 Conditional probability

Does having one of these infections affect the chances of having the other? For example, what is the probability of having HIV, given that the person has HBV? How does this compare with the probability of HIV if he or she doesn't have HBV? These are the conditional probabilities, $p(\text{HIV}+ \mid \text{HBV}+)$ and $p(\text{HIV}+ \mid \text{HBV}-)$, and can be calculated from Table 2.3. To obtain $p(\text{HIV}+ \mid \text{HBV}+)$ we look only at the HBV+ column of the table, and note that 500 of the 1860 cases have HIV, or 27%. Similarly, to obtain $p(\text{HIV}+ \mid \text{HBV}-)$ we look only at the HBV− column of the table and note that 40 of the 342 cases have HIV, or 12%.

These are conditional probabilities because they express the probability of an outcome under the condition that the other outcome has occurred. You could also think of it as the probability within a particular subset. For example, $p(\text{HIV}+ \mid \text{HBV}-)$ is the probability of HIV in the subset known to be negative for HBV. Since the probability of HIV depends on which subset we are referring to (the overall group (25%), the HBV+ group (27%), or the HBV− group (12%)), the HIV and HBV statuses are considered dependent events. Conversely, if these three probabilities turned out to be the same, then the events would be considered statistically independent.

2.6.3 Dependence and independence

Generalizing the above example, we can formally define *probabilistic independence*.

Clearly, in any data set some difference may occur between the conditional and unconditional probabilities merely by chance. We will not develop the statistical methods to examine this issue in this book. You will encounter several methods that statisticians use to determine the probability that an observed difference in the data could have resulted from random chance. For example, in the data in Table 2.3 the difference in HIV probability between the HBV+ and HBV− groups is: 27% − 12% = 15%. Several methods may be used to calculate the probability that this difference could have resulted by chance if there were truly no difference in the underlying probabilities; in our example, this p-value is less than 0.0001, that is, a highly statistically significant difference. Another frequently used statistical method is to calculate a *confidence interval* for the difference; in this case, such a confidence interval may be calculated as 10–20%, which does not include zero. Thus, the difference in the conditional probabilities is not explained by chance. This is not surprising. Those IV drug users engaged in unsafe practices such as needle sharing are more likely to get both infections; those engaged in safe practices such as needle exchange and cleaning are more likely to avoid both infections. Statistical independence in a data set can be tested using the chi-squared test for independence, which can be found in any statistics book.

DEFINITION   When the conditional probability of an event E, given another event F, is the same as the unconditional probability of event E, we say that events E and F are *probabilistically independent*. That is, if $p(E \mid F) = p(E)$, then E and F are independent events.

While commonly used, p-values and their close relatives, confidence intervals, have limitations as guides to decision making. Many statisticians and decision analysts object to the use of p-values because they do not tell us anything that would help us assess the probabilities of interest. In our example, a p-value of <0.0001 does *not* mean that the probability that HBV and HIV are independent is >0.9999! Similarly, a 95% confidence interval (as defined by frequentists) for a probability estimate does *not* imply that the true probability has a 95% chance of being inside the interval! The distinction we are drawing here is beyond the scope of this book, and it lies at the heart of the difference between the 'frequentists' and 'Bayesians.' Even the authors of this book align themselves at different points along this philosophical spectrum! It is a testament to the power of decision analysis as a method that it can be couched comfortably within either outlook on chance and probability.

2.6.4 Multiplying probabilities

When we wish to combine probabilities, as when obtaining the chance of a sequence of events, the exact method used will depend on whether the events are dependent or independent. If the events are independent, we can multiply the probabilities of each of the events in the sequence. If the events are dependent, we need to know the probabilities for each event conditional on the previous events in the sequence. Figure 2.6 shows the chance tree for the HIV and HBV probabilities.

To obtain the probability of having both HBV and HIV requires multiplying the probability of having HBV, $p(\text{HBV}+)$, by the probability of HIV given HBV, $p(\text{HIV}+ \mid \text{HBV}+)$.

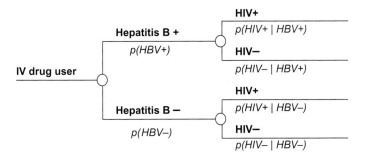

Figure 2.6   The chance tree for the human immunodeficiency virus (HIV) and hepatitis B virus (HBV) probabilities.

The calculation of the joint probability is performed as follows:

$$p(E \text{ and } F) = p(F) \times p(E \mid F) = p(E) \times p(F \mid E) \tag{2.4}$$

Note that if E and F are independent this simplifies to $p(E \text{ and } F) = p(E) \times p(F)$. Verifying this relation is a test for independence.

Important conditional probabilities that we will consider in the next chapters are the probability of an outcome given different treatments and the probability of a test result given different diseases. These probabilities are crucial to rational diagnostic testing and treatment decisions.

> **DEFINITION**   The probability of the concomitant occurrence of any number of events is called the *joint probability* of those events. The joint probability of two events, E and F, is written in probability notation as $p[E \text{ and } F]$ or as $p[E, F]$.

2.7 Expected value

So far we have been concerned with situations where each outcome at a chance node can be represented as the probability of a single event, such as HIV infection. Events are combined by applying the basic laws of conditional and joint probability discussed in this chapter. This process is called *averaging out*. However, the concepts of expected value and averaging out can be generalized to outcomes which are not probabilities but are some other number, such as the number of seizures, migraine attacks, days of illness, years of life, or costs. In Chapter 4 we will show how a special scale, called a utility scale, can be constructed so that it is just as appropriate to apply averaging out to utilities as to probabilities. First, however, we shall look further at averaging out and describe its application to problems that involve expected fixed-term outcomes.

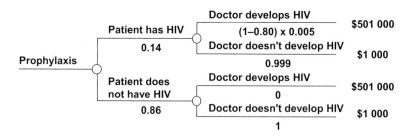

Figure 2.7   Chance tree of prophylaxis for the needlestick example with costs (in dollars) as outcome.

EXAMPLE (cont.)   Suppose we are interested in the expected future health-care resource costs of needlestick injuries, including the cost of prophylaxis and later costs of treatment. Not all health-care workers will take prophylaxis, and whether they do or do not, only a few will develop an HIV infection. Given these uncertainties, how can we calculate the expected future costs? The chance tree for prophylaxis (Figure 2.7) outlines the uncertainties and costs involved for that particular option.

Suppose that the cost of prophylaxis (including tests, visits, and drugs) is $1 000 and the cost of long-term treatment $500 000. Furthermore, assume that the effectiveness of prophylaxis in preventing HIV is 80% (relative risk = 0.80), so the proportion who will still develop HIV in spite of the prophylaxis is (1–80%) = 20%. To find the expected costs, we repeat the same averaging-out procedure as before, except now we multiply each path probability by the dollar values. The expected cost of prophylaxis is then:

$0.14 \times [((1 - 0.80) \times 0.005 \times \$501\ 000) + (0.999 \times \$1\ 000)] +$
$0.86 \times [(0 \times \$501\ 000) + (1 \times \$1\ 000)] = \$1070$

Thus, the expected cost is $1070. But note that no single case will have this particular cost. The expected value is a weighted average of costs representing our prediction of the average over a large series of similar cases.

DEFINITION   Suppose that an uncertain quantity X may have different values denoted by $X_1, X_2 \ldots X_n$ with probabilities $p_1, p_2 \ldots p_n$. Then we define its *expected value* as:

$$E[X] = p_1 \cdot X_1 + p_2 \cdot X_2 + \ldots p_n \cdot X_n. \tag{2.5}$$

The notation $E[X]$ is read as 'the expected value of X.' The expected value is also called the mean of the distribution of the possible values of the quantity.

2.7.1 Averages, expected values, and the law of large numbers

The expected value is closely related to the usual notion of a weighted average, and the relationship is more than coincidental. Suppose that we observe 100 patients undergoing the same procedure, as in our example, and then compute the average number of days of hospitalization. Keep in mind that the average is simply the sum of all the days of hospitalization divided by the number of patients. You know intuitively that if you observe enough patients and the probabilities are correct, the average will tend to be very close to the expected value. Statisticians call this property the law of large numbers. As the number of independent, identical replications becomes very large, their empirical average is likely to get very close to the expected value. A more familiar example involves a coin-tossing game with a fair coin. If you win one dollar when heads come up but lose one dollar when tails comes up, your winnings on a single toss are values of one dollar (with a probability of 0.5) or minus one dollar (with a probability of 0.5). The expected value of this is:

$$[(1/2)\ (\$1)] + (1/2)\ (-\$1)] = \$0 \tag{2.6}$$

You will never get $0, the expected value, on a single toss; you either get – $1 or + $1. However, the law of large numbers states that in the long run the average winnings per coin toss will be approximately zero.

2.8 Summary

Verbal expressions of uncertainties create two kinds of problems:
- There is wide variation in the interpretation of probabilistic terms. People can assign very different probability estimates to common verbal expressions such as 'likely,' 'possibly,' 'rarely,' and 'occasionally.' Hence, while it may seem that using these terms facilitates communication and understanding, we believe that their use can conceal important disagreements.
- If verbal expressions are assigned to different uncertainties in a complex problem, there is no agreed-upon, conventional, or normatively correct method for combining them into a single expression. This paves the way for still more misunderstanding and error.

Using probabilities and related numerical expressions to talk about uncertainty solves both problems: first, numbers are more precise than words and are therefore less likely to be misunderstood. Second, there are well-defined rules for combining probabilities mathematically. There are no rules for how verbal expressions should be combined, so there will be great variability in the conclusions drawn from a chain of verbal expressions.

We have identified three major types of uncertainties in health care:

- Diagnostic uncertainty is about the true underlying causes of illness. What is wrong with this patient?
- Prognostic uncertainty is about the future course of events. What may happen?
- Treatment uncertainty is about the consequences of treatment. Does the treatment lead to more benefit than harm?

All of these uncertainties can be expressed as chance events in a balance sheet or chance nodes in a decision tree.

The probability of a sequence of events is calculated by multiplying the probability of each event, conditioned on the previous events in the sequence. A decision tree or probability tree is a convenient way of displaying the probabilities to be multiplied. These tools help the decision maker keep track of the relevant uncertainties and calculate the probability of clinically relevant outcomes.

REFERENCES

1. Panlilio AL, Cardo DM, Grohskopf LA, Heneine W, Ross CS. *Updated US Public Health Service Guidelines For The Management Of Occupational Exposures To HIV And Recommendations For Postexposure Prophylaxis*. US Department of Health and Human Services, Centers for Disease Control and Prevention; 2005.
2. Shaw N, Dear P. How do parents of babies interpret qualitative expressions of probability? *Arch Dis Child*. 1990;65(5):520–3.
3. Woloshin KK, Ruffin M, Gorenflo DW. Patients' interpretation of qualitative probability statements. *Arch Fam Med*. 1994;3(11):961.
4. Timmermans D. The roles of experience and domain of expertise in using numerical and verbal probability terms in medical decisions. *Med Decis Making*. 1994;14(2):146–56.
5. Fleming KA. Evidence-based pathology. *Evidence Based Medicine*. 1997;2(5):132–3.
6. Des Jarlais DC, Bramson HA, Wong C, et al. Racial/ethnic disparities in HIV infection among people who inject drugs: an international systematic review and meta-analysis. *Addiction*. 2012;107(12):2087–95.
7. Pierorazio PM GT, Han M, et al. Long-term survival after radical prostatectomy for men with high Gleason sum in the pathological specimen. *Urology*. 2010;76(3):715–21.
8. Armitage P, Berry G, Matthews JNS. *Stat Methods Med Res*. Wiley-Blackwell; 2008.
9. Kannel WB. The Framingham Study: ITS 50-year legacy and future promise. *Journal Of Atherosclerosis And Thrombosis*. 1999;6(2):60–6.
10. Baker S, Priest P, Jackson R. Using thresholds based on risk of cardiovascular disease to target treatment for hypertension: modelling events averted and number treated. *BMJ*. 2000;320(7236):680.
11. Jackson R. Updated New Zealand cardiovascular disease risk–benefit prediction guide. *BMJ*. 2000;320(7236):709–10.
12. Levine OS, Vlahov D, Koehler J, et al. Seroepidemiology of hepatitis B virus in a population of injecting drug users: Association with drug injection patterns. *Am J Epidemiol*. 1995;142(3):331–41.

Choosing the best treatment

Firstly, do no (net) harm.

(adapted from) Hippocrates

3.1 Introduction

Some treatment decisions are straightforward. For example, what should be done for an elderly patient with a fractured hip? Inserting a metal pin has dramatically altered the management: instead of lying in bed for weeks or months waiting for the fracture to heal while blood clots and pneumonia threatened, the patient is now ambulatory within days. The risks of morbidity and mortality are both greatly reduced. However, many treatment decisions are complex. They involve uncertainties and trade-offs that need to be carefully weighed before choosing. Tragic outcomes may occur no matter which choice is made, and the best that can be done is to minimize the overall risks. Such decisions can be difficult and uncomfortable to make. For example, consider the following historical dilemma.

3.1.1 Benjamin Franklin and smallpox

Benjamin Franklin argued implicitly in favor of the application to individual patients of probabilities based on previous experience with similar groups of patients. Before Edward Jenner's discovery in 1796 of cowpox vaccination for smallpox, it was known that immunity from smallpox could be achieved by a live smallpox inoculation, but the procedure entailed a risk of death. When a smallpox epidemic broke out in Boston in 1721, the physician Zabdiel Boylston consented, at the urging of the clergyman Cotton Mather, to inoculate several hundred citizens. Mather and Boylston reported their results (1):

> Out of about ten thousand Bostonians, five thousand seven hundred fifty-nine took smallpox the natural way. Of these, eight hundred eighty-five died, or one in seven. Two hundred eighty-six took smallpox by inoculation. Of these, six died, or one in forty-seven.

Though at first skeptical, Franklin eventually saw the advantages of inoculation and advocated the practice. After presenting statistics such as those just given, Franklin said (1):

> In 1736, I lost one of my sons, a fine boy of 4 years old, by the smallpox taken in the common way. I bitterly regretted that I had not given it to him by inoculation. This I mention for the sake of parents who omit that operation, on the supposition that they should never forgive themselves if a child died under it. My example shows that the regret may be the same either way, and that therefore the safer should be chosen.

Whichever strategy is chosen, there is a risk of dying from smallpox. That is unavoidable. So Franklin urged adoption of the strategy with the lowest probability of death, having derived the probability for an individual patient from observed frequencies in other patients.

Clearly these probabilities depend on several factors, including risk of dying from smallpox inoculation and that from natural smallpox, as well as the risk of catching smallpox during an epidemic. If the risk of catching smallpox is sufficiently low, as during non-epidemic periods, then the inoculation would clearly not be worthwhile. At some critical level of risk, the inoculation becomes the better strategy. This risk is known as an *action threshold*. This chapter will focus on treatment decisions with trade-offs, and by explicitly describing and analyzing the complex risks and benefits, will provide insight into the central dilemmas of the problem. In particular we will look at the treatment threshold. This threshold provides a simple summary of a decision analysis which saves us from repeating the analysis for every new case. The treatment threshold can assist in providing rational guidelines for individual clinical decision making and for health policy.

3.2 Choosing the better risky option

Let us examine more closely the probabilities in Mather and Boylston's description. Of the 10 000 Bostonians, 286 chose inoculation; the remaining 9714 chose no inoculation. What were the consequences of these choices? Figure 3.1 shows the path probabilities emanating from each of the two choices. These paths contain two stages: first, the risk of smallpox, which in the case of inoculation is certain. Second, there is the risk of death given smallpox, with the risk being lower for smallpox from inoculation.

To calculate the averaged out probabilities of survival, we have given 'survive' a value of 1 and 'die' a value of 0 in the tree (Figure 3.1). (Had we wanted to calculate probabilities of death we would have reversed these values). The tree in Figure 3.2 shows the calculated overall chances of survival

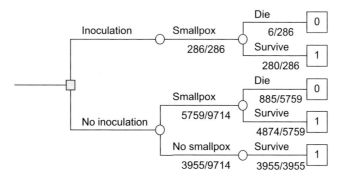

Figure 3.1   Decision tree for smallpox inoculation.

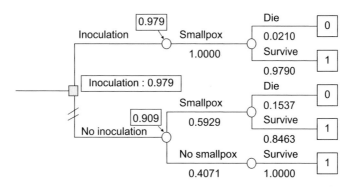

Figure 3.2   Averaging out the probabilities of survival for the smallpox inoculation problem. Note that the probabilities have been converted from absolute numbers to proportions.

based on the path probabilities following each of the two options. For inoculation the averaged out survival is 0.979 and for no inoculation it is 0.909. The absolute risk difference is thus 0.07 or 7%. We could also express this as the 'number-needed-to-inoculate,' which would be $1/0.07 = 14$, that is, for every 14 people inoculated, one smallpox death would be averted.

The proportions cited by Mather and Boylston overstate the advantage of inoculation, as they compared the risk of death from smallpox caused by inoculation with the risk of death from smallpox caught naturally. The tree clarifies that the risk of catching smallpox during the epidemic should also be considered. There are two further caveats on their analysis. First, the advantage of inoculation is not based on a randomized trial, so we cannot exclude another reason for the apparent difference, such as the relative ages or nutritional state of the groups, as an explanation for the apparent better survival of the inoculated group. Second, the risk of developing smallpox is based on the rates known *after* the epidemic was over, but you would have needed to make the decision about inoculation at the beginning of the epidemic. The appropriate choice of data might have been frequencies seen in previous epidemics.

This decision problem is a variant of one that we will encounter frequently, a decision between treating now versus expectant management ('watchful waiting'). The recurring trade-off problem is this: if we treat now (in this case, give smallpox by inoculation), there is a small but measurable risk of harm that might be avoided by expectant management. If expectant management is selected (in this case, no inoculation), there is a chance (40%) that the patient will not become infected and will survive. Under these circumstances, the patient will be better off with watchful waiting. But watchful waiting has its own risks: if the patient contracts smallpox 'in the common way,' the probability of mortality is much higher than with smallpox by inoculation. If that outcome occurs, we will wish that we had inoculated earlier, as Franklin expressed. The best action is determined by three factors: the chance of getting community-acquired smallpox, the associated probability of death, and the probability of death from smallpox after inoculation. Even in a simple problem as this, it may not be immediately apparent whether a risky preventive measure is preferable to watchful waiting; considering all relevant probabilities in a decision tree and averaging out the probability of survival clarifies the trade-offs. A moment's reflection will show that an increase in the mortality due to inoculation or a lower rate of community-acquired smallpox or a lower mortality from community-acquired smallpox would make the preventive strategy less attractive.

3.3 The best treatment option under diagnostic uncertainty

Sometimes treatment must be initiated before a clear diagnosis is reached. Of course, the usual order of medical management is to make a diagnosis, then select treatment based on this diagnosis. However, as we will discuss in detail later (Chapters 5–7), you will usually need to manage trade-offs in treatment options together with trade-offs due to the inaccuracy inherent in most diagnostic tests. In other words, despite our diagnostic efforts, a residual diagnostic uncertainty will often remain and we need to choose the best treatment option conditional on this uncertainty. There are some specific circumstances where this is a major problem.

1. Emergency conditions. In some urgent problems there may not be adequate time to obtain a firm diagnosis before starting treatment. For example, meningococcal meningitis (bacterial infection of the membranes that envelop the brain) can kill within hours, and hence we often need to treat, e.g., with intravenous penicillin, before the diagnosis can be

confirmed. In this and other examples, the expected benefit to those with the disease needs to be weighed against the expected harm of 'unnecessary' procedures in those without the disease.

2. Invasive diagnostic procedures. Even if there is sufficient time, the toll of some diagnostic procedures may outweigh the potential benefit. For example, a pulmonary nodule on a CT scan needs to be evaluated for malignancy, which may require a biopsy or even partial thoracotomy. If the probability of malignancy is high, radiation without biopsy may be preferred.

3. Residual uncertainty. Sometimes no cause of an illness will be found, even after thorough investigation. For example, no cause will be found for most cases of microscopic hematuria (blood in the urine); similarly, it is often difficult to find the cause of a chronic cough without use of empirical treatments for asthma or esophageal reflux (backflow of stomach contents into the esophagus).

The aim of diagnostic testing is to improve treatment decisions when the diagnosis is in doubt. Hence first understanding the treatment decision is important in devising a diagnostic strategy. This is the reverse order to practice: when seeing an individual patient, diagnosis precedes treatment; when analyzing diagnostic strategies, treatment decisions precede diagnosis. For example, when diagnosing a common cold, it does not help to identify the precise virus involved (there are over 200), because it does not affect the choice of treatment. An understanding of the treatment options thus guides the diagnostic process.

Let us begin by addressing the issue of when treatment is warranted despite an uncertain diagnosis. We then look at how and when the results of a diagnostic test should alter the treatment chosen and hence reduce the proportion of patients treated inappropriately.

EXAMPLE   **Suspected pulmonary embolism:**

A 30-year-old, seven-month-pregnant woman presents at your clinic with right-sided chest pain that gradually increased overnight. She is breathing faster than usual (tachypneic) with 20 breaths/min and has a mildly increased pulse rate (88 beats/min). An electrocardiogram shows no signs of right heart strain (ventricular overload). She has no clinical signs of blood clot in the legs (deep venous thrombosis, DVT). There is no family history of venous thromboembolism (VTE). A sensitive D-dimer test (blood test) yields a positive result. You suspect that she has a blood clot in her lungs (pulmonary embolism [PE]), but the diagnosis is uncertain.

In discussing the problem we will use a proactive approach.

3.3.1 Step 1: PROactive

P   Define the *problem*

R   *Reframe* from multiple perspectives

O   Focus on the *objective*

Given the patient's history, signs, symptoms, and positive D–dimer test result, you are concerned that she may have PE, but the diagnosis is uncertain. Clinical prediction rules and further diagnostic testing can address the diagnostic uncertainty (2, 3), which we will address in Chapters 5–7. First we will address the treatment decision.

Pulmonary embolism is a life-threatening event. Treatment with anticoagulation is effective in preventing further PE and hence in reducing the fatality probability. Anticoagulation, however, carries a risk of major bleeding which can be fatal and therefore one would like to avoid anticoagulation if it is unnecessary. Anticoagulation in a pregnant woman would mean subcutaneous injections of low molecular weight heparin (LMWH), temporarily stopping anticoagulation during delivery and oral anticoagulation with vitamin K antagonists post-partum depending on the patient's history (4).

The main objective of management is to avoid a recurrent PE, which may be fatal or lead to morbidity. From the perspective of the physician, he or she should try to maximize the survival chances for both the patient and her unborn child. Clearly the fetus's chances of survival are directly related to the woman's chances of survival. By optimizing the patient's survival chances we will concurrently be optimizing the chances of survival of the unborn child and both their chances of avoiding morbidity. In this example we will therefore focus on survival of the pregnant woman.

The problem then is whether or not to anticoagulate this pregnant woman in order to avoid the possible mortality of recurrent PE. In deciding, we need to take into account that we are uncertain whether PE is present and that anticoagulation has a small risk of fatal hemorrhage. From the perspective of both the woman and her unborn child, the objective is to maximize the survival chances of the woman.

3.3.2 Step 2: ProACTive

A   Consider all relevant *alternatives*

C   Model the *consequences* and estimate the *chances*

T   Identify the *trade-offs*

As we indicated in Chapter 1, the management alternatives are intervention (treatment with anticoagulation), wait-and-see (withholding anticoagulation),

Alternatives ⟶ Consequences ⟶ Outcomes

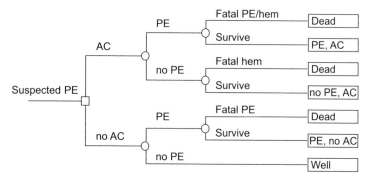

Figure 3.3   Decision tree comparing two strategies for suspected pulmonary embolism (PE). AC, anticoagulation. Hem, hemorrhage.

or getting more diagnostic information. At this point we have decided that obtaining more information is too risky because it would entail the use of X-rays (CT pulmonary angiography) or radioactive isotopes (ventilation–perfusion (V/Q) scan), which is considered contraindicated because of the pregnancy. Although this contraindication may be debatable, for this example we would like to focus solely on the choice between anticoagulation and no anticoagulation.

In considering the consequences it is convenient to structure the problem in the form of a decision tree (Figure 3.3). The decision tree starts on the left with the decision node and decision options. For our example these are 'anticoagulate' (AC) or 'do not anticoagulate' (no AC). Following each option the consequences are modeled to represent all the possible states (e.g., diagnoses) that may exist and events that may occur. Under both treatment options PE may or may not be present. The chance node is used to represent the uncertainty of the underlying true disease status and this probability reflects one of the unknowns for this particular decision problem. If PE is present, it may be fatal. The probability of death is conditional on whether PE is present and on whether anticoagulation is given. With anticoagulation the risk of death from PE is reduced. Anticoagulation, however, has a risk of fatal hemorrhage, which may occur whether PE is present or not.

The decision tree represents the chronological order of events from left to right: first the management options leading from the decision node (the square) and subsequently the chance events leading from the chance nodes (the circles). At the end of each path of events in the tree we visualize the outcome of that path. For example, at the end of the path 'AC → PE → fatal

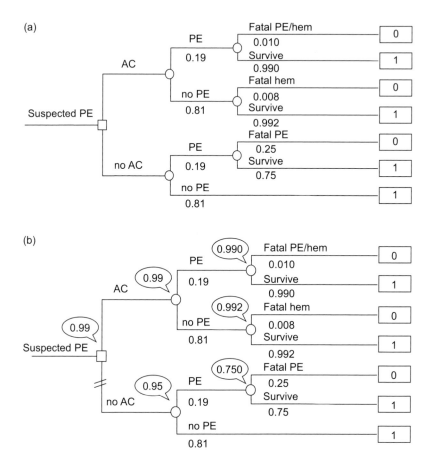

Figure 3.4   Decision tree comparing anticoagulate (AC) and do not anticoagulate (no AC) for suspected pulmonary embolism (PE) with (*a*) the event probabilities and outcome values filled in, and (*b*) the rolled-back tree. Hem, hemorrhage.

PE/hemorrhage,' the outcome is 'dead.' In this tree we combined the events fatal PE conditional on PE and fatal hemorrhage conditional on AC because both would result in death and because we do not have estimates of the probabilities of these events separately.

After formulating the problem, considering all the possible alternatives, and structuring the consequences in the form of a decision tree, we need to assign probabilities to the events and values to the outcomes (Figure 3.4*a*). The probabilities related to this problem are tabulated in Table 3.1. An important point to keep in mind when filling in the event probabilities is that each probability should be determined conditional on all the events that preceded it, i.e., on the events to the left of the index event in the decision tree. For example, the probability of a fatal PE or fatal hemorrhage in our

Table 3.1 Balance sheet for treatment options for a patient with suspected pulmonary embolism (PE)

	Anticoagulate (AC)	Do not anticoagulate (no AC)
Risk of death from PE or hemorrhage	1% if PE 0.8% if no PE	25% if PE 0% if no PE
Morbidity	Reduced quality of life in the event of non-fatal PE or non-fatal hemorrhage	Reduced quality of life in the event of non-fatal PE
Other benefits/ downsides	Medication: subcutaneous injections of LMWH during pregnancy, consider 6 weeks of oral vitamin K antagonists post-partum	No medication
Costs	Costs of AC	Avoids cost of AC

LMWH: low molecular weight heparin
Data from the literature (4, 5)

decision tree is conditional on whether PE is present and whether anti-coagulation is given or not.

From the balance sheet in Table 3.1 we see that there are risks and benefits to both options. The main trade-off is between the risk of death due to untreated PE and the risk of death due to hemorrhage caused by anticoagulation. The risk of a fatal bleed with anticoagulation is 0.008. Withholding anticoagulation, we assume that the risk of a fatal bleed is practically zero. The mortality risk (combined fatal PE or fatal hemorrhage) if PE is present is 0.25 if anticoagulation is withheld and is reduced to 0.01 if anticoagulation is given.

In this example the values assigned to the outcomes are fairly straightforward because we have chosen to optimize survival and not to include morbidity or costs explicitly in our decision model, even though we did consider them in our balance sheet. Therefore we use a very straightforward outcome value, namely alive or dead, alive being assigned a value of 1.0 and dead a value of 0.0. Alternatively we could value the outcomes with life expectancy, quality-adjusted life years, costs, or some other values that reflect our preferences. Whatever we use, the unit of outcome should represent the outcome we wish to optimize and should include any trade-offs we wish to capture in evaluating the problem. This will, in turn, be determined by the perspective we are taking in analyzing the decision problem and by our objective. We will return to the subject of valuing outcomes in Chapter 4.

One of the trade-offs in this decision is the possible harm of anticoagulation vs. the benefit that can be gained from the medication. Clearly here the harm from treatment is much smaller than the foregone benefit if we do not start treatment. Notice that comparing the harm of the treatment to its benefit reflects this trade-off, which we will expand on in Step 3.

3.3.3 Step 3: ProactIVE

I   *Integrate* the evidence and values
V   Optimize expected *value*
E   *Explore* the assumptions and *evaluate* uncertainty

The next step in the decision-making process is to integrate the evidence and the values. Based on the decision tree we calculate the average outcome value that we can expect (the expected value) for each option by averaging out the evidence-based probabilities and integrating the value of the outcomes. As we did in the previous chapter, to find the expected value we work backwards from the right-hand side of the tree, successively averaging out at each chance node until we have folded back the entire tree to the decision node. *Averaging out* refers to this process of multiplying the probabilities for each of the events leading from a chance node and doing this successively from right to left. Averaging out and calculating the expected value in fact calculates the weighted average of the outcome values (the numbers at the tips of the branches) with each outcome value weighed for the probability that it will occur (the path probability of that branch). In this simplified example the outcome values are simply 0 or 1, 0 being equivalent to dead and 1 being alive. Thus, multiplying the outcome values by probabilities will yield the probability of being alive.

After repeating the above procedure for all the possible options at the decision node, we need to decide which option is best. If we have used a positive (desirable) outcome value such as survival or life expectancy, we will want to maximize the expected value. If we have used a negative (undesirable) outcome value, such as mortality or costs, we will want to minimize the expected value. This process of removing less optimal alternatives from further consideration is called *folding back*. Averaging out and folding back are together referred to as *rolling back* the decision tree.

In our example, the overall expected survival chances are 99% with anti-coagulation and 95% without anticoagulation (Figure 3.4*b*). Therefore, given the case as presented and given the problem as we have defined it, and given all the assumptions we have made, and given the simplifications we have used, and assuming we want to optimize survival, we would, on average, choose to anticoagulate. But notice all the caveats we made: to be really confident about our decision we need to explore how our assumptions will affect the decision in a 'what-if' analysis – a *sensitivity analysis*.

DEFINITION	A *sensitivity analysis* is any test of the robustness of the conclusions of an analysis over a range of structural assumptions, probability estimates, or outcome values.

We may justifiably doubt the validity and generalizability of our analysis for several reasons. We may, for example, be unsure of the accuracy of the probability estimates or the applicability of the outcome values. To evaluate whether our results apply under other assumptions, we can repeat the analysis substituting a range of estimates for the probabilities or outcome values in question to see whether this alters the conclusion of the analysis. This is called a 'what-if' or sensitivity analysis. If the conclusion does not change over a range of estimates around the initial estimate, this should reassure us. If, on the other hand, the conclusion is sensitive to small alterations in a key probability, this may lead us back to the literature or to experts in search of a more refined estimate.

For example, we might ask how the results of our analysis would change if the probability of PE were higher or lower than initially estimated. In Figure 3.5 we have plotted the survival probability for both the 'anticoagulate' and 'do not anticoagulate' options over the full range of probabilities of PE from 0 to 1. Both options demonstrate a decrease in expected value with an increasing probability of PE; however the 'do not anticoagulate' strategy is far more sensitive to this probability because the mortality risk given PE is far larger without anticoagulation. For extremely low probabilities of PE, withholding anticoagulation yields a higher expected value because the harm of anticoagulation outweighs the benefit. For high probabilities of PE, anticoagulation yields a higher expected value because the benefit of anticoagulation outweighs the harm. Hence there must be a probability where we switch between the two options. This is the *treatment threshold (treat–do not treat threshold)*. Below this threshold, withholding treatment is better; above the threshold, treatment is better, and at the threshold, treatment and no treatment are exactly equal (6, 7).

DEFINITION	The *treatment (treat–do not treat) threshold* is the probability of disease at which the expected value of treatment and no treatment are exactly equal, and neither option is clearly preferable.

There are several different ways to perform sensitivity analysis and find the treatment threshold. We can use a numerical, algebraic, or graphical method.

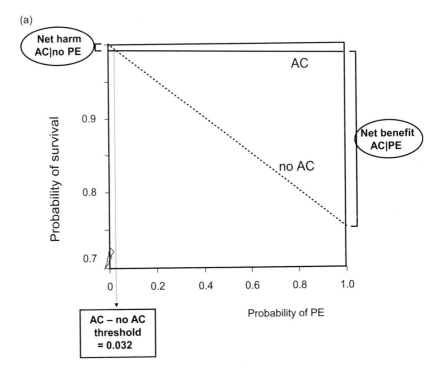

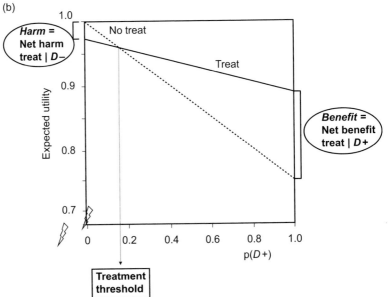

Figure 3.5   Graphical presentation of the ratio of harms to benefits of treatment and how this affects the associated treatment (treat–do not treat) threshold (*a*) for a young pregnant woman with suspected pulmonary embolism and (*b*) the generic graph for the treatment decision considering disease D (*D*+ *disease, D*– *no disease*). Notice how the treatment threshold increases as the ratio of harm to benefit increases. AC, anticoagulate; no AC, do not anticoagulate.

(a)

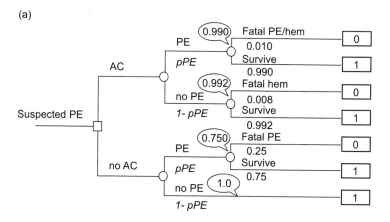

(b)

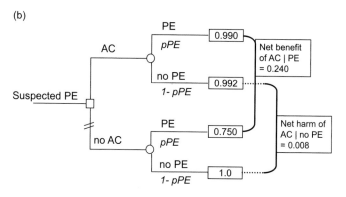

Figure 3.6   The decision tree comparing anticoagulate (AC) and do not anticoagulate (no AC) for suspected pulmonary embolism (PE), with an unknown prior probability of pulmonary embolism of *pPE(a)*. In (*b*) the last branches have been replaced with the partially rolled back numerical results that represent the probability of survival for the four possible situations determined by whether or not AC is given and whether or not PE is present. The *net benefit of treatment* is the difference in survival between patients with PE who receive AC and similar patients who do not receive AC. The *net harm of treatment* is the difference in survival between patients without PE who do not receive AC and similar patients who do receive AC.

All these methods are useful to have in your decision analysis toolkit, as they will each be useful in different circumstances. We will look at each in turn.

3.3.3.1 Numerical sensitivity and threshold analysis

Sensitivity analysis can be performed numerically by constructing a decision tree and inserting the uncertain variable, in this case the disease probability, as a variable (e.g., call it *pPE*). We then either plot or tabulate the expected value for all values of this probability. For example, in Figure 3.4a we could replace the disease probability with a variable name *pPE* (Figure 3.6a) and

Table 3.2A Sensitivity analysis on the probability of disease (pPE) for the range 0 to 0.10

pPE	AC	No AC	Optimal decision
0	0.9920	1.0000	No AC
0.01	0.9920	0.9975	No AC
0.02	0.9920	0.9950	No AC
0.03	0.9919	0.9925	No AC
0.04	0.9919	0.9900	AC
0.05	0.9919	0.9875	AC
0.06	0.9919	0.9850	AC
0.07	0.9919	0.9825	AC
0.08	0.9918	0.9800	AC
0.09	0.9918	0.9775	AC
0.10	0.9918	0.9750	AC

AC, anticoagulate; no AC, do not anticoagulate.

subsequently we can calculate the expected value over a range of values of this probability (Table 3.2). For obvious reasons this is preferably done using computer programs.

From Table 3.2A we can conclude that for probabilities of PE of 0.03 or lower, withholding anticoagulation is best, whereas for probabilities of PE of 0.04 or higher, anticoagulation is best. The treatment threshold is therefore somewhere between 0.03 and 0.04. Rerunning the analysis for the range of values between 0.03 and 0.04 (Table 3.2B) we find a more precise estimate of the threshold variable, which is (rounded-off) 0.032. Clearly these repeated calculations are tedious (and best done by computer), but for many problems there are some simple formulas for finding thresholds, which we will now examine.

3.3.3.2 Algebraic sensitivity and threshold analysis

To perform sensitivity analysis algebraically, we construct the decision tree and insert the disease probability as a variable (e.g., call it pPE). Subsequently we average out algebraically. For example, for the young pregnant woman the option 'anticoagulation' has an expected value of (Figure 3.6b):

$$\text{Expected value}(AC) = 0.990 \times pPE + 0.992 \times (1 - pPE) \tag{3.1}$$

Table 3.2B Sensitivity analysis on the probability of disease (*pPE*) for the range 0.03 to 0.04

pPE	AC	No AC	Optimal decision
0.030	0.9919	0.9925	No AC
0.031	0.9919	0.9923	No AC
0.032	0.9919	0.9920	No AC
0.033	0.9919	0.9918	AC
0.034	0.9919	0.9915	AC
0.035	0.9919	0.9913	AC
0.036	0.9919	0.9910	AC
0.037	0.9919	0.9908	AC
0.038	0.9919	0.9905	AC
0.039	0.9919	0.9903	AC
0.040	0.9919	0.9900	AC

AC, anticoagulate; no AC, do not anticoagulate.

For the option withholding anticoagulation, the expected value is:

$$\text{Expected value(no AC)} = 0.750 \times pPE + 1.0 \times (1 - pPE) \tag{3.2}$$

Setting the expected values of the options to be equal, we can solve for the unknown threshold probability of *pPE*:

$$0.990 \times pPE + 0.992 \times (1 - pPE) = 0.750 \times pPE + 1.0 \times (1 - pPE)$$

$$0.240 \times pPE = 0.008 \times (1 - pPE)$$

$$0.240 \times pPE + 0.008 \times pPE = 0.008$$

$$pPE = 0.008/(0.240 + 0.008) \tag{3.3}$$

To express the treatment threshold in formula form, we first define both net benefit and net harm.

DEFINITION   The *net benefit* of a treatment is the difference in outcome in patients with the disease who receive treatment and similar patients who do not receive treatment. That is,

Net benefit = utility(treatment | disease) − utility (no treatment | disease) (3.4)

We shall formally define *utility* in the next chapter, but for now we just need to interpret it as the value of the outcomes to the patient. Note that *net benefit* here refers to the clinical benefit, which needs to be distinguished from net proportional benefit (introduced in Chapter 7), and net health benefit and net monetary benefit (discussed in Chapter 9 and 12). A net benefit is usually expressed as a utility, that is, a desirable outcome (e.g., survival). A net benefit may alternatively be expressed as a disutility, that is an undesirable outcome (e.g., mortality). For example, in our patients with suspected PE the net benefit of treatment in terms of utility is the difference in survival between anticoagulation vs. withholding anticoagulation in those with PE. For our patients this is $(1 - 0.01) - (1 - 0.25) = 0.99 - 0.75 = 0.24$, that is, an increase in survival chances of 0.24. Alternatively, we may express the results in terms of a disutility, which in this case would be $0.01 - 0.25 = - 0.24$, that is, a reduction (negative sign) in mortality of 0.24.

DEFINITION   The *net harm* of a treatment is the difference in outcome between patients without the disease who do not receive treatment and similar patients who do receive that treatment. That is:

$$Net\ Harm = utility(no\ treatment\mid no\ disease)$$
$$- utility(treatment\mid no\ disease) \qquad (3.5)$$

For example, in our patient the net harm of treatment is the difference in outcome between withholding anticoagulation vs. anticoagulation in those without PE. This is $(1 - 0) - (1 - 0.008) = 0.008$, i.e., no treatment increases survival by 0.008 compared to treatment, which is the same as saying treatment decreases survival by 0.008. Recognize that the 0.24 and 0.008 in equation 3.3 represent the net benefit and net harm, respectively.

Following the same algebraic derivation as above but now with the utilities expressed as variables, it follows that at the treatment threshold:

$$Odds\ at\ treatment\ threshold = \frac{p}{1-p} = \frac{Harm}{Benefit} \qquad (3.6)$$

Note that *harm* and *benefit* refer to the net harm and net benefit as defined above. We convert from odds to probability by adding the numerator to the denominator on both sides of the equation, which gives the treatment threshold probability:

$$Probability\ at\ treatment\ threshold = p = \frac{Harm}{Harm + Benefit} \qquad (3.7)$$

3.3.3.3 Graphical sensitivity and threshold analysis

A simple and helpful method for determining the treatment threshold is to compare the benefits and harms of treatment directly and visualize them graphically. The smaller the harm relative to the benefit, the lower the treatment threshold should be. Conversely, the larger the harm relative to the benefit, the higher the treatment threshold should be. To illustrate this, Figure 3.5a presents the results of our analysis for the presented example. In our example the harm of anticoagulation is relatively small compared with the benefit and the treatment threshold is therefore low.

Now consider another similar case of suspected PE. A 67-year-old woman who two days ago underwent hysterectomy and lymph node dissection for sarcoma presents with a similar picture of chest pain, faster breathing, increased pulse rate, no clinical signs of blood clot in the legs (deep venous thrombosis), and an indeterminate result on diagnostic testing. This patient has a different ratio of benefit to harm because her chances of a fatal bleed are much higher, given that she has just undergone major abdominal surgery. In fact, we would expect her chances of a fatal bleed to be approximately 0.04. The combined probability of mortality from a bleed or fatal PE if she has PE and receives anticoagulation will be approximately 0.05. If she has PE but anticoagulation is withheld, we would expect a similar probability of mortality as before of 0.25. The net harm of treatment is thus larger and the net benefit of treatment with anticoagulation is less than for the young pregnant woman. The treatment threshold therefore shifts to higher values (Figure 3.5b).

Figure 3.5 can be seen as analogous to a scale where the harms and benefits are weighed. The harms are indicated on the left axis, the benefits on the right axis, and the treatment threshold is the pivot point. As the ratio of harms to benefits increases, the scale becomes heavier on the left in comparison to the right, and in so doing the pivot point representing the treatment threshold increases.

The precise treatment threshold can be calculated from the graph. The benefit and harm can be marked on the vertical axes of the sensitivity analysis figure (Figure 3.5). Benefit is marked on the right-hand axis by indicating the expected outcomes with and without treatment in a group with the disease (that is, $pPE = 1$). Similarly, harm is marked on the left-hand vertical axis by indicating the expected outcomes with and without the treatment in those without the disease (that is, $pPE = 0$). The line joining the value of treating the nondiseased (at probability 0) and the value of treating the diseased (at probability 1) represents the expected value of treatment over the range of values from 0 to 1. Similarly, the expected value of no treatment is the line joining the value of withholding treatment from the non-diseased (at probability 0) and the value of withholding treatment from the diseased

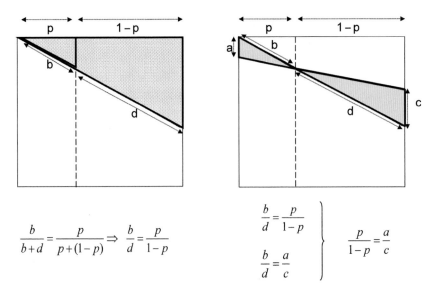

$$\frac{b}{b+d} = \frac{p}{p+(1-p)} \Rightarrow \frac{b}{d} = \frac{p}{1-p}$$

$$\left.\begin{array}{c} \dfrac{b}{d} = \dfrac{p}{1-p} \\[2mm] \dfrac{b}{d} = \dfrac{a}{c} \end{array}\right\} \quad \dfrac{p}{1-p} = \dfrac{a}{c}$$

Figure 3.7   Geometric proof of the formula for the treatment threshold: the ratio of p to $(1 - p)$ is the same as the ratio of a (harm) to c (benefit).

(at probability 1). These two lines cross at the treatment threshold, where the expected value of the two options is equal.

Our intuition, the algebraic formula, and the graphical presentation, all tell us that if the harm is much smaller than the benefit, the treatment threshold should be low. Conversely, if the harm is large compared with the benefit, then the treatment threshold should be high. And if benefits and harms are equal, the treatment threshold is 0.5.

3.3.3.4 Geometric proof of the threshold formula

A simple geometric proof of the threshold formula can be seen from Figures 3.5b and 3.7. Observe that the bases on the y-axes of the benefit and harm are the bases of similar triangles. Figure 3.7 illustrates that the ratio b/d equals the ratio $p/(1 - p)$. Also, the ratio a/b equals the ratio c/d. Thus, $a/c = b/d$ and therefore $p/(1 - p) = a/c$. Hence, at the point of indifference between treatment and no treatment, the harm and benefit are in the same ratio as the threshold probability p and its complement $(1 - p)$, that is, $p/(1 - p) = harm/benefit$. Adding the numerator to the denominator on both sides of the equation, which is equivalent to converting from odds to probabilities on both sides, gives the treatment threshold probability:

$$Treatment\ threshold = \frac{Harm}{Harm + Benefit} \tag{3.7a}$$

Notice that this is exactly the same formula (3.7) we derived algebraically. For our example cases, we can calculate the treatment thresholds using this formula. For the young pregnant woman the ratio of harm to benefit is 0.008:0.24, or 1:30, and the treatment threshold is therefore low:

$$\text{Treatment threshold} = 0.008/(0.240 + 0.008) = 1/31 = 0.032 \qquad (3.8)$$

Hence, we would prefer to anticoagulate the young pregnant woman if the probability of PE is higher than 0.032 and withhold anticoagulation if it is lower. If the probability is exactly 0.032 we are indifferent as to whether we anticoagulate or not. For the elderly woman the ratio of harm to benefit is 0.04:0.20, or 1:5, and the treatment threshold therefore shifts to higher values, as can be seen graphically in Figure 3.5:

$$\text{Treatment threshold} = 0.04/(0.04 + 0.20) = 1/6 = 0.167 \qquad (3.9)$$

3.3.4 Subjective treatment threshold estimates

When there is insufficient time for the type of formal analysis described above, a quick approximate and subjective alternative would be to ask: 'How many times worse is not treating a case of true disease (foregone benefit) compared to unnecessarily treating a case without the disease (iatrogenic harm)?' If your answer is N times, then the harm to benefit ratio is $1/N$ and thus the corresponding treatment threshold is $1/(N + 1)$. For example, you might ask for treatment of suspected meningococcal meningitis (an infection that is often rapidly fatal if not treated): 'How many times worse is failing to treat a case of meningococcal meningitis compared to the harm of giving parenteral penicillin to a child who does not have meningococcal meningitis?' The treatment threshold here is clearly very low. You might consider it 100 times worse, in which case the treatment threshold is $1/(100 + 1) \cong$ 1%. This does not mean that only 1:100 patients you might treat will turn out to have meningitis. The actual patients will have a range of presenting features and hence a range of chances of meningitis. Among these maybe a few are near the 1:100 threshold, while others may have much higher probabilities.

3.3.5 One-way, two-way, three-way, and *n*-way sensitivity analysis

Thus far we performed one-way sensitivity analysis: the value of one probability was varied while the other probability and outcome values remained constant. After exploring the effect of a change in the variable values one at a time, one may question the effect of simultaneous changes in the variables. In two-way sensitivity analysis the effect of simultaneous changes in two variable values is evaluated. For example, for our case example we could question what the threshold probability of PE would be if the risk of a fatal recurrent PE without anticoagulation were to be lower than the initially estimated value of

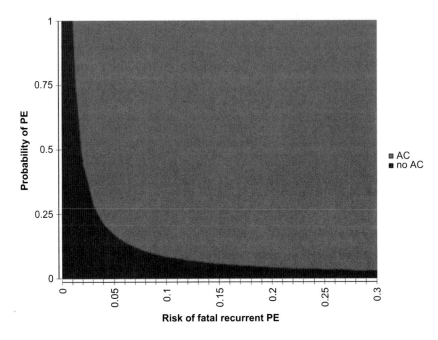

Figure 3.8   Two-way sensitivity analysis determining the threshold probability of pulmonary embolism (PE) for different values of the risk of a fatal recurrent PE without anticoagulation (AC). AC indicates the combinations of the two variable values for which anticoagulation has the highest expected value and no AC indicates the combinations of the two variable values for which withholding anticoagulation has the highest expected value.

0.25. Varying the two variables simultaneously yields a graph that shows for which combinations of values of the two variables treatment with anticoagulation is preferred and for which values withholding anticoagulation is preferred (Figure 3.8). If we repeat the two-way sensitivity analysis for various values of a third variable we get a three-way sensitivity analysis.

In n-way sensitivity analysis we vary multiple variable values at the same time. An n-way sensitivity analysis is useful to evaluate the results for a different setting, for different types of patients, and for best- and worst-case scenarios. In best- and worst-case scenarios we would pick extreme values for the variables, biasing towards and subsequently against the program under consideration. Evaluating variability and uncertainty is discussed in more detail in Chapter 12.

3.4 The decision to obtain diagnostic information and the do's and don'ts of tree building

Whereas we felt that a CT pulmonary angiogram was contraindicated in the case of the young pregnant woman, in the elderly woman we may want to consider obtaining more diagnostic information by performing a CT

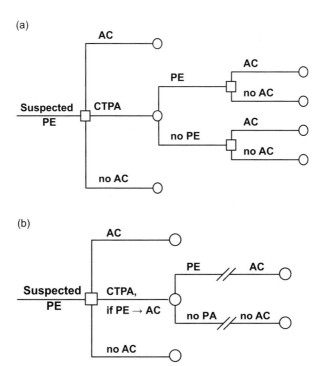

Figure 3.9

The decision to treat with anticoagulation (AC), withhold anticoagulation (no AC), or perform a CT pulmonary angiogram (CTPA) in suspected pulmonary embolism (PE). (*a*) Extensive form of the tree with embedded decision nodes and (*b*) strategic form of the decision tree.

pulmonary angiogram. The aim of obtaining more diagnostic information would be to shift our probability assessment across the treatment threshold. In other words, performing a diagnostic test to obtain additional information is worthwhile only if at least one decision would change by the test results and if the risk to the patient associated with the test is less than the expected benefit that would be gained from the subsequent change in the decision.

We can model the decision to obtain diagnostic information by adding this option in the decision tree (Figure 3.9). Strictly speaking, after performing the CT pulmonary angiogram we are again faced with the choice of whether or not to give anticoagulation (AC vs. no AC) and thus the decision tree contains embedded decision nodes. After performing a CT pulmonary angiogram, however, we will know whether or not the patient actually has a PE. If she has a PE, anticoagulation is clearly the better option. If she does not have a PE, withholding anticoagulation is clearly better. It would be perfectly permissible at this point to *prune* the tree by eliminating the branches that would never apply anyway. The branches that can be pruned even before calculating the expected value are withholding anticoagulation if PE is definitely present and giving anticoagulation if PE is definitely absent. In this simple case, pruning the tree has changed it from a decision tree in *extensive form* (Figure 3.9*a*) to one in *strategic form* (Figure 3.9*b*).

DEFINITION	A decision tree in *strategic form* contains no embedded decision nodes but instead all options are strategies.

In strategic form the options are expressed as strategies in terms such as 'do *A*; if *X*, then do *B*; if *Y*, then do *C*.' In the strategic form of a decision tree that, for example, models diagnostic strategies, the next management decision given the test result would be included in defining the overall diagnostic strategy.

To illustrate the difference between the extensive and strategic form of a decision tree modeling diagnostic workup, consider the first case example (the young pregnant woman) but now prior to a decision whether or not to apply a clinical prediction rule, prior to deciding whether or not to anticoagulate. Several clinical prediction rules exist that provide the probability of pulmonary embolism based on demographics, signs and symptoms, and lab tests (such as the D-dimer test). Figure 3.10*a* presents the decision tree in extensive form. It has been pruned to eliminate the branches that are clearly irrelevant but it still contains embedded decision nodes. We can redraw the tree in strategic form (Figure 3.10*b*) by bringing all the decisions up front and, instead of only letting the immediate decision lead from the initial decision node, we define the entire set of complete strategies up front. Note that in the example the strategies are defined by the chosen positivity of the clinical prediction rule (PR), above which the patient will be anticoagulated, a topic we will revisit in Chapter 7. Trees in strategic form can be particularly useful when analyzing cost-effectiveness, performing sensitivity analysis, and determining the thresholds between strategies.

In building decision trees one needs to be careful about sequencing decision nodes and chance nodes in the correct order. Going from left to right, a decision tree generally depicts the sequence of events as they may occur over time, i.e., in chronological order. For example, one would first do the non-invasive test (such as the prediction rule for suspected PE) and only after doing the reference test (the CT pulmonary angiogram in this case) will we know whether the disease is present or not. To model this chronologically we would model the test result first and then the true disease status (Figure 3.10).

Sometimes, however, it can be convenient to model it the other way around – that is, model disease status first followed by the test result. But watch out when

(a)

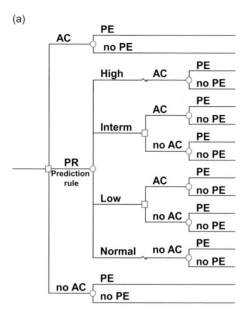

(b)

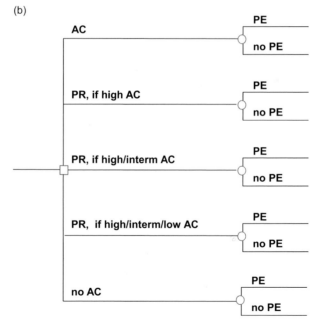

Figure 3.10   The decision to treat with anticoagulation (AC), withhold anticoagulation (no AC), or apply the clinical prediction rule (PR) in the young pregnant woman with suspected pulmonary embolism (PE). (*a*) Extensive form of the tree with embedded decision nodes and (*b*) strategic form of the decision tree. The strategies are defined by the chosen positivity of the prediction rule above which the patient will be anticoagulated.

you do this! Modeling disease status first and then the test result is only permissible if there are no intervening decisions or events that may influence the course of the disease or affect probabilities thereafter. Most important is that you need to remember to let the next management decision depend on the test result, which you observe, and not on the true disease status, which is the underlying truth but unknown to the decision maker as long as a reference test has not (yet) been performed. You can think of it as follows: there are two worlds. The one is the observable perceived reality, and the other is the underlying truth which you will never know with absolute certainty unless you have performed the reference test (if there is such a test for the disease). We model both the observable reality and the underlying truth but our decisions can only be based on the observable world. We will return to the sequencing of events in the decision tree in the context of interpreting diagnostic test information when we invert diagnostic decision trees in Chapter 5. In Chapter 6 we will discuss the threshold probabilities for the choice between no treatment and performing a test and between performing a test and treatment.

3.5 Summary

Every decision problem should first be defined from the relevant perspective and the objective should be formulated. A decision tree is useful to visualize and structure the alternatives, the consequences of each alternative and the associated chances, and the value trade-offs for a decision problem. The evidence and values are integrated by calculating the expected value of each option, which equals the sum of the outcome values of that option, each outcome value weighed for the probability that it will occur. We choose the option that maximizes the expected value if value is expressed as a desirable outcome and minimizes expected value if it is expressed as an undesirable outcome. Finally, we explore our assumptions and evaluate the uncertainty of our probability and value estimates through sensitivity analysis.

In choosing whether or not to treat a patient in the face of diagnostic uncertainty, a threshold probability exists for the probability of disease below which withholding treatment is better and above which treatment is better. At the treatment threshold the expected value of treatment and withholding treatment are exactly equal. The treatment threshold is determined by the ratio of net harm incurred by treating patients without the disease and the net benefit gained by treating patients with the disease. The smaller the harm relative to the benefit, the lower the treatment threshold should be. Conversely, the larger the harm relative to the benefit, the higher the treatment threshold should be.

REFERENCES

1. Schmidt WM. Health and welfare of colonial American children. *Am J Dis Child.* 1976;130(7):694–701.
2. Mos IC, Klok FA, Kroft LJ, et al. Safety of ruling out acute pulmonary embolism by normal computed tomography pulmonary angiography in patients with an indication for computed tomography: systematic review and meta-analysis. *J Thromb Haemost.* 2009;7(9):1491–8.
3. Lucassen W, Geersing GJ, Erkens PM, et al. Clinical decision rules for excluding pulmonary embolism: a meta-analysis. *Ann Intern Med.* 2011;155(7):448–60.
4. Bates SM. Pregnancy-associated venous thromboembolism: prevention and treatment. *Semin Hematol.* 2011;48(4):271–84.
5. van Erkel AR, Pattynama PM. Cost-effective diagnostic algorithms in pulmonary embolism: an updated analysis. *Acad Radiol.* 1998;5 Suppl. 2:S321–7.
6. Pauker SG, Kassirer JP. Therapeutic decision making: a cost–benefit analysis. *N Engl J Med.* 1975;293(5):229–34.
7. Pauker SG, Kassirer JP. The threshold approach to clinical decision making. *N Engl J Med.* 1980;302(20):1109–17.

4

Valuing outcomes

Values are what we care about. As such, values should be the driving force for our decision making. They should be the basis for the time and effort we spend thinking about decisions. But this is not the way it is. It is not even close to the way it is.

Ralph Keeney

4.1 Introduction

Value judgments underlie virtually all clinical decisions. Sometimes the decision rests on a comparison of probability alone, such as the probability of surviving an acute episode of illness. In such cases, there is a single outcome measure – the probability of immediate survival – that can be averaged out to arrive at an optimal decision. In most cases, however, decisions between alternative strategies require not only estimates of the probabilities of the associated outcomes, but also value judgments about how to weigh the benefits versus the harms, and how to incorporate other factors like individual preferences for convenience, timing, who makes decisions, who else is affected by the decision, and the like. Consider the following examples.

EXAMPLE 1 **Genetic susceptibility for breast cancer:**

A 25-year-old woman has a strong family history of breast cancer, including a sister who developed the disease at age 35. Her sister has undergone genetic testing for cancer predisposition and has been found to carry a mutation in the BRCA1 breast cancer gene. The woman is concerned about her own risk of breast cancer and chooses to be tested. She is found to have the same mutation, and is told that her lifetime risk of developing breast cancer is approximately 65%. If she does nothing at all with this information, her chance of surviving to age 70 is 53% (compared with all women's survival probability of 84%). She has a number of options open to her: (1) careful surveillance, including regular mammography and magnetic resonance imaging (MRI), which would increase her chance of surviving to age 70 to 59%; (2) prophylactic mastectomy – surgical removal of both breasts – which would increase her chance of surviving to age 70 to 66%; (3) prophylactic mastectomy now plus prophylactic oophorectomy (PO) – surgical removal of the ovaries – when she turns 40, which would increase her chance of surviving to age 70 to 79%. Both surgical options increase her chance of survival beyond that of

---

surveillance, but carry some personal costs – mastectomy can affect sexual function and body image, oophorectomy causes early-onset menopause and prevents child bearing. Does the benefit of risk reduction with surgery outweigh the personal costs of these interventions?

EXAMPLE 2   **Childhood vaccination:**

A mother brings her 6-month-old daughter for a well-baby visit to her pediatrician, and is told the daughter is perfectly healthy and is due for hepatitis B, rotavirus, *haemophilus* influenza type b, influenza, pneumococcal, polio, and pertussis vaccines. All six vaccinations are recommended by the Centers for Disease Control and Prevention for this age child, and all prevent diseases that can have serious and possibly fatal complications. There is a small elevated risk of febrile seizures from simultaneous administration of pneumococcal and influenza vaccines, of about an additional 17 seizures/100 000 doses. The influenza vaccine could be delayed to an interim visit when the parent would bring the child back for that vaccination alone, between this one and the next scheduled well-child visit at 12 months. But there are risks to delaying vaccinations, including missing doses because return visits are missed or postponed, and the extra visit adds inconvenience for the mother and stress for the child. Is the risk of febrile seizures from multiple vaccinations at one visit high enough to outweigh the inconvenience and stress of returning at a separate visit for it alone?

In both these examples, a decision requires value judgments, either for treatment or prevention. In both cases, we are concerned not only with the probabilities of surviving or dying from either the intervention or the disease, but also we are concerned with the effect of the decision on the quality of life and well-being of the patient and the surrounding individuals (e.g., the child's mother, the woman's future children). All interventions carry a chance of non-fatal harms that may reduce the quality of the patient's life, in large or small ways. Clearly a choice will vary depending on one's values. Value judgments are especially relevant when a disease cannot be definitively cured and a patient may live many years in an impaired or compromised state, or when a treatment or intervention, even if ordinarily quite effective, carries some risk of severe side effects. In such cases, are explicit, quantitative valuations of each of the possible outcomes required for optimal decision making? The answer depends on how the benefits and harms are valued, and by whom.

In this chapter we will first describe two decision-making perspectives, the individual's and society's, then discuss how these have different applications and require different styles of valuation. We will then look at the methods and validity of several ways of measuring the individual's (i.e., the patient's) values, and how and when they may be used in different decision-making settings.

4.2 Decision-making paradigms

In considering each of the following decision-making paradigms, it may be helpful to ask yourself the following questions. First, who is the decision maker? Is it the doctor, the patient, the caregiver, the insurer, the policy maker? Second, what information does the decision maker need? And third, how can the decision maker be helped to clarify his or her values relevant to the decision? The answers to these questions provide a framework for value clarification in each setting.

4.2.1 The clinical encounter

In this decision-making setting, a doctor and patient (plus sometimes the family or caregivers) face choices among alternative treatment strategies. Their goal is to choose the best treatment for that particular patient. It has been well documented that most patients in this situation want to be provided with information about their medical condition and options for managing it. However, they vary widely in the degree of decision-making autonomy they wish to exercise (1). Decision-making preferences range from a somewhat 'old school' approach where the patient cedes all responsibility to the physician, to a more current 'shared decision-making' approach in which the patient/ family and physician work as a team to evaluate options and reach a decision. Decision models and aids are increasingly being developed and used to assist both patients and physicians in the decision-making process. In some cases, responsibility for decision making is delegated to a caregiver, such as a parent, spouse, or an adult child of an elderly patient. Caregivers have the dual role of trying to anticipate the patient's decision preferences and integrating their own into the process, regardless of whether decision making is shared with the physician. Regardless of their preferred role, it is known that well-informed patients adhere better to treatment plans than those who do not participate in decision making at all, so the question arises of what do patients and caregivers want and need to know to make the best decisions for themselves (2, 3).

Like all decision makers, patients and caregivers need to know the list of the possible outcomes associated with each strategy under consideration, the probability that each outcome will occur, and the likely impact of those outcomes on their lives. They can then apply their own values in weighing the benefits and harms of each strategy, and choose the option that maximizes the outcomes that matter most to them.

Let's return to the example of the woman considering alternative strategies for managing her elevated breast cancer risk. Screening with regular mammography and MRI does nothing to change her baseline 65% risk of developing breast cancer. Surgery, either prophylactic mastectomy or prophylactic oophorectomy, or both, would reduce her risk of breast and ovarian cancer substantially, but would require that she undergo the irrevocable step of having both breasts and possibly ovaries surgically removed. What information does she need to make this decision? The expected effect of each option on her survival is well described in the scenario. However, the way the information is presented reflects the nature of the clinical studies that have been done addressing this question, and may not include the information needs of patients.

Most women considering this choice would want to know how much each option would help them to live a normal life span, compared to women who do not have the BRCA1 genetic mutation. Because there have not been (and probably never will be) any randomized trials of prophylactic surgery, this information is not available from a single source. However, information from observational studies combined with clinical trials can provide estimates of the survival benefits associated with surgery. These numbers, from a decision analysis of survival alone, are shown in Table 4.1.

Thinking purely about her chance of living a normal life span with different treatment options, a woman could use this table to inform her choice of strategy, and the timing of that choice, considering the survival probability if she chose that option. She would notice that prophylactic mastectomy (PM) combined with prophylactic oophorectomy (PO) has the largest benefit, regardless of when the mastectomy is performed. Moreover, earlier PM is slightly better than later PM, though delaying the PM does not have a substantial effect on her survival. An individual woman considering prophylactic mastectomy and/or oophorectomy could turn to these data to obtain estimates about one of the potential benefits of the intervention: gain in expected survival. She is then in a better position to apply her own values in deciding whether that benefit outweighs the harm, in impact on body image, sexuality, and reproductive function, for her personally.

Presented with all the requisite information, active decision makers are in a position to apply their own values to choose the best treatment for them. This process can be facilitated with decision aids, that clearly and often visually present the trade-offs involved in choosing between treatments (see for example, decision aids for BRCA1/2 carriers considering mastectomy 5–7, 8). Decision aids may use decision 'boards,' interactive videodiscs, and/or

Table 4.1 Survival probabilities to age 70 and 80 years for a 25-year-old BRCA1+ patient for prophylactic mastectomy (PM) and prophylactic mastectomy plus prophylactic oophorectomy (PO) at different ages compared with breast preservation

Clinical strategies	Survival probability to age 70*	Survival probability to age 80*
No screening or surgeries	53%	33%
Regular screening with mammography and MRI	59%	38%
No screening, PM at age 25	66%	44%
Regular screening with mammography and MRI, PM at age 30	66%	44%
Regular screening with mammography and MRI, PM at age 40	64%	43%
Regular screening with mammography and MRI, PM at age 50	61%	41%
Regular screening with mammography and MRI, PM at age 30 and PO at age 40	79%	61%
Regular screening with mammography and MRI, PM at age 40 and PO at age 40	77%	59%
Regular screening with mammography and MRI, PM at age 50 and PO at age 40	75%	58%
**survival probability for general US female population*	84%	66%

Adapted from Kurian et al. (4)

websites, and many have been tested for their effectiveness in assisting with the decision process (8).

Whether or not the decision-making process is facilitated by decision aids, in this paradigm the choice is essentially made in a 'black box.' Information on the nature and probabilities of various outcomes is supplied by the physician, a decision aid, the internet, or family and friends, and the patient applies his or her own values to weight those outcomes, meaning to choose which factors are more or less important, to generate a decision about which choice is best for him or her. In this decision-making model, the process of combining the relevant probabilities and values is intuitive (in the black box, or the individual's own mind), not explicitly articulated.

However, not all patients want to be active decision makers. It is not uncommon for patients presented with a choice between two options to turn to the physician and ask, 'What would you do if you were me?' This is often not a simple question to answer. To generate a recommendation, the physician must not only know the probabilities of various outcomes, but also weight them according to someone's values. Only by applying value judgments can the physician determine whether the morbidity of a toxic therapy is justified by a small resulting increase in life expectancy, or whether it is worth the inconvenience of a return visit to reduce a very small chance of a particular side effect, such as febrile seizure.

Whose values should apply in making these choices? Obviously, the physician's goal in counseling the patient wanting guidance should be to identify the best option for that individual patient. The relevant values are the patient's, not the physician's. Often, simple questioning techniques are sufficient to guide this process. Several directed questions to patients to elicit their feelings about the key outcomes affected by the choice may be enough to allow the physician to make a tailored recommendation. These conversations can be guided by a myriad of decision aids available for choices, ranging from vaccinations to weight loss surgery (see the Patient Decision Aids Research Group at the Ottawa Hospital Research Institute, University of Ottawa, for a comprehensive listing and assessment of available aids: http://decisionaid.ohri.ca). There are even generic decision aids that can be used across types of decisions, and Facebook applications to make and share decisions ('iShould') (9). Formal decision analysis can play a key role in focusing these discussions by identifying (through sensitivity analysis) the one or two critical values that are needed to determine the optimal treatment for an individual. For more complex decisions, it may sometimes be helpful to go one step further, and actually elicit quantitative values from the patient, using one of the methods described later in this chapter (Figure 4.1).

4.2.2 Societal decision making

Many health-care decisions must be made at the level of populations. Examples include immunization programs, food and transportation safety regulations, and health education activities. Increasingly, medical decisions are made for classes or groups of patients, at a level removed from the encounter between the individual patient and physician. For example, clinical practice guidelines specify how patients in particular clinical circumstances should be treated. Guidelines are designed to eliminate variation in patterns of care that represent deviations from what is believed to be the most effective therapy for a given disease. Insurers and policy makers allocating limited

Ottawa Personal Decision Guide

1. Clarify the decision   Date _____

What decision do you face? _____

When do you need to make a choice? _____

How far along are you with making a choice?   ☐ not thought about options   ☐ close to making a choice
                                            ☐ thinking about options   ☐ already made a choice

Are you leaning toward one option?   ☐ No   ☐ Yes, which one? _____

2. Explore the decision.
A. List the options and main benefits and risks that you already know.
B. <u>Underline</u> the benefits and risks that you think are most likely to happen.
C. Use stars [★] to show how much each benefit / risk matters to you: 5 stars means it matters 'a lot'; No star means 'not at all.'

	Benefits (reasons to choose this option)	How much it matters (★)	Risks (reasons to avoid this option)	How much it matters (★)
Option #1		★ ★ ★ ★ ★		★ ★ ★ ★ ★
		★ ★ ★ ★ ★		★ ★ ★ ★ ★
		★ ★ ★ ★ ★		★ ★ ★ ★ ★
Option #2		★ ★ ★ ★ ★		★ ★ ★ ★ ★
		★ ★ ★ ★ ★		★ ★ ★ ★ ★
		★ ★ ★ ★ ★		★ ★ ★ ★ ★
Option #3		★ ★ ★ ★ ★		★ ★ ★ ★ ★
		★ ★ ★ ★ ★		★ ★ ★ ★ ★
		★ ★ ★ ★ ★		★ ★ ★ ★ ★

Which option do you prefer?   ☐ #1   ☐ #2   ☐ #3   ☐ Unsure

Support

Who else is involved? (name)			
Which option does this person prefer?			
Is this person pressuring you?	☐ Yes ☐ No	☐ Yes ☐ No	☐ Yes ☐ No
How can this person support you?			

What role do you prefer in making your choice?
   ☐ I prefer to share the decision with _____
   ☐ I prefer to decide myself after hearing the views of _____
   ☐ I prefer that someone else decides. Who? _____

3. Identify the decision making needs.

	Knowledge	Do you know the benefits and risks of each option?	☐ Yes	☐ No
	Values	Are you clear about which benefits and risks matter most to you?	☐ Yes	☐ No
	Support	Do you have enough support and advice to make a choice?	☐ Yes	☐ No
	Certainty	Do you feel sure about the best choice for you?	☐ Yes	☐ No

The SURE Test © O'Connor & Légaré, 2008.

4. Plan the next steps based on the needs.

Knowledge (If you feel you do not have enough facts)
   ☐ Find out about the chances of benefits and risks.
   ☐ List your questions.
   ☐ List where to find answers.
     (e.g. library, health professionals, counsellors)

Values (If you are not sure what matters most to you)
   ☐ Review stars in the balance scale to see what matters to you.
   ☐ Find people who know what it's like to experience the benefits and risks.
   ☐ Talk to others who have made the decision.
   ☐ Read stories of what mattered most to others.
   ☐ Discuss with others what matters most to you.

Support
(If you feel you do not have enough support)
   ☐ Discuss your options with a trusted person.
     (e.g. health professional, counsellor, family, friends)
   ☐ Find help to support your choice. (e.g. funds, transport, child care)

(If you feel pressure from others)
   ☐ Focus on opinions of others who matter most.
   ☐ Share your guide with others.
   ☐ Ask others involved to complete this guide. Find areas of agreement. When facts disagree, agree to get more information. When you disagree on what matters most, respect the other's opinion. Take turns to listen and then mirror back what the other has said that matters most to them.
   ☐ Find a neutral person to help you and others involved.

Other plans
   ☐ Describe

Figure 4.1   Ottawa Personal Decision Guide. Copyright 2011. O'Connor, Stacey Jacobsen. Ottawa Hospital Research Institute and University of Ottawa, Canada. All rights reserved.

health-care resources face the even more difficult task of determining not only whether an intervention is effective, but also whether they can afford to offer it to their constituents. Public health decision makers must consider effectiveness, cost, and acceptability of policies, such as school-required vaccinations or aerial spraying for mosquito control. Medical decisions are made in the formulation of both guidelines and resource allocation decisions, but they are made on behalf of groups of people, such as members of a particular health plan, or members of society.

Whose values should be reflected in these decisions? Framed in this way, the answer seems obvious. The relevant values are those of the members of the group whom the decision makers are charged to represent. For insurers, the goal should be to write guidelines and set coverage policies that reflect the values of their subscribers. For governmental policy makers, charged with making decisions about how to allocate tax dollars, the relevant values are those of the society as a whole. But it is also clear that this type of decision making cannot rely on the 'black box' model that is both useful and appropriate for the clinical encounter with a single patient. A strategy is needed that weighs the harms and benefits of competing alternatives explicitly in accordance with the values of the population to whom the decisions will apply. This kind of strategy facilitates comparisons of the net benefits generated by alternative uses of health-care resources across a variety of medical conditions, and compared with non-health uses of those resources. To understand the net benefits of alternatives, we must consider the values of the group as a whole: society, insurance subscribers, etc., and apply the group's values to the decision. Assessing a group's values is a complicated task, generally approached as an aggregation of individual group members' values (as is commonly done with health indices, discussed in more detail in section 4.8). Alternately, group values can be directly assessed by asking individuals to consider the group as a whole, though this is clearly a hard task for any one person to perform (see section 4.5.4 for discussion of the 'person trade-off' technique). Regardless of the approach taken, for credibility and accuracy, it is paramount that values used in societal decision making be explicit, elicited from the relevant constituency, and based on a valid method of measurement.

The remainder of this chapter presents methods for incorporating the preferences of patients and other stakeholders explicitly and quantitatively into decision analyses. These methods may be useful both in guiding individual clinical decisions, whether or not formal preference values are elicited from patients, and in decisions affecting populations.

4.3 Attributes of outcomes

The first step in valuing outcomes is to recognize that some decisions involve more complicated outcomes than others. Consider the following taxonomy of outcome measures.

4.3.1 Two possible outcomes

The first and simplest kind of value problem is one in which there are only two possible outcomes. Examples might be such dichotomies as survive or die, cure or no cure, success or failure, or patient satisfaction or dissatisfaction. The pulmonary embolism problem as presented in simplified form in Chapter 3 is an example of a value problem with two outcomes, survival or death. In such cases the need for explicit value assessment does not arise. The criterion for decision making is simply to choose the strategy that gives the highest probability of the better outcome or, equivalently, the lowest probability of the worse outcome. In these cases, the method of averaging out is equivalent to the process of combining probabilities according to the principles developed in Chapter 3 to arrive at the overall probability of the outcome of interest for each strategy.

4.3.2 Many possible outcomes: the single-attribute case

The second and more complex type of value problem occurs when there is a spectrum of possible outcomes, ranging on a scale from least preferred through somewhat preferred up to most preferred. Often in this class of problems there is an underlying scale associated with the outcomes, which might naturally serve as the values we are seeking. The most commonly used single-attribute outcome is survival time. For example, if one were willing to accept that the only important outcome to consider in the genetic breast cancer susceptibility example was survival, then the optimal treatment at any age might be identified from Table 4.1 by choosing the option that maximizes the chance of surviving to an advanced age. But suppose the probability of surviving to one age (e.g., 70 in the breast cancer example) was greatest for one strategy, but the probability of surviving to a different age (e.g., 80) was greatest for another strategy. Which strategy is better? A simple averaging of survival chances could fail to reflect a patient's preferences about risk or the timing of benefits. For example, a patient might prefer nine years of survival over a 50–50 chance between 20 years of survival and immediate death. Notice that the expected value of the latter gamble is ten years, but the patient might still prefer to have nine years for certain. We might, therefore, wish to modify this underlying scale to account for the possibility that a person might be risk-averse, and/or place greater importance on outcomes occurring in the near term than later in the future. We will return to the topics of risk aversion and time preference in Section 4.12.

4.3.3 Many possible outcomes: the multiattribute case

In the third and most complex class of value problems, there are two or more dimensions or values. In the breast cancer susceptibility case, for example, the outcomes of both therapeutic alternatives (prophylactic mastectomy vs.

prophylactic mastectomy plus oophorectomy) have two basic components: survival probability and quality of life. The decision is challenging because one must decide how to make trade-offs between the competing values associated with the two dimensions, or attributes. For example, to consider the trade-off very bluntly, one must decide whether a life that is longer, but spent without breasts and/or ovaries, is better or worse than a life that is somewhat shorter but with one's natural breasts and ovaries. Decisions about such trade-offs are made much easier if the outcomes can be measured on a single scale that reflects the importance of both attributes, meaning in this example, a scale that equates chance of living to a certain age with breasts and/or ovaries to chance of living to that age without breasts/ovaries. And if this scale is generic rather than disease-specific, it could serve as the basis for comparisons of benefits across conditions.

4.4 Quality-adjusted survival

How might one go about constructing a scale that measures both length and quality of life? Consider the plot in Figure 4.2. This figure shows quality of life scores on the vertical axis, with lower being worse and higher being better, and time on the horizontal axis. It depicts serial quality-of-life measures for a patient presenting with a symptomatic disease that is associated with less than perfect quality of life, who then receives a toxic therapy that further decreases his quality of life temporarily, but then enjoys a transient remission of his disease and symptoms such that his quality of life improves, and who then goes on to progressively worsening disease and symptoms, and eventually dies (quality of life is considered zero when dead).

What's interesting about this figure is that the area under the 'curve' (actually a step function) is a function of both the levels of quality of life

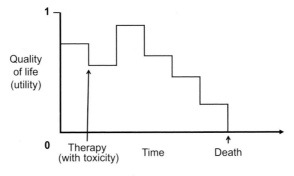

Figure 4.2   Quality-of-life score for a patient with a symptomatic disease, showing transient remission due to toxic therapy, subsequent progressive worsening of disease and symptoms, and eventually death.

experienced by this patient and the lengths of time lived at each particular level of quality of life. Therefore, the area under the curve might serve as a metric for valuing the two attributes of length and quality of life on a single scale, and maybe even in units that are generic and common to all conditions, rather than disease-specific, depending on how quality of life is measured. But there's a catch: this only works if quality of life is measured in such a way that the product of length of life and quality of life is meaningful. For example, one year of life at a quality of life 'x' must be exactly as desirable as six months of life at a quality of life of '$2x$.'

What are the characteristics of a quality-of-life measure that satisfies this condition? First, it must be a global evaluation of a state of health, reflective of all aspects of the state of health being assessed. A more focused measure, that only considers some of the attributes of quality of life and leaves others unspecified, will not fully capture the nature of the trade-off between length and quality of life represented by the area under this curve. Second, it must be measured on a ratio scale, between extremes of perfect health and death. This means that if perfect health is represented by the number 1 and death by 0, then a value of 0.5 is exactly half as desirable as perfect health, and a value of 0.25 is exactly half as desirable as that. And finally, it must use length of life as the metric for measuring the subject's preference for the quality of life in a given health state. This last condition is the most difficult to satisfy, but follows directly from the way in which we are using this quality-of-life measure as a factor for weighting length of life.

It is no coincidence that we have just described a *utility*, defined as the quantitative measure of the strength of a person's preference for an outcome. This concept has its origins in expected-utility theory (10, 11). The notion of quality-adjusted survival, measured in quality-adjusted life years (QALY; pronounced kwah′lē), was later developed from this theoretical groundwork, rather than the reverse (12). Nonetheless, we have introduced utilities by using quality-adjusted survival to provide a more intuitive context for understanding what utilities are, as well as a motivation for trying to measure them.

4.5 Techniques for valuing outcomes

Utilities are clearly different from more familiar, descriptive quality-of-life measures. Generic quality-of-life instruments such as the 36-Item Short Form developed in the Medical Outcomes Study (SF-36) (13, 14) or disease-specific instruments such as the Beck Depression Scale (15) capture information on the nature of the quality-of-life impairments of respondents. These scales are often summarized into scores for several different quality-of-life domains, like physical functioning, emotional functioning, pain, and others. Most do not measure global quality of life directly or indirectly, and when they do, they do not capture preferences for a given state of health on a scale that lends itself to being averaged out. Rather, they provide a summary measure of functioning or limitations as reported by the individual. Utility measures are fundamentally different; they reflect how a respondent *values* or *feels* about a state of health, not just the characteristics of that health state or how the state affects their ability to function.

This difference is best illustrated with an example. Imagine that you and your best friend both injure your right knees in a car accident. The result of the injury is the same for both of you: you have some chronic discomfort in the knee, and this is relieved by non-steroidal anti-inflammatory medications. Both of you are able to run 1 km, but not longer distances. You are both avid distance runners and are very distressed by this limitation. However, you believe that it will be possible for you to find other athletic pursuits that you will enjoy, while your friend does not. It is likely that you and your friend would score nearly identically on quality-of-life instruments measuring physical functioning, pain, and even distress. However, your utilities for this health state would likely differ. Your friend might consider a somewhat shorter life without this disability to be as desirable as a longer one with it, while you would probably not be willing to make this trade-off. Simply put, your *preferences* for this health state are different.

Utilities can also be defined functionally. A true utility scale is one that can be averaged out in a decision tree without distorting the preferences of the individual whose preferences are represented. In the example of life span or life expectancy, if each time interval of survival were assigned a value equal to its duration (i.e., 20 years = 20, ten years = 10, 0 years = 0), then the expected value of a 50–50 gamble between 20 years and 0 years would be ten. Since the patient in the example used earlier prefers nine years over the gamble, this cannot be a utility scale for this patient. But other functions could serve as value scales for this patient. For example, a value scale which assigns to each life span the square root of the length of life would be consistent with this ranking of options, because:

$$0.5\sqrt{20} + 0.5\sqrt{0} < \sqrt{9} \tag{4.1}$$

The inequality in (4.1) means that, under this value scale, the patient prefers nine years for sure over the gamble between 0 and 20 years. A scale of QALYs is frequently used in decision analysis and in economic evaluations as a utility measure. But it is not guaranteed that quality-adjusted life expectancy (i.e., averaged-out quality-adjusted survival) will reflect a decision maker's preferences regarding decisions under uncertainty, unless particular conditions apply. We will return to these conditions later in this chapter.

There are several different strategies for capturing such preference-based measures of quality of life. They vary in their theoretical underpinnings, conceptual difficulty, and practical feasibility. It is important to be familiar with all the techniques. The best one to use for a particular application may depend on the goals and nature of the study being done.

DEFINITION   A *utility* scale (or *utility function*) is an assignment of numerical values to each member of a set of outcomes, such that if the expected value of the utilities assigned to the outcomes in one chance tree is greater than the expected value of the utilities assigned to the outcomes in another chance tree, then the first chance tree is preferred to the second chance tree, and vice versa.

4.5.1 Rating scale

The simplest approach to measuring a subject's preference for a given state of health, whether it's the subject's own state of health or a hypothetical one, is a *rating scale*. An example of a verbal rating scale is:

'On a scale where 0 represents death and 100 represents perfect health, what number would you say best describes your current state of health over the past 2 weeks?'

Very similar results are obtained with visual stimuli such as 'feeling thermometers,' as shown in Figure 4.3, and visual analog scales (oriented horizontally).

The rating scale is a global measure that captures a subject's valuation of a particular state of health, including all elements that an individual incorporates into thinking about one's own health. A rating scale in this context is anchored at 0 and 100 if described verbally, and implies a 0–100 scale if depicted pictorially or in a horizontal, unmarked scale. This approach is easily explained to most people and it is relatively easy to administer. However, it is not a true utility because it isn't a ratio scale between perfect health and death. That is, a health state rated as 90 is not necessarily twice as good as one rated as 45. Moreover, there is no reason to think that a subject who rates an impaired state of health at '50' would be willing to trade away half of his or her life expectancy to be relieved of that impairment, in other words, to improve that state of health to '100.' As a result, the rating scale does not necessarily satisfy the criterion of expected value. A certain life span of 20 years in a health state whose rating is 40 is not necessarily less desirable than a 50–50 chance of living those 20 years in perfect health (rating = 100), with the alternative of death (rating = 0). Several 'transformations' of rating scale scores have been proposed to try to approximate true utilities, however, and will be discussed in Section 4.7.

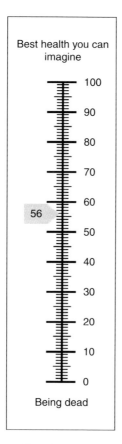

Figure 4.3   Feeling thermometer: a visual aid used to elicit a rating scale score for the current state of health.

The rating scale is the first of three 'direct' methods for valuing outcomes that we will discuss. These will be contrasted with 'indirect' methods that will be presented later in the chapter.

4.5.2 Standard (reference) gamble

The approach to direct utility assessment most firmly grounded in expected-utility theory is the *standard gamble* (or *reference gamble*). The essence of the standard gamble is that it assesses the utility for a health state by asking what risk of death one would accept to improve it. This is done by asking a respondent to choose between life in a certain (compromised) health state and a gamble between death and perfect health. The utility of the health state is then represented by the probability of perfect health in the gamble such that the respondent is indifferent between the gamble and the certain health state.

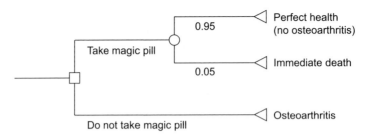

Figure 4.4   Chance tree to illustrate the standard (reference) gamble for a hypothetical
                    state of osteoarthritis.

Let's illustrate this process with an example. Consider the following health
state: Imagine that you have osteoarthritis that affects your hips. You need a
walker when you are out of your home, and you cannot run at all. You have
moderate pain that is partially relieved by daily non-steroidal medications.
Now imagine that a genie offers you a 'magic pill.' If you take this pill, there is
a 50% probability that you will be completely relieved of your arthritis forever
and will live out your natural life expectancy. However, the pill has one severe
side effect. There is a 50% probability that it will cause immediate and painless
death. Would you take the pill? If the answer is no, would you consider taking
the magic pill if there were a 99% probability that you would be relieved of
your arthritis and a 1% probability of immediate painless death? If the answer
to this question is yes, would you consider taking the magic pill if there were a
75% probability that you would be relieved of your arthritis and a 25%
probability of immediate painless death?

In the standard gamble, this iterative process is repeated, varying the
probabilities in the gamble, until the respondent feels that the two options,
taking the magic pill (with the associated uncertainty of the pill's outcome)
and not taking the pill, are equally desirable. This is called the 'point of
indifference,' because at that point the subject no longer expresses a preference for one of the two options, and he is thus 'indifferent' about the options.
At the point of indifference, the respondent's utility for the health state,
osteoarthritis in this example, is indicated by the probability that the magic
pill will restore the person to perfect health. So if you reached the point of
indifference when offered a magic pill associated with a 95% probability of
perfect health and a 5% probability of immediate death (as shown in
Figure 4.4), your utility for the health state would be 0.95. In other words,
on a utility scale of 0–1, where 0 equals being dead and 1.0 equals being in
perfect health, living with osteoarthritis as described in this scenario is valued
at 0.95. The *dis*utility of this health state, defined as 1 minus the utility, would
therefore be 0.05.

Now let's describe the process we just went through a bit more rigorously
(as shown in Figure 4.5). Consider a choice between life in a given health state

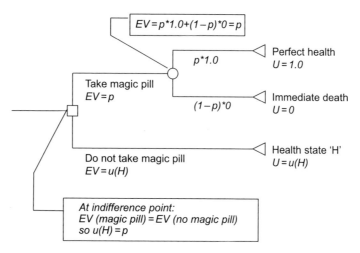

Figure 4.5   Chance tree to illustrate the standard (reference) gamble in general form.

H and a gamble between perfect health (with probability p) and death (with probability $= 1 - p$). Suppose that we arbitrarily assign a value of 1.0 to perfect health and of 0 to death. Then the expected value of this gamble $= [p \cdot 1.0 + (1 - p) \cdot 0] = p$. We recognize this expected value as the probability of getting perfect health in the gamble. If the respondent considers the gamble equally desirable as a health state H, then the utility of that health state must be equal to p. We denote this by $u(H) = p$. By varying the probability p in the standard gamble until the respondent declares himself or herself indifferent between the gamble and the health state, we can find the utility of any health state that is valued between perfect health and death by a series of choices between gambles and that health state.

A variant of the standard gamble that uses a slightly different set-up can be used when valuing very mild or temporary health states, called a *chained gamble* (16, 17). The chained gamble procedure establishes an anchor state that is better than death but still worse than the certain state being evaluated, so that the gamble is now between perfect health and this better-than-death health state. In order to calculate the expected value of the gamble we need to know the utility of this new health state, call it C; the expected value of the chained gamble $= p \cdot 1.0 + (1 - p) \cdot u(C)$. So the chained gamble procedure must also value state C using the standard reference gamble, with the typical anchor states of perfect health and death, to arrive at $u(C)$. The utility of C can then be used in the chained calculations for all other certain states. Another use for a chained gamble procedure is to avoid repeated valuations involving consideration of a risk of death, which in some limited circumstances may be discomforting to respondents. At this point, two comments on terminology are in order. First, it is customary in decision analysis to use the word 'indifferent' to reflect a situation in which an individual is equally happy (or unhappy) with two outcomes or gambles. It does not mean that the person does not care about the choice; it does mean that the person has no preference one way or the other. Second, we use the term 'gamble,' despite its frivolous connotations, to refer to any chance tree involving outcomes of interest. The use of this word in decision theory has a long history, and we apologize to any readers who take our use of this word to imply anything less than the greatest respect for the seriousness of life-and-death choices.

A critical feature of the standard gamble is that it reflects decision making under uncertainty. When faced with the choice between living in the certain health state or taking the gamble, you do not know for sure which of the two outcomes in the gamble you will experience, only the probability that each will occur. As a result, your utility measured with a standard gamble reflects not only your preferences about life in that certain state of health, life in perfect health, and death, but also your attitudes toward risk taking.

4.5.3 Time trade-off

The third approach to direct measurement of preference for states of health is the *time trade-off*. In this case, the utility for a health state is assessed by asking how much *time* one would give up to improve it. This is done by asking a respondent to choose between a set length of life in a given (compromised) health state and a shorter length of life in perfect health. The respondent's utility for the compromised health state is indicated by the ratio of the shorter to the longer life expectancy at which the respondent finds the two health states equally desirable.

Consider the osteoarthritis health state once again: Assume that you have osteoarthritis and your natural life expectancy is 40 years. Now imagine that you are offered a choice: live your life as is, for 40 more years with osteoarthritis, or instead, live in perfect health but for only 20 more years. Would you choose your normal life expectancy or the shorter one? If your choice would be to live your normal 40 years with osteoarthritis, would you change your decision if the choice was between your normal 40 years with osteoarthritis and 39 years in perfect health? If you would choose the shorter 39 years in perfect health, would you still choose it if the life with perfect health was instead for only 30 years? In the time trade-off, this iterative process is repeated, varying the length of life in perfect health, until the respondent feels that the two options, the longer life in the compromised health state and the shorter life in perfect health, are equally desirable. As in the standard gamble, this is called the 'point of indifference.' This person is indifferent between 30 years lived in perfect health and 40 years lived with osteoarthritis. The

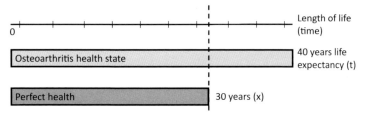

Utility (osteoarthritis) = x/t = 30/40 = 0.75

Figure 4.6   Illustration of the time trade-off for osteoarthritis at point of indifference.

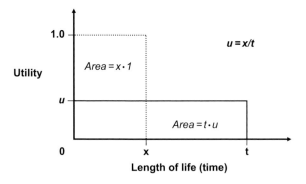

Figure 4.7   Utility calculation for time trade-off in general form.

respondent's utility for the health state, osteoarthritis in this example, is given by the ratio of the length of life in perfect health (30 years) to the length of life in the compromised health state (40 years), or 0.75. This concept is illustrated graphically in Figure 4.6.

At the point of indifference, the subject believes that the life characterized by time t spent in health state with utility u is equivalent to the life with length x, spent in perfect health with utility '1.0.' Assuming this subject does not have a time preference (as will be discussed in Section 4.12), then the area of the rectangle for the longer life, t times u, is equal to the rectangle for the shorter life, x times 1.0. Hence, $t \cdot u = x$, and u equals x/t. So if you reached this point of indifference when offered a magic pill associated with a reduction in your life expectancy from 40 to 30 years, your utility for the health state would be 30/40 or 0.75 (Figure 4.7).

In contrast to the standard gamble, the time trade-off represents decision making under certainty. Whichever option you choose, you know exactly what your outcome will be (the length of your life and your health state). Therefore, the utility it generates is unaffected by your attitude toward risk. It is however affected by your preference for time now versus sometime in the future, as will be discussed in Section 4.12. Because it does not incorporate the element of uncertainty included in the standard gamble, the time trade-off is not technically a utility but rather an approximation thereof. Though experts in the field debate the technical and procedural merits of the time trade-off versus the standard gamble (18), in practicality the techniques are used interchangeably to elicit utilities. As you will have noticed, the main difference between the two techniques is that the time trade-off measures values for health states in terms of time as a valuation metric, while the standard gamble uses risk of death as a metric.

4.5.4 Other techniques for valuing outcomes

It is worth noting briefly that several other techniques are sometimes used to quantify values for states of health. Though none of these result in utilities *per se*, they are useful methods for specific circumstances and applications. Assessments of *willingness to pay* (WTP) ask how much the respondent would be willing to pay in financial terms to improve a state of health, avoid a particular outcome, or reduce the chance of death (19, 20). Alternatively, the question can be framed to ask how much the respondent would want to receive to remain in an impaired state of health (termed 'willingness to accept'). The result puts a monetary value on a health outcome, and is used largely for cost–benefit analysis. Cost–benefit analyses are economic evaluations in which all outcomes are expressed in monetary terms, in contrast to cost-effectiveness (or cost–utility) analyses, in which health outcomes are expressed in terms of (quality-adjusted) life years, and results are expressed in terms of cost per (quality-adjusted) life year. We will return to cost–benefit analysis in Chapter 9, although most of the attention will be devoted to cost-effectiveness analysis. Though WTP can indicate the value one individual places on different outcomes, it is difficult to use as a valuation method across individuals because it is highly dependent on an individual's monetary resources (i.e., a dollar is more valuable to a poor person than to a wealthy one). The WTP is therefore infrequently used in decision making for health and medicine.

Equivalence measures (also called *person trade-off*) ask the respondent to indicate how many people would have to be cured of one impaired health state to be equivalent to curing 100 people in another impaired health state. It asks about the social worth of alternative health-care interventions, and is generally viewed as better suited for policy making than for clinical decision making (21). The person trade-off has been criticized, however, for integrating a paternalistic attitude because it assesses preferences for 'other people' which may differ from those for oneself. Moreover, it has proved challenging to implement on a practical level because the trade-off is difficult for respondents to make.

Ranking health states is increasingly being promoted as a useful valuation method in low-literacy or low-numeracy populations, and for administrative ease. Ranking involves placing at least two (and often more) states on a relative scale, though without assigning a numerical value to either (as is done in a rating scale). In practice, ranking is often conducted with paper cards including a description of the health state on the front, which are placed on a table or board in order from 'best' to 'worst.' Ranking can also be presented quite simply on a computer screen. Ranking lends itself to valuing hypothetical health states more so than in clinical decision making, as by definition it involves the comparison between states. Methods to infer utility values from these rankings are under development and not yet widely accepted, though the simplicity of the method is obvious (22, 23).

All of the methods described thus far fall into the broad category of *stated preference* methods for valuing health states, which includes all approaches in which an individual *articulates* his or her value for the state. An alternative approach, called *revealed preference*, infers preferences from actual real-world decisions, such as through a purchase, as could be done with a choice of car or insurance policy – or surgical procedure – for example. A widely used method, called *discrete choice experiments*, simulates real decisions by asking a respondent to make hypothetical choices between two or more alternatives. The 'DCE' as these are called, is a method in which preferences for a certain good or item (or in this case a health state) are attached to the attributes that contribute to the value a person assigns to it. Values are then inferred through a series of choices between different 'bundles' of those attributes. The DCE methods can be useful in determining individual preferences in clinical decision making, and are being explored for their usefulness in estimating utilities (24, 25).

For example, recall our osteoarthritis health state discussed above. If there were two possible treatments available for osteoarthritis between which a patient was choosing, the 'attributes' of the treatments could be described as (1) effect on mobility, (2) side effects, and (3) cost to patient. Each of these attributes could in turn be described in different levels, such as restoring 100% or 80% of prior mobility, side effects that are mild, moderate or severe, and costing $10/month or $50/month. A DCE would present combinations of these three attributes at different levels and ask the person to choose between them, such as: 'treatment A restores 80% of mobility, has mild side effects and costs $50/month, versus treatment B that restores 100% of mobility, has severe side effects, and costs $10/month.' Over a series of choices a person's relative preferences for each of the attributes associated with those treatments are 'revealed', and the resulting value weights (deduced by statistical analysis) can assist in decision making.

Finally, a different approach is advocated by the World Bank and World Health Organization to determine societal health priorities, using the Global Burden of Disease framework (26). 'Disability-Adjusted Life years', or DALYs, describe the burden that a particular disease places on a society or country by tallying two elements: the years of life lost (i.e., premature mortality) due to the disease, and the years lost due to disability resulting from the disease. It is notable that both of these elements measure losses due to a disease – loss of length of life and loss of abilities – so a DALY reflects the burden imposed on society by a disease, or the loss of life and ability due to a disease. The DALYs are conceptually (though not technically) opposites of QALYs: QALYs represent years of life gained (though adjusted for quality), while DALYS are years of life and ability lost. Furthermore, technical differences exist in how the quality/disability weights are derived for each. In general, DALYs are used to describe disease burden at the population level while QALYs are used to evaluate the benefits associated with specific interventions, but the reach of both metrics is expanding as the importance of systematic analysis of resource allocation decisions is increasingly recognized.

These alternative techniques have advantages and disadvantages in comparison with utilities, and may be useful in particular settings or applications.

4.6 Comment on nomenclature

Often the terms 'preferences,' 'values,' 'utilities' are used interchangeably. However, there are subtle but important differences among them. The most generic of the three terms is *preferences*. All of the techniques described in the previous section measure preferences for different states of health. Purists would limit use of the term *utility* to describe the results of a standard reference gamble, arguing that a true utility must reflect decision making under uncertainty (27). They would argue that the term *values* should be used to describe the results of measurements done under conditions of certainty, including rating scales and time trade-offs, and the alternative techniques mentioned. However, most experts in the field are willing to grant the status of 'utility' to the results of a time trade-off (particularly if adjusted for the time preference rate: see Section 4.12).

4.7 Relationships among techniques for valuing outcomes

Ideally, the three major techniques for valuing outcomes – the rating scale, the standard gamble, and the time trade-off – would yield the same numbers, or at worst, would yield scores that are easily transformable from one scale to another, as we can do with the Fahrenheit and Celsius scales. As our discussion should have made clear, reality is more complex. The techniques measure somewhat different but related concepts. Not surprisingly, when the same subjects are asked to evaluate a health state using each of the measures, the results are not identical. In general, the utilities elicited with the standard gamble are the highest. Most subjects are reluctant to accept a risk of immediate death, even if the impaired health state involves serious compromise in quality of life. Hence standard gamble utilities tend to be high compared to those elicited using other valuation methods. The time trade-off tends to yield somewhat lower values, suggesting that a known, limited decrease in life expectancy is a more acceptable 'price' to pay for being relieved of a quality-of-life impairment than a low probability of immediate death, even if the overall life expectancies are equivalent. Given errors of measurement and the psychological differences between risky and riskless choices, the scores or utilities elicited are not easily transformable. Nonetheless, standard gamble and time trade-off utilities are often used interchangeably.

Rating scale values tend to be considerably lower than utilities generated by either of the other two techniques. This makes sense, because there is no 'penalty' associated with assigning a health state a rating scale value lower than that of perfect health. Respondents who would not be willing to accept any risk of death, or any decrease in the length of their life, to be relieved of a mild impairment in quality of life, might well assign it a less than perfect score on a rating scale (meaning a score below 100). So the different techniques would result in different values, though ostensibly measuring the same thing. Because rating scales are considerably easier to administer than either of the other two techniques, there has been a longstanding interest in finding a way to 'transform' the values they generate into utility scores. One commonly used strategy is to increase the rating scale value according to an empirically derived statistical relationship. One such relationship that has been found to fit the data rather well is a power function. For example, Torrance *et al.* (28) observed the following relationship between the rating scale values and standard gamble utilities for the same states of health:

$$Utility = 1-(1-value)^r \tag{4.2}$$

where the exponent r has been estimated consistently in the range from about 1.6 to 2.3.

Similarly, a number of comparisons have been made between the results of preference measures and conventional quality-of-life or health status measures. The literature describing this 'cross-walking' process is growing because of the increasing frequency with which quality of life and health status measures are included in clinical trials, and the relative ease of administering these measures compared with utility instruments (29). One widely used health status scale, the SF-36, has been mapped or cross-walked onto a utility scale to allow the estimation of utilities from SF-36 data. This process involves developing an 'SF-6D,' which is a sub-set of the responses from questions on the SF-36, from which a utility score can be derived (30). An SF-6D can also be developed from responses to questions on the SF-12, itself a subset of questions from the SF-36 (31). These mapping functions have greatly expanded investigators' ability to estimate preferences for health states from clinical trials and other studies that collect quality of life data. The method by which preferences are derived for the SF-6D will be discussed further in Section 4.8 below, on health indices.

4.8 Health indices

A 'health index' is in some ways a hybrid between descriptive quality-of-life measurement and utility assessment. The EuroQol with five dimensions (EQ-5D), the Health Utilities Index (HUI) and the Short-Form 6 dimensions (SF-6D) are widely used examples of these so-called health indices or multi-attribute utility measures (28, 30–34). As shown in Figure 4.8, health indices include two components: a health state classification instrument, and a formula for assigning a utility to any unique set of responses to that instrument.

The health state classification instrument measures health-related quality of life and, as a result, generates descriptive data regarding the quality of life of the patient who completes it. The instrument is administered, usually in paper form, to people who have experience with a health state – generally 'patients.' These descriptive data result in a classification of the health state along certain 'domains' or 'dimensions.' The EQ-5D questionnaire leads to a classification along five dimensions (hence, '5D' in the name): mobility, self care, usual activities, pain/discomfort, and anxiety/

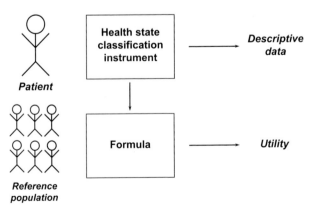

Figure 4.8   Health indices and their components.

depression (35). The HUI questionnaire leads to a classification of a health state along eight domains, or dimensions, or attributes: ambulation, dexterity, cognition, emotion, pain and discomfort, vision, hearing, and speech (28, 33). Quality of life or health status is described according to different possible levels of each dimension/domain. For example, in the EQ-5D, pain/discomfort could be described as none, moderate, or extreme. The EQ-5D describes each dimension in terms of three levels of disability or limitation, while the HUI offers up to six levels per domain. The SF-6D is a special case of a health index. As described above in Section 4.7, the SF-6D was developed specifically to translate SF-36 and SF-12 quality-of-life data into utilities. Unlike the HUI and EQ-5D, the SF-6D is not itself an instrument that can be administered to a patient, but rather it is a compilation of questions from the SF-36 or SF-12 used exclusively to arrive at a utility score for that SF-36/12-described health state.

These descriptions, however, are not utilities. Utilities are derived through a 'mapping rule' that assigns preferences, or utilities, to the health state that was described by the health state classification instrument. These preferences are elicited by polling members of a 'reference population' to elicit their utilities for all of the states of health that can be described by possible combinations of levels of domains in the health state classification instrument. The reference population is often comprised of members of the general public from which the subject originates. The EQ-5D's mapping rule is based on time trade-offs, and 'valuation sets' are available for many different reference populations from many different countries. In the case of the HUI, the mapping rule is based on utilities assessed by a combination of standard gambles and adjusted rating scales (by a power function transformation), from a sample of the population in one city in Canada. The mapping rule for the SF-6D is based on standard gambles conducted with a population sample from the United Kingdom. Because the utility for each possible health state described by the health state classification instrument is elicited from a population sample, most (but not all) members of which do not have experience with the health state itself, utilities from health indices are societal or community perspective values. They are arrived at through a process that involves a 'patient' describing his or her health state on the classification instrument, to which a utility from a population sample is assigned, and the result is a societal value for that state. The two principal advantages of health indices are that they are easily completed by patients in a clinical trial or other clinical study, and that the utilities they generate represent community or societal preferences. There are, however, circumstances in which health indices are inadequate or unsuitable for the health state being valued, and direct measures are preferred (36).

Some research is being conducted to develop mapping rules to estimate utilities from condition-specific health status instruments, such as for asthma, but these efforts are still in the early stages and are not yet commonly used.

4.9 Off-the-shelf utilities

For decision analyses in which the analyst has neither the time nor resources to administer a utility survey, or to administer a health state classification instrument such as the HUI or EQ-5D, or have access to SF-36 or SF-12 data to transform into an SF-6D, it is possible to turn to published utilities from other sources. While health states may be described in terms not exactly equivalent to what is needed for the analysis, either in very general or exceedingly detailed terms (such as 'asthma' or 'contralateral tumor associated with breast cancer: year one after recurrence'), these sources may be serviceable approximations. Examples of such 'off-the-shelf' utilities are available from individually published studies accessible through an online, searchable database of cost–utility analyses ('Tufts CEA Registry' available at https://research.tufts-nemc.org/cear4/) (37), as well as published studies using US and other countries' data (38).

4.10 Health states worse than dead

Thoughtful readers may have been asking whether it is possible to accommodate a preference that a particular health state is worse than being dead. While this possibility raises difficult ethical questions, such as the sometimes conflicting responsibilities of the physician to respect a patient's wishes and to preserve life, the technical answer to the question is 'yes,' it is possible to have utilities less than zero. Indeed, health states that involve chronic, severe pain, or severe mental dysfunction such as dementia, may be considered by some people to be worse than being dead, which would imply a negative utility value (39). The elicitation procedures for such states, using the rating scale, time trade-off, and standard gamble, all require modification, but it can be done (39, 40). In the HUI mapping function, for example, several health states have utilities less than zero, the minimum being – 0.34 for the health state corresponding to the worst level of all eight attributes. The EQ-5D also has a specific method for valuing health states considered 'worse than dead.' The concept of 'maximum endurable time' has been developed to capture an individual's tolerance for existing in a health state considered worse than being dead, with the recognition that the value assigned to these states may be a function of their duration – for example, severe pain may be tolerable for a matter of weeks but not indefinitely (41).

4.11 Practical considerations in utility measurement

Perhaps because utility techniques are grounded in theoretical rather than empirical considerations, they are challenging to administer. Utility elicitation requires that respondents consider hypothetical situations, grasp the nature of probabilities, and imagine experiencing sometimes unrealistic outcomes, including cure from a chronic illness or immediate death. There is general consensus that, while rating scale values can be elicited reliably in self-administered surveys, utility measurement with standard gambles and time trade-offs is best done in an interactive format, either with an interviewer or in a computerized format. A major advantage of these methods is that they allow the questions to be administered as a series of dichotomous choices. So, instead of asking a single open-ended question about what risk of death or amount of life expectancy the subject might accept to be relieved of the impairments in a given state of health, the question is approached iteratively, with systematic variation in the probability of death in the gamble or time alive in the time trade-off until the point of indifference is reached, as demonstrated in the examples in Section 4.5.

It is also very helpful to provide the subject with visual aids describing the nature of the health states being evaluated, and the specific characteristics of the choices being presented. The visual depiction of probabilities has been thoughtfully studied to best relay this often confusing concept. In the standard gamble, probabilities are often depicted as rectangles of dots of two colors indicating the proportion representing the chance of perfect health and death in the gamble. In the time trade-off, the visual aids often depict graphically the time spent in impaired and perfect health states as horizontal bars of different lengths for the subject to consider (as in Figure 4.6). Visual aids can range in sophistication from simple diagrams on pieces of paper given to subjects being interviewed in person or over the phone, to boards with sliding or rotating sections to represent lengths of life and probabilities, to interactive computerized utility assessment programs with pop-up screens and embedded prompts. One advantage of computerized programs is that they insure greater standardization of the format of the utility elicitation interview across respondents in any particular survey. The choice of survey format is usually dependent on other administrative constraints of the study and the subject characteristics. Such constraints include: the number of people to be interviewed (a small sample can be interviewed in person while a national sample may be better surveyed in an online format); study resources (on a per-person basis, in person interviews are far more costly than internet administered surveys); and subject literacy and numeracy (e.g., elderly subjects with functional constraints are better interviewed in person than via computer). No matter what method is used, direct utility elicitation is generally time-consuming and resource-intensive.

4.12 Risk preference and time preference

Some additional concepts need to be considered when eliciting and interpreting utilities. These include risk preference and time preference.

Imagine that you have the opportunity to play the following game. I flip a coin and you call it heads or tails in the air. If you're right, I give you $100. If you're wrong, you win nothing. Not a bad opportunity! If you play repeatedly, you will make $50 per game, on average. But I am only offering you the opportunity to play once, and there is a 50% chance you will win nothing. Now, what is the minimum amount of money you would be willing to take as a one-time payment *instead* of playing this game? If you answered that you would forego playing the game for $50, the average value of the game, you are said to be *risk-neutral*. However, you may be willing to accept a payment of as little as $30 rather than play the game. Many individuals would opt for a smaller amount of money, offered with certainty, over a gamble with a higher value on average. These individuals are said to be *risk-averse*. In other words, they prefer a certain outcome of lower value over a gamble with a higher average value, but a risk of a poor outcome (not winning anything). These preferences are said to be 'with respect to money' because they are made in the context of gambles that involve monetary payments.

The utilities of an individual who is risk-neutral with respect to money would lie along the straight diagonal line in Figure 4.9. Risk-neutral individuals value each amount of money provided with certainty, shown on the x-axis to be equivalent to the percent chance of winning $100, as indicated on the y-axis. So a risk-neutral person would consider $50 given with certainty to be equivalent to a 0.50 probability of winning $100. The utilities of an individual who is risk-averse would form a concave curve, above and to the left of the diagonal. For this person, $30 given with certainty would be equivalent to a 0.50 probability of winning $100 – he is averse to taking the risk of not receiving any money, so would accept a certain payment smaller than the expected value of the gamble. An individual who prefers a gamble with a small probability of a very large payoff over a certain outcome with the same expected value is said to be *risk-seeking*. Gamblers are often risk-seeking because they find utility in the gamble itself, and seek out such situations over certain ones. For such an individual, the utility curve would lie below the diagonal.

The same concepts can be applied to non-monetary outcomes, including health outcomes such as years of life spent in a particular health state

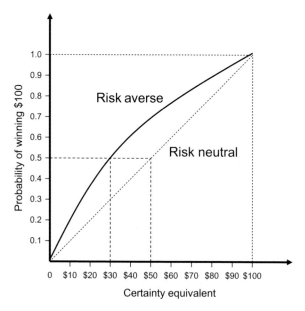

Figure 4.9   Utility curve illustrating risk attitude (risk neutral and risk averse). The curve for someone who is risk seeking would be below the diagonal.

(including one's current health, a better health state, or an ill health state). Consider a gamble in which you have a 50% probability of 40 years of life and a 50% probability of 0 years of life. If you would consider a certain alternative of 20 years of life to be equivalent to this gamble, you are risk-neutral with respect to years of life. However, if you are risk-averse with respect to life years, you will prefer a shorter, but certain, length of life over the gamble. In general, risk attitudes are inferred from expressed choices, just as values are. It is important to note that risk attitude is not necessarily a stable personality trait; an individual might be risk-seeking with respect to money (a gambler) and risk-averse with respect to years of life. The context of the attitude should be specified.

For a person to have a risk-neutral utility function, the 'certainty equivalent,' or the certain amount (of money, of years, etc.) that the person considers equal to the gamble, is equal to the expected value of the gamble. For a risk-averse utility function, the certainty equivalent is less than the expected value. For a risk-seeking utility function, the certainty equivalent is greater than the expected value.

The concept of risk preference comes into play in the standard gamble because people are considering choices that involve certain outcomes and gambles. So their preferences will include both how they feel about the options and how they feel about risk. Risk preference does not apply to the time trade-off since this technique does not involve uncertainty. However,

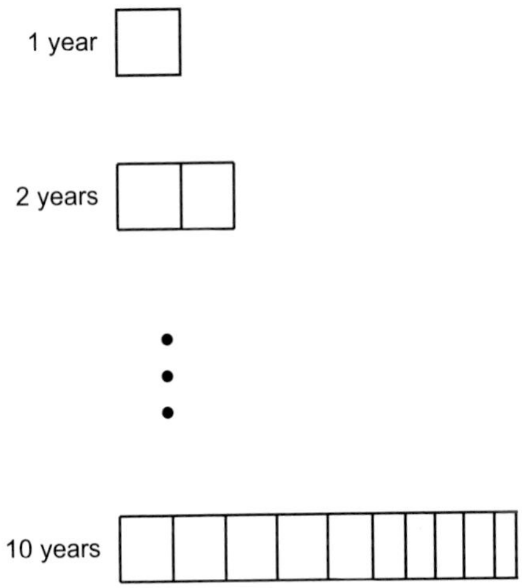

1 year

2 years

10 years

Figure 4.10   Diminishing incremental value of additional time.

the related concept of *time preference* does. As shown in Figure 4.10, the incremental value of an additional year may not be constant.

Most people would favor an intervention that increased life expectancy from one year to two, over one that increased life expectancy from nine years to ten, for example. In other words, a year in the near future is *worth* more than a year in the distant future. This has implications for the interpretation of utilities generated with a time trade-off. Consider Figure 4.7 once again. If future years are valued less than those in the near term, the value of u will depend on the value of t. All else being equal, the longer the life expectancy in impaired health, the higher the proportion of that life expectancy one might be willing to give up in exchange for perfect health. This follows from the fact that years of life farther in the future are valued less, and a longer life expectancy includes more of those far-off years. Consequently, the longer the life offered in the time trade-off, the lower the utility for the impaired state of health. It is possible to adjust time-trade-off utilities for time preference, but only if you have an independent estimate of the rate of time preference (i.e., the rate at which the length of the rectangles in Figure 4.10 is diminishing (42)).

DEFINITION	Consider a gamble in which each possible outcome is expressed on some numerical scale (such as dollars or years of life). The *certainty equivalent* of a gamble is the outcome along the scale such that the decision maker is indifferent between the gamble and that certain outcome.

4.13 Quality-adjusted life expectancy as a utility

We have seen that in order to be amenable to being averaged out in a decision tree, health-state utilities must reflect preferences under uncertainty in the sense implied by the standard gamble. We have also seen that, in order to be amenable to being used as the weights in quality-adjusted survival (i.e., in QALYs), they must reflect time trade-offs. In order to use averaged-out life span as a utility (i.e., life expectancy), preferences must be risk-neutral with regard to longevity. In sum, *all three* of these criteria must be met in order to be able to use quality-adjusted survival to reflect preferences in a decision analysis. While this may seem to be an insurmountable hurdle, it has been shown that if an individual's preferences satisfy only two conditions, then quality-adjusted survival can represent his or her preferences:

1. Constant proportional trade-off: the proportion of life span that an individual would give up in order to improve health from an impaired health state to perfect health does not depend on the length of life, and
2. Risk neutrality on survival: a gamble involving length of life in a given health state is equivalent to the expected value of the gamble in the same health state (43–45).

While the conditions for utility may not be met precisely, studies have shown them to be met approximately enough so that rankings of gambles on quality of life and survival are not unduly distorted and can be used with confidence in decision analysis (42). Finally, as we shall see in Chapters 9 and 10, an adjustment can be made for time preference (i.e., condition 1) by using discounting.

4.14 Other psychological issues in utility assessment

Whether or not a formal utility assessment technique is used, the focus on values emphasizes that eliciting and clarifying a patient's preferences is inherently a psychological process. We may use methods that have a foundation in a formal mathematical theory, but in another sense, the issues that arise are related to some recurrent issues in psychological scaling. The following are some of the issues to consider in the elicitation and use of these values. Some of these topics are also the focus of ongoing research that is advancing the methods of the valuation field.

1. In many cases, decision making must be made prospectively, before the patient has experience with the outcome of the treatment intervention, such as, for example, prophylactic mastectomy. While we can advise patients on what others have experienced, we know that prospective values differ from retrospective ones, with the latter often reflecting adaptation to

a health state that may have seemed fearsome ahead of time (called 'hedonic adaptation'). There is a known temporal aspect to values that depends on anticipation and experience among other things, and we should integrate this knowledge as much as possible into our assessments with patients and with societal values (46).

2. Knowing that people gradually adapt to their current reality and what was anticipated to be a very unpleasant situation becomes at least bearable, a utility assessment of a yet-to-be-experienced outcome may judge it to be worse than it will subsequently prove to be. Alternately, for a minority of patients, the new reality may turn out to be worse than they had feared. In either case, sensitivity analysis of the relevant utilities is crucial, because there is some reason to believe that either set of numbers (prospective or concurrent utilities) may be valid estimates of the patient's 'true' values.

3. All the methods of utility assessment that we have described assume that the people being assessed have pre-existing preferences, either well known to themselves or buried deep within themselves, that are simply being uncovered by the elicitation procedure. In some situations, however, people may not have pre-existing preferences at all, and their responses to questions may be generated 'on the fly' in response to the implicit pressure of the interview situation. We, and the individuals themselves, often don't know if these preferences are easy or difficult to access and articulate. The utility assessment technique therefore must be conducted with care to not overly influence or bias responses that are not 'fully formed' at the time of questioning. Some investigators take efforts to help respondents 'construct' their preferences during the survey process so that they can provide thoughtful and considered values (47).

4. It is well known that utility elicitation is subject to framing effects, in which the format or wording of the questions asked of subjects may influence their responses. In the standard gamble and time trade-off methods, values are inferred from choices. While these choices should be stable over minor changes in the wording of the problem (which is termed 'procedural invariance') this is not always the case. When preferences change as a function of minor changes in the wording of the task, of the 'framing' of the question, the assumption of procedural invariance has been violated. Systematic framing effects have been documented in a variety of utility elicitation situations for a variety of underlying reasons (48–50). Since we are striving to know a person's 'true' preference for a health state, which should not be subject to how the question is asked (or, moreover, the metric used to measure it), framing is a worrisome problem in utility elicitation. Some investigators utilize methods to identify respondents who are seemingly subject to framing effects and omit or correct their responses

before analysis (51). Most spend considerable effort designing, developing, and testing utility surveys to minimize these effects.

5. Finally, expected-utility theory is a *prescriptive* theory, not a *descriptive* one. It describes how people *ought* to make decisions under uncertainty if they wish to satisfy certain axioms and principles, not necessarily how they actually make decisions in an imperfect world. It is also a 'small world' theory, since any decision model inevitably omits some factors from the decision that another decision maker may find critical. There is a large and growing field devoted to the study of how people actually make decisions, when they do not use decision analysis, called decision psychology or behavioral decision theory (see Chapter 13). Behavioral economics is a neighboring field that combines psychology and economics to explain people's decision making under different circumstances and in different settings. These fields are advancing our understanding of how values are integrated into decisions in health and in other fields, which also informs how best to elicit or measure those values. These approaches will not replace expected utility theory but rather will help explain the divergences from the 'rational' behavior that is expected in a 'clean,' perfect world.

4.15 Discussion: decision-making paradigms revisited

With these new tools in hand, let us return to the decision-making paradigms introduced at the beginning of the chapter. When and how should values be measured and incorporated into the decision-making process in each setting?

4.15.1 The clinical encounter

Most medical decisions require some value judgments. The information needs of patients on the autonomous end of the spectrum include a thorough understanding of the nature, likelihood, and timing of the outcomes associated with each intervention under consideration. This patient may then weigh those alternatives, applying his or her own values in an internal process alone or with family, but private from the clinician. For this type of patient there is no need to supply them with information on other patients' utilities or values, or for any kind of formal or informal elicitation of their values.

The only caveat in this autonomous scenario is that competent patients may occasionally make decisions that seem to the clinician to be unconventional or even unreasonable. This may reflect uncommon but deeply held beliefs or values. Thoughtful and informed decisions based on unconventional or unusual underlying values should be accepted and honored similarly to those that are more conventional. However, if decisions reflect difficulty processing complex medical information, and/or inordinate fear of certain outcomes or medical procedures, fear that could be alleviated with further education, it may be appropriate to intercede. It is the physician's responsibility to help patients avoid making decisions that are inconsistent with their (the patient's, and sometimes their family's and caregivers') underlying goals and values. A formal analysis of the risks and benefits of alternative strategies, and perhaps an 'off-the-shelf' or back-of-the-envelope decision analysis, including utility elicitation, could help achieve this goal in two ways. First, the process of making the expected harms and benefits explicit can be useful in educating the patient about the choices. Second, this utility elicitation process helps to ensure that the patient's choice reflects underlying values rather than a misunderstanding of the nature or probabilities of the various outcomes.

For patients who prefer more input from their clinician, a different approach is called for. In any approach, someone's preferences must be used to weigh the outcomes associated with alternative strategies. While physicians are uniquely qualified to integrate the complex clinical data relevant to medical decision making, their values may be poor proxies for those of patients. The ideal of shared medical decision making can only be achieved if the individual patient's preferences are somehow brought to bear on the choice among alternatives. On some occasions, formal utility elicitation and incorporation of those utilities into a decision analysis can be the best way to achieve this goal. But often, simpler strategies are sufficient. A formal decision analysis can identify the critical utility values to which the choice of the preferred strategy is sensitive, and the thresholds of those values at which the preferred strategy changes. These results can then be used to structure informative but less conceptually complex questions for patients that allow them to express where their preferences fall relative to that threshold.

Some patients, such as those who are cognitively impaired or very young children, may not be able to supply any information at all about their preferences. In this situation, the experiences of other patients who have faced similar choices may provide some guidance. Sometimes a proxy can provide preference data that they think would reflect the patient's preferences, to the best of their knowledge. These preferences can be in the form of reported decision choices or quantitative values – utilities – to be used in a decision process. Parents are generally proxies for children, and family caregivers are usually proxies for impaired patients. While proxies may have deep familiarity and knowledge of patients' wishes and values, it is often difficult to separate the proxy's preferences from the patient's. In a caregiving relationship these preferences may be so tightly intertwined that separating them is counter to good decision making – both may be important inputs to the optimal decision. If such values are considered biased, unreliable, or are unavailable, explicit quantitative data on other patients' values for the relevant health states can instead form the basis for judgments about the optimal strategy for the typical patient. Such utility data are available in the literature for a large number of health states, collected in a wide range of cross-sectional surveys or from participants in clinical trials.

4.15.2 Societal decision making: clinical guidelines

As discussed earlier, value judgments are embedded in most clinical guidelines. Those judgments should reflect the preferences of the population served by the guideline. But exactly who is in that population? Consider the example of a guideline about whether to use adjuvant chemotherapy in women with node-negative breast cancer. One could argue that the relevant values are those of patients facing that particular clinical decision, for example, women newly diagnosed with node-negative breast cancer. But these women are less knowledgeable about the outcomes of treatment than are women who have a history of treated node-negative disease; perhaps the preferences of that group are more informative and more relevant. But this may be too narrow a view. Since this guideline will affect women diagnosed in the future, too, one might want to solicit and incorporate the preferences of all women in the population, including those who do not now have any disease but may get it sometime later. But men may be affected by this guideline as well, through its impact on the women in their lives, and the diversion of resources into treatment for breast cancer that might otherwise be available to fund programs targeted to men. Should their preferences be reflected in the guidelines?

The question of *whose* preferences and values should be included in decision making for clinical guidelines continues to be a matter of debate in the field. One particularly difficult issue is how to reflect in guidelines the fact that different patients have different preferences and, therefore, that the clinical strategy that is best for some patients may not be best for others. With that in mind guidelines ought, in principle, to consider patient preferences among the patient characteristics that determine the best course of action, just as age, genetic markers, clinical risk factors, and co-morbidity are considered. There is near consensus, however, that guidelines should include preference assessment in some form as one of the steps. This is especially important for choices that are toss-ups with respect to survival outcomes, but involve important differences in quality of life.

4.15.3 Societal decision making: resource allocation

The most widespread application of quantitative utility assessment is decision making for resource allocation. Judgments about how to spend limited health-care resources should take into account the full range of the expected health benefits of alternative programs, including both length and quality of life, and should use units that allow comparisons across conditions. The first consensus declaring quality-adjusted survival as the preferred outcome measure for cost-effectiveness analysis (CEA) was issued in the mid-1990s (52), and continues to serve as the gold-standard of guidelines for CEA. In subsequent years, many countries have integrated this outcome into their national health care resource allocation processes, including the United Kingdom, the Netherlands, Canada, and Australia (53). These decision-making approaches in turn require the assessment of quantitative utility weights for the calculation of QALYs, with the accompanying methodological questions of what methods to use and from whom to elicit the values.

Guidance on these questions has been forthcoming from national sources in the countries that advocate the integration of quality adjustment into outcomes. Specific instruments have been recommended for use in obtaining utility weights in some countries, whereas specific approaches have been recommended in others. For example, the National Institute for Health and Clinical Excellence in the United Kingdom recommends the use of the EuroQol-5D to collect weights, or alternately the time trade-off technique for direct elicitation (54). Other countries are less specific in their guidance and recommend consistency in comparisons and validity in methods (such as Australia (55) and Canada (56)). In the United States, federal guidelines prohibit the consideration of costs in resource allocation decisions, yet non-governmental bodies have issued recommendations on the approach to preference measurement, including the Institute of Medicine (57).

In cost-effectiveness analysis conducted for societal decision making, there is a relatively firm consensus that societal values be used in the analysis. To quantify these values, the views of a representative sample of members of the general public are needed, which can be elicited using the direct techniques described in this chapter, such as the standard gamble, or using a health index instrument (as described in Section 4.8) which relies on underlying community values. It is important to remember that these community values that underlie the health index-derived utilities are themselves a function of a sample of individuals recruited to value the spectrum of health states. We know that populations from different countries value the same health states differently; for example, the states that make up the EuroQol-5D are valued differently by the UK population than they are by a population sample of the US (58), although the differences between countries are not as large as some might expect. Country-specific 'valuation sets' have been collected from population samples in different countries to provide country-specific values for some instruments, and work on this front continues for others.

From a methodological point of view, careful consideration of the appropriateness of the method used to elicit utilities, as well as the relevance of the sample providing the values *vis a vis* the decision question being addressed, will result in the most valid values for integration into a decision analysis. It is the analyst's responsibility to consider these choices and to conduct the appropriate sensitivity analyses because decision makers often fail to look 'under the covers' at the details of the analysis to understand the implications of different choices.

Finally, it is important to remember that not all analyses require high-quality empirical utility data. If the results of the decision analysis or cost-effectiveness analysis are insensitive to the utility values, resources should not be spent on collecting them. None the less, it is important that all decision analysts understand the strengths and limitations of alternative methods of eliciting and quantifying preferences, and exercise judgment about how and when to undertake this challenging task. We return to the role of utilities in cost-effectiveness analysis in Chapter 9.

4.16 Summary

Most decisions regarding alternative strategies require some value judgment about how to weigh the benefits versus the harms. The value of the outcomes may have several (competing) attributes such as length and quality of life. To compare strategies we need a scale that combines the important attributes in one metric. Quality-adjusted survival, measured in QALYs, provides such a scale. Furthermore, QALYs fulfill the criteria of a utility, that is, they can be considered a quantitative measure of the strength of a person's preference for an outcome.

Commonly used techniques for valuing outcomes include direct-elicitation methods (the rating scale, the standard reference gamble, and the time trade-off), health indices, and non-preference based methods such as stated preference techniques (willingness to pay, discrete choice experiments, etc.). Other factors that may affect outcome values are risk-aversion and risk-seeking attitudes and time preference. The choice of method to value outcomes is important to the validity of a decision analysis, as these values contribute building blocks to the analysis that can solidify or weaken the entire structure.

REFERENCES

1. Pauker SG. Medical decision making: how patients choose. *Med Decis Making.* 2010;30(5 Suppl):8S–10S.
2. Epstein RM, Alper BS, Quill TE. Communicating evidence for participatory decision making. *JAMA.* 2004;291(19):2359–66.
3. Trevena LJ, Davey HM, Barratt A, Butow P, Caldwell P. A systematic review on communicating with patients about evidence. *Eval Clin Pract.* 2006;12(1): 13–23.
4. Kurian AW, Sigal BM, Plevritis SK. Survival analysis of cancer risk reduction strategies for BRCA1/2 mutation carriers. *J Clin Oncol.* 2010;28(2):222–31.
5. Schwartz MD, Valdimarsdottir HB, DeMarco TA, et al. Randomized trial of a decision aid for BRCA1/BRCA2 mutation carriers: impact on measures of decision making and satisfaction. *Health Psychology.* 2009;28(1):11–9.
6. Kaufman EM PB, Lawrence WF, Shelby R, et al. Development of an interactive decision aid for female BRCA1/BRCA2 carriers. *J Genet Couns.* 2003;12:109–29.
7. Kurian AW, Munoz DF, Rust P, et al. Online tool to guide decisions for BRCA1/2 mutation carriers. *J Clin Oncol.* 2012;30(5):497–506.
8. O'Connor AM, Bennett CL, Stacey D, et al. Decision aids for people facing health treatment or screening decisions. *Cochrane Database of Systematic Reviews (Online).* 2009(3):CD001431.
9. Wilcox E. Decisions for dummies. *CMAJ.* 2009;181(5):E78.
10. Raiffa H. *Decision analysis: introductory lectures on choices under uncertainty.* 1st ed. New York: Random House; 1968.
11. Von Neumann J, Morgenstern O. *Theory of games and economic behavior.* Princeton, NJ: Princeton University Press; 1944.
12. Pliskin J, Shepard D, Weinstein M. Utility functions for life years and health status. *Oper Res.* 1980;28(1):206–24.
13. McHorney CA, Ware JE, Jr., Raczek AE. The MOS 36-Item Short-Form Health Survey (SF-36): II. Psychometric and clinical tests of validity in measuring physical and mental health constructs. *Med Care.* 1993;31:247–63.
14. Ware JE, Jr., Sherbourne CD. The MOS 36-item short-form health survey (SF-36). I. Conceptual framework and item selection. *Med Care.* 1992;30:473–83.
15. Beck AT, Ward CH, Mendelson M, Mock J, J. E. An inventory for measuring depression. *Archives of Gen Psych.* 1961;4:53–63.
16. Wright DR, Wittenberg E, Swan JS, Miksad RA, Prosser LA. Methods for measuring temporary health states for cost-utility analyses. *PharmacoEconomics.* 2009;27(9):713–23.
17. Jansen SJ, Stiggelbout AM, Wakker PP, et al. Patients' utilities for cancer treatments: a study of the chained procedure for the standard gamble and time tradeoff. *Med Decis Making.* 1998;18(4):391–9.
18. Dolan P, Gudex C, Kind P, Williams A. Valuing health states: a comparison of methods. *J Health Econ.* 1996;15(2):209–31.
19. Bayoumi AM. The measurement of contingent valuation for health economics. *PharmacoEconomics.* 2004;22(11):691–700.

20. O'Brien B, Gafni A. When do the "dollars" make sense? Toward a conceptual framework for contingent valuation studies in health care. *Med Decis Making.* 1996;16(3):288–99.

21. Richardson J, Nord E. The importance of perspective in the measurement of quality-adjusted life years. *Med Decis Making.* 1997;17(1):33–41.

22. Craig BM, Busschbach JJ, Salomon JA. Modeling ranking, time trade-off, and visual analog scale values for EQ-5D health states: a review and comparison of methods. *Med Care.* 2009;47(6):634–41.

23. Salomon JA. Reconsidering the use of rankings in the valuation of health states: a model for estimating cardinal values from ordinal data. *Population Health Metrics.* 2003;1(1):12.

24. Flynn TN, Louviere JJ, Marley AA, Coast J, Peters TJ. Rescaling quality of life values from discrete choice experiments for use as QALYs: a cautionary tale. *Population Health Metrics.* 2008;6:6.

25. Lancsar E, Louviere J. Conducting discrete choice experiments to inform healthcare decision making: a user's guide. *PharmacoEconomics.* 2008;26(8):661–77.

26. Salomon J, Vos T, Hogan D, et al. Common values in assessing health outcomes from disease and injury: Global Burden of Disease 2010 disability weights measurement study. *Lancet.* in press.

27. Torrance GW. Measurement of health state utilities for economic appraisal. *J Health Econ.* 1986;5(1):1–30.

28. Torrance GW, Feeny DH, Furlong WJ, et al. Multiattribute utility function for a comprehensive health status classification system. Health Utilities Index Mark 2. *Med Care.* 1996;34:702–22.

29. Brazier JE, Yang Y, Tsuchiya A, Rowen DL. A review of studies mapping (or cross walking) non-preference based measures of health to generic preference-based measures. *Eur J Health Econ.* 2010;11(2):215–25.

30. Brazier J, Roberts J, Deverill M. The estimation of a preference-based measure of health from the SF-36. *J Health Econ.* 2002;21(2):271–92.

31. Brazier JE, Roberts J. The estimation of a preference-based measure of health from the SF-12. *Med Care.* 2004;42(9):851–9.

32. Dolan P. Modeling valuations for EuroQol health states. *Med Care.* 1997;35(11):1095–108.

33. Feeny D, Furlong W, Boyle M, Torrance GW. Multi-attribute health status classification systems. Health utilities index. *PharmacoEconomics.* 1995;7:490–502.

34. Torrance GW, Furlong W, Feeny D, Boyle M. Multi-attribute preference functions. Health Utilities Index. *PharmacoEconomics.* 1995;7(6):503–20.

35. The EuroQol Group. EuroQol--a new facility for the measurement of health-related quality of life. *The EuroQol Group. Health policy (Amsterdam, Netherlands).* 1990;16(3):199–208.

36. Prosser LA, Grosse SD, Wittenberg E. Health utility elicitation: is there still a role for direct methods? *PharmacoEconomics.* 2012;30(2):83–6.

37. Bell CM, Chapman RH, Stone PW, Sandberg EA, Neumann PJ. An off-the-shelf help list: a comprehensive catalog of preference scores from published cost-utility analyses. *Med Decis Making.* 2001;21(4):288–94.

38. Franks P, Hanmer J, Fryback DG. Relative disutilities of 47 risk factors and conditions assessed with seven preference-based health status measures in a national U.S. sample: toward consistency in cost-effectiveness analyses. *Med Care.* 2006;44(5):478–85.

39. Patrick DL, Starks HE, Cain KC, Uhlmann RF, Pearlman RA. Measuring preferences for health states worse than death. *Med Decis Making.* 1994;14:9–18.

40. Tilling C, Devlin N, Tsuchiya A, Buckingham K. Protocols for time tradeoff valuations of health states worse than dead: a literature review. *Med Decis Making.* 2010;30(5):610–9.

41. Stalmeier PF, Lamers LM, Busschbach JJ, Krabbe PF. On the assessment of preferences for health and duration: maximal endurable time and better than dead preferences. *Med Care.* 2007;45(9):835–41.

42. Johannesson M, Pliskin JS, Weinstein MC. A note on QALYs, time tradeoff, and discounting. *Med Decis Making.* 1994;14:188–93.

43. Bleichrodt H, Gafni A. Time preference, the discounted utility model and health. *J Health Econ.* 1996;15(1):49–66.

44. Bleichrodt H, Johannesson M. The validity of QALYs: an experimental test of constant proportional tradeoff and utility independence. *Med Decis Making.* 1997;17(1):21–32.

45. Wakker P. A criticism of healthy-years equivalents. *Med Decis Making.* 1996; 16(3):207–14.

46. Dolan P. Thinking about it: thoughts about health and valuing QALYs. *Health Econ.* 2011;20(12):1407–16.

47. Payne J BJ, Schkade D. Measuring constructed preferences: toward a building code. *J Risk Uncertainty.* 1999;19(1–3):243–70.

48. Kahneman D, A. T. Choices, values and frames. *Amer Psychologist.* 1984;39:341–50.

49. Kuhberger A. The influence of framing on risky decisions: a meta-analysis. *Org Behav Hum Decis Processes.* 1998;75:23–55.

50. McNeil BJ, Pauker SG, Sox J, H.C., Tversky A. On the elicitation of preferences for alternative therapies. *N Engl J Med.* 1982;306:1259–62.

51. Wittenberg E, Prosser LA. Ordering errors, objections and invariance in utility survey responses: a framework for understanding who, why and what to do. *Applied Health Econ Health Policy.* 2011;9(4):225–41.

52. Gold MR, Siegel JE, Russell LB, Weinstein MC. *Cost-effectiveness in health and medicine.* 1st ed. New York: Oxford University Press; 1996.

53. Grosse SD, Prosser LA, Asakawa K, Feeny D. QALY weights for neurosensory impairments in pediatric economic evaluations: case studies and a critique. *Expert Rev Pharmacoecon Outcomes Res.* 2010;10(3):293–308.

54. National Institute for Health and Clinical Excellence. *Guide to the Methods of Technology Appraisal.* London: NICE 2008.

55. Pharmaceutical Benefits Advisory Committee. *Guidelines for Preparing Submissions to the Pharmaceutical Benefits Advisory Committee*. Canberra ACT: Department of Health and Aging 2008.

56. Canadian Agency for Drugs and Technologies in Health. *Guidelines for the economic evaluation of health technologies*. Ottawa, Canada 2006.

57. Miller W, Robinson L, Lawrence R, editors. Valuing Health for Regulatory Cost-Effectiveness Analysis. Washington, DC: Institute of Medicine, National Academies Press; 2006.

58. Nan L, Johnson JA, Shaw JW, Coons SJ. A comparison of EQ-5D index scores derived from the US and UK population-based scoring functions. *Med Decis Making*. 2007;27(3):321–6.

Interpreting diagnostic information

The interpretation of new information depends on what was already known about the patient.

Harold Sox

5.1 Diagnostic information and probability revision

Physicians have at their disposal an enormous variety of diagnostic information to guide them in decision making. Diagnostic information comes from talking to the patient (symptoms, such as pain, nausea, and breathlessness), examining the patient (signs, such as abdominal tenderness, fever, and blood pressure), and from diagnostic tests (such as blood tests, X-rays, and electrocardiograms (ECGs)) and screening tests (such as Papanicolaou smears for cervical cancer or cholesterol measurements).

Physicians are not the only ones that have to interpret diagnostic information. Public policy makers in health care are equally concerned with understanding the performance of diagnostic tests. If, for example, a policy maker is considering a screening program for lung cancer, he/she will need to understand the performance of the diagnostic tests that can detect lung cancer in an early phase of the disease. In public policy making, other types of 'diagnostic tests' may also be relevant. For example, a survey with a questionnaire in a population sample can be considered analogous to a diagnostic test. And performing a trial to determine the efficacy of a treatment is in fact a 'test' with the goal of getting more information about that treatment.

Obtaining information may be expensive, risky, or both. The purpose of information, however it is obtained, is to aid in deciding on the best further management. Most of this information is, however, subject to some degree of error. Both false positives and false negatives are possible, the rates of which will differ between different pieces of information. Hence we must examine how to interpret and select information to minimize the impact of such errors. Let us consider an example.

EXAMPLE   A 50-year-old man presents with fatigue, and the initial workup shows an iron-deficiency anemia. You do an immunochemical fecal occult blood test (FOBT), to check whether gastrointestinal bleeding, particularly from a colorectal cancer, is present and this is found to be positive. You are aware, however, that the FOBT is not perfectly accurate in detecting cancers: some cancers are not bleeding and are missed (false negatives), and there are other causes of apparent bleeding (false positives). How do you interpret the FOBT?

This chapter will be concerned with the process of using such imperfect diagnostic information to reassess the probability that a patient has one of several possible diseases. When a test result is 'positive' we are interested in 'the probability of a disease given a positive test result', also known as the positive predictive value or post-positive-test probability of disease (Figure 5.1). In probability notation, this is written as $p(D+\,|\,T+)$. When a test result is 'negative,' we are interested in 'the probability of no disease given a negative test result,' the negative predictive value or post-negative-test probability of no disease. In probability notation, this is written as $p(D-\,|\,T-)$. Sometimes the patient may have one of more than two diseases (D_1, D_2, D_3 ... D_i...), and the possible test results (R_1, R_2, R_3 ... R_j ...) may not be easily characterized as 'positive' and 'negative.' An example might be a patient with acute abdominal pain who presents with a constellation of symptoms and signs, white blood cell count, and other test results, and who may have appendicitis, cholecystitis, gastritis, pancreatitis, diverticulitis, or other causes of pain. In such cases, we are interested in $p(D_i\,|\,R_j)$, the probability of each diagnosis given the test results.

Usually, estimates of probabilities of disease, conditional upon test results, are not readily available. Instead, one is more likely to have an assessment of

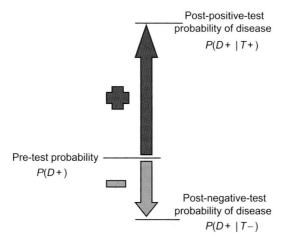

Figure 5.1   Probability revision: the pre-test probability is revised upward if the test is positive or downward if the test is negative.

the probability of a test result among patients with or without the disease. For example, there may be a study which reports $p(T+\,|\,D+)$, the probability of a positive test given the presence of disease, and $p(T+\,|\,D-)$, the probability of a positive test given the absence of disease. This chapter is concerned with the process of converting probabilities of this latter type (test results given disease status) to probabilities of the type we usually want to help guide decision making (disease status given test results). We discover quickly that this process also depends on assessing the pre-test (prior) probability of the disease, $p(D+)$. The process of taking the test result into account by converting the pre-test (prior) probability, $p(D+)$, to a post-test (posterior) probability of disease, $p(D+\,|\,T+)$ or $p(D+\,|\,T-)$, is called probability revision.

The post-test probability will depend both on the pre-test probability and the information obtained from the test. The aim of this chapter is to introduce both the methods of calculation and theory behind calculating the post-test probability.

We begin with a discussion on pre-test probabilities, then discuss how test performance is measured, and subsequently explain how to calculate post-test probability. Although it is important to understand how the calculations are done for purposes of formal decision analysis, the concepts themselves can be very helpful in the clinical setting even without explicit calculation. This chapter will emphasize tests with two possible outcomes, and Chapter 6 will look at how and when such tests should alter clinical decisions. Chapter 7 expands upon the material in this and the next chapter, assisting the decision maker to assess more generally the value of diagnostic test information when there are more than two possible test results, and when there is more than one test available.

DEFINITIONS   The *pre-test (prior) probability of disease* is the probability of the presence of the target disease conditional on the available information prior to performing the test under consideration.

The *post-test (posterior) probability of disease* is the probability of the presence of the target disease conditional on the pre-test information and the test result.

Probability (Bayesian) revision is the process of converting the pre-test probability to the post-test probability, taking the test result and test characteristics into account.

5.1.1 Prevalence and pre-test (prior) probability

If a patient were chosen at random from a given population, the pre-test probability of disease for the patient would be the disease prevalence in that population. However, patients are not selected at random. Even candidates for screening are not selected at random. Each person who presents for a possible test has specific characteristics, including history, physical findings, and previous test results. These characteristics, along with the disease prevalence, determine the probability that an individual has a given disease at any point in time. This probability is conditional upon available information and may be taken as the pre-test probability with respect to a subsequent test. For example, the pre-test probability that a patient has colorectal cancer before the FOBT level has been determined will be adjusted based on age, gender, clinical history, and family history. In that sense, the prior probability is actually a posterior probability that is conditional upon all of these factors (for example, the probability of colorectal cancer in a 50-year-old male whose mother had colorectal cancer) while it is still a prior probability with respect to the FOBT test. The prior probability here reflects the proportion of patients with similar characteristics in whom colorectal cancer would be expected. This chapter will focus on diagnostic tests that have only two outcomes, positive ($T+$) or negative ($T-$), and a single disease so that we may divide the tested group into those with the disease ($D+$) and those without the disease, the non-diseased ($D-$).

5.1.2 The 2 × 2 table for the FOBT and colorectal cancer

How will you interpret positive and negative FOBTs in the example? First, we need to understand the accuracy of the test by quantifying the error rates. To obtain the error rates, you might consult the literature. You find a study of an immunochemical FOBT, the results of which are shown in Table 5.1(1). Although a somewhat older study, the results are still relevant and consistent with later similar studies as reviewed by the US Preventive Services Task Force (2).

The table clearly demonstrates that the FOBT is imperfect. Using the terms in Table 5.1B, there were five false negatives, that is, five patients with colorectal cancer whose FOBT was negative; there were 271 false positives, that is, people without colorectal cancer who showed a positive FOBT. We shall use Table 5.1 to define some important probabilities that describe the rates of these errors. Using these probabilities we will introduce the concept of probability revision. Specifically, we will calculate the probability that a patient has colorectal cancer (CRC) given a positive fecal occult blood test result (FOBT), or $p(CRC+|FOBT+)$. In the process we will also calculate several other probabilities that we will find useful for decision making. One of these is the probability that a patient has colorectal cancer despite a negative FOBT, or $p(CRC+|FOBT-)$. Since a patient either has or does not have colorectal cancer, we can apply the summation principle to calculate the

Table 5.1 (A) Results of 7211 screens for colorectal cancer with an immunochemical test for fecal occult blood (FOBT) in 'high-risk' but asymptomatic patients. (B) Terms for the four cells of the 2 × 2 table

(A) FOBT	Disease status			(B) General	Disease status	
FOBT result	Colorectal cancer	No colorectal cancer	Totals	Test result	Disease	No disease
Positive	24	271	295	Positive	True positive TP	False positive FP
Negative	5	6911	6916	Negative	False negative FN	True negative TN
	29	7182	7211		Total disease TP + FN	Total no- disease FP + TN

(A) Based on(1).

probabilities of *not* having colorectal cancer, conditional upon the test results, as 1.0 minus the corresponding probability of having cancer.

Also of interest, and a byproduct of the process of probability revision, is the probability that the FOBT will be positive, or $p(T+)$. As we will demonstrate, the probability of a positive test result is not necessarily the same as the probability that disease is present, $p(D+)$. Why might we be interested in the probability of a positive test? There may be follow-up tests and procedures induced by positive tests, which have risks and costs associated with them. In the case of a positive FOBT, patients may then undergo colonoscopy (endoscopic procedure of the large intestine) to confirm the presence of cancer, a procedure that not only has a modest risk of morbidity and mortality, but also causes discomfort and anxiety (loss of quality-of-life-related utility). And from the viewpoint of a health-care payer or society, a positive FOBT induces the cost of a colonoscopy.

5.1.3 Two important conditional probabilities: sensitivity and specificity

Consider the proportion of patients with colorectal cancer who have a positive FOBT test result. This proportion is 24/29, or about 0.83 (83%). This is the probability of a positive test result given that the disease is present; it may be expressed symbolically as $p(T+|D+)$. We call this probability the *sensitivity* or *true-positive ratio* (*TPR*) of the test. Similarly, the proportion of patients without the disease who have a negative test result is 6911/7182 or about 0.96 (96%). This probability of a negative test result given that the disease is absent is denoted by $p(T-|D-)$ and is called the *specificity* or *true-negative ratio* (*TNR*) of the test.

Sensitivity and specificity describe how often the test is correct (in the diseased and non-diseased groups respectively); they are two independent values. The complement of the sensitivity, that is $(1.0 - TPR)$, is the proportion of patients with disease who have a negative test result, or $p(T-|D+)$; this is called the *false-negative ratio* (*FNR*) of the test. In the example the false-negative ratio is 5/29, which equals 0.17 (17%). We could have obtained the *FNR* as $1 - TPR$, or $100\% - 83\% = 17\%$. The complement of the specificity, that is $(1.0 - TNR)$, is the proportion of patients without the disease who have a positive test result, or $p(T+|D-)$; this is called the *false-positive ratio* (*FPR*) of the test and, for the FOBT in Table 5.1, is equal to 271/7182, which equals 0.04 (4%). We could have obtained the *FPR* as $1 - TNR$, or $100\% - 96\% = 4\%$.

Thus, we have derived four proportions from the 2×2 table: sensitivity and specificity which are two independent values to describe how often the test is correct, and the false-negative and false-positive ratios which are two independent values to describe how often the test is in error. The formal definitions of these terms are as follows:

DEFINITIONS   Consider a test with two results, positive $(T+)$ and negative $(T-)$, used to distinguish between two disease states, $D+$ (disease present) and $D-$ (disease absent).

The *sensitivity* or *true-positive ratio* (*TPR*) is the proportion of patients with the target disease who have a positive test result. In probability notation this is $p(T+|D+)$.

The *specificity* or *true-negative ratio* (*TNR*) is the proportion of patients without the target disease who have a negative test result. In probability notation this is $p(T-|D-)$.

The *false-positive ratio* (*FPR*) is the proportion of patients without the target disease who have a positive test result. In probability notation this is $p(T+|D-)$.

The *false-negative ratio* (*FNR*) is the proportion of patients with the target disease who have a negative test result. In probability notation this is $p(T-|D+)$.

A sensitive test, one with a high true-positive (and low false-negative) ratio, is good at detecting patients with the target disease (sensitive to the presence of disease, unlikely to miss the diagnosis) and thus good at *ruling out* the disease.

A specific test, one with a low false-positive (and high true-negative) ratio, is good at screening out patients who do *not* have the disease (specific to that disease) and thus good at *ruling in* the disease. Remember that test sensitivity applies to patients with the disease; test specificity applies to patients without the disease.

Observe that the true-positive ratio and the false-negative ratio sum to 1.0, or 100%, and that the true-negative ratio and false-positive ratio also sum to 1.0, or 100%. An ideal test has a true-positive ratio of 1.0 (and therefore a false-negative ratio of 0.0) and a false-positive ratio of 0.0 (and therefore a true negative ratio of 1.0). The definitions of these probabilities and others to be introduced in this chapter are summarized in Table 5.2.

5.1.4 Post-test (posterior) probabilities: the post-positive-test and post-negative-test probabilities

Although sensitivity and specificity are important characteristics of a test, they are not the probabilities we need to decide how to treat a patient. Sensitivity and specificity are the probabilities of test results given the presence or absence of disease, respectively. However, in health-care practice we do not know whether or not someone has the disease, but rather we find a test result is positive or negative, and from this information we wish to infer the probability of disease. Thus we usually need to know the probabilities of disease given positive or negative test results, which, as we shall see, may turn out to be very different.

For an individual selected randomly from the study population upon which the estimates of sensitivity and specificity were based (Table 5.1), the probability of disease given a positive test result, $p(D+ \mid T+)$, may be obtained from the 2×2 table. This probability is calculated as $TP/(TP + FP)$, which is the proportion of those with positive test results $(TP + FP)$ who also have the disease (TP). We call this the *post-positive-test probability of disease* or *positive predictive value* of the test. (Some authors use other terms for this proportion, and the same is true for many other concepts defined in this book. Since there are no universally recognized conventions, we have tried to adopt the most widely used nomenclature.) In our study population the post-positive-test probability of disease would be 24/295, which is approximately 0.08 or 8%. *The post-negative-test probability of disease* is the conditional probability of having the disease given a negative test result, or $p(D+ \mid T-)$. It may be calculated as $FN/(FN + TN)$ from Table 5.1B. In the example the post-negative-test probability in the study population is 5/6916, or approximately 0.0007 or 0.007%.

Table 5.2 Various probabilities related to diagnostic tests

Common name	Meaning	Probability notation	Equivalent probability	Estimate from 2 × 2 table from study sample
Sensitivity (true-positive ratio (*TPR*))	Probability of positive test results in those with the target disease	$p(T+\,\vert\,D+)$	$1 - p(T-\,\vert\,D+)$	$TP/(TP+FN)$
False-negative ratio (*FNR*)	Probability of negative test results in those with the target disease	$p(T-\,\vert\,D+)$	$1 - p(T+\,\vert\,D+)$	$FN/(TP+FN)$
Specificity (true-negative ratio (*TNR*))	Probability of negative test results in those without the target disease	$p(T-\,\vert\,D-)$	$1 - p(T+\,\vert\,D-)$	$TN/(TN+FP)$
False-positive ratio (*FPR*)	Probability of positive test results in those without the target disease	$p(T+\,\vert\,D-)$	$1 - p(T-\,\vert\,D-)$	$FP/(TN+FP)$
Pre-test (prior) probability of disease	Probability of target disease in the population of interest	$p(D+)$	$1 - p(D-)$	Requires independent estimate
Pre-test probability of non-disease	Probability of absence of target disease in the population of interest	$p(D-)$	$1 - p(D+)$	Requires independent estimate
Post-positive-test probability of disease (positive predictive value)	Probability of target disease in those with positive results	$p(D+\,\vert\,T+)$	$1 - p(D-\,\vert\,T+)$	Requires knowledge of pre-test probability
Post-positive-test probability of non-disease	Probability of absence of target disease in those with positive results	$p(D-\,\vert\,T+)$	$1 - p(D+\,\vert\,T+)$	Requires knowledge of pre-test probability
Post-negative-test probability of disease	Probability of target disease in those with negative results	$p(D+\,\vert\,T-)$	$1 - p(D-\,\vert\,T-)$	Requires knowledge of pre-test probability
Post-negative-test probability of non-disease (negative predictive value)	Probability of absence of target disease in those with negative results	$p(D-\,\vert\,T-)$	$1 - p(D+\,\vert\,T-)$	Requires knowledge of pre-test probability
Ratio of test positives	Probability of positive test results in the population	$p(T+)$	$1 - p(T-)$	Requires knowledge of pre-test probability

A related term is the *negative predictive value*, which is the probability that a patient with a negative test does not have the target disease, that is, $p(D- | T-)$. In terms of the discussion at the beginning of the chapter, the positive predictive value and the negative predictive value are both examples of post-test (posterior) probabilities.

DEFINITIONS   The *post-positive-test probability of disease* or *positive predictive value* is the probability that a patient with a positive test result has the target disease. In probability notation it is written as $p(D+ | T+)$.

The *post-negative-test probability of non-disease* or *negative predictive value* is the probability that a patient with a negative test result does not have the target disease. In probability notation it is written as $p(D- | T-)$.

We have seen that patients in the study population who have a positive FOBT have an 8% probability of colorectal cancer. But recall that this study population was asymptomatic. In that population 29 persons had colorectal cancer and 7182 persons did not have colorectal cancer. Would these post-test probabilities also apply to patients with iron-deficiency anemia, as in our clinical example? Would they apply to a more generally selected population, such as in mass screening? In general, the answer is no to both questions. The estimates of the post-test probabilities obtained directly from Table 5.1 apply only to the study population. Unless the proportion of patients with the disease in the study population equals the proportion of patients with the disease in the population in which the test will be applied, these post-test probabilities will not apply. In general, the test characteristics sensitivity and specificity are conditional on whether disease is present or not and are usually generalizable across settings. The post-test probabilities are not test characteristics and are not generalizable because they depend on the pre-test probability of disease.

To interpret the test result for our specific patient we need to estimate the post-test probabilities based on an independent estimate of the pre-test probability of the disease in the population from which our patient is selected. That is, we require a procedure that will permit us to carry over the information from the study population to the target population of interest. One way to do this, as we shall now see, is to construct a hypothetical table as if the study had been done in a population with the pre-test probability in which we are interested.

5.1.5 Probability revision: using the 2 × 2 table

Let us return to the clinical example of the man with iron-deficiency anemia. In the study population of Table 5.1, 24 of 295 positives had cancer, and hence the post-positive-test probability was 24/295 or about 8.1%. Because this study

Table 5.3 The steps in probability revision for the fecal occult blood test (FOBT) for the diagnosis of colorectal cancer (CRC) for a patient with a pre-test probability of CRC of 8%

FOBT result	CRC	No CRC	Total by row
Step 1: Use pre-test probability to fix column totals: 8% × 10 000 = 800			
Positive			
Negative			
Total by column	*800*	*9200*	*10 000*
Step 2: Use sensitivity to fill in disease column: 83% × 800 = 664			
Positive	*664*		
Negative	*136*		
Total by column	800	9200	10 000
Step 3: Use specificity to fill in non-disease column: 96% × 9200 = 8832			
Positive	*664*	*368*	
Negative	*136*	*8832*	
Total by column	800	9200	10 000
Step 4: Compute row totals: 664 + 368 = 1032 and 136 + 8832 = 8968			
Positive	*664*	*368*	*1032*
Negative	*136*	*8832*	*8968*
Total by column	800	9200	10 000

was in an asymptomatic population, however, this estimate would be incorrect, because it assumes that the pre-test probability of the disease in the population from which our patient was selected is the same as the pre-test probability in the study population (0.4%). For patients presenting with iron-deficiency anemia, three studies showed cancer in 19 of 170, 11 of 100, and two of 114 patients. Pooling these results suggests a rate of 32 per 384 or about 8%, which is already almost as high as that among the FOBT positives in Weller's group.

The first step is to modify the column totals of Table 5.1 so that they reflect the pre-test probability in the population of concern. This is shown in Step 1 of Table 5.3, where the probability of colorectal cancer is fixed at 8% of a hypothetical cohort of 10 000 similar patients. The second step is to use the known true-positive ratio, or test sensitivity, to fill in the first column of the table. Since the sensitivity is 83%, this means that 83% of the 800 colorectal cancers, or 664 members (6.64%) of the hypothetical population, have the disease *and* a positive test result.

Similarly, 17% of those with colorectal cancer have a negative test result; hence, 17% of the 800, or 136 members (1.36%) of the population have the disease *and* a negative test result.

The third step (Table 5.3) is to use the known true-negative ratio, or test specificity, to fill in the second column of the table (i.e., the joint probabilities of no colorectal cancer and each possible test result). Since the true-negative ratio is 96%, this means that 96% of 9200 or 8832 members (88.32%) of the population have no colorectal cancer and a negative test result and that 4% of 9200 or 368 members (3.68%) of the population have no colorectal cancer and a positive test result.

Finally, we complete the 2 × 2 table by filling in the numbers and proportions of test positives and test negatives. Those are simply the totals across the rows. Notice that the probability of a positive test is 10.32%, even though the pre-test probability of cancer is only 8%. Evidently the false positives outnumber the false negatives. This is true even though the false-positive ratio of the test (4%) is less than its false-negative ratio (17%). Do you understand how this can be? (Hint: There are many more people without the disease than with the disease.)

With the 2 × 2 table completed, we can compute the probability of colorectal cancer given a positive FOBT test result in this population. Of the 1032 with positive test results, 664 have colorectal cancer and the remaining 368 do not. Therefore, 664/1032, or approximately 64%, of patients with iron-deficiency anemia and a positive FOBT test result actually have colorectal cancer. Contrast this result with the 8% that was obtained by implicitly assuming a disease pre-test probability of 0.4% (Table 5.1) rather than a pre-test probability of 8%. Clearly, the pre-test probability makes a difference!

The process we have just worked through is called probability revision. We start with a pre-test probability of colorectal cancer, which in this case is 0.08. We observe a test result, which in this example is a positive FOBT test result. We revise the probability to obtain a post-test probability of colorectal cancer given the positive test result. In this example the post-test probability is 0.64.

The method shown in Table 5.3 can also be used to compute the post-negative-test probability of colorectal cancer. In Table 5.3, Step 4, the total number of patients with a negative test result is 8968. Included among these patients with a negative test result are 136 who have colorectal cancer. Therefore, the post-negative-test probability of colorectal cancer in this population is 136/8968 or approximately 0.015. This leaves a probability of not having colorectal cancer, given a negative test result, of 1.0 minus 0.015 or 0.985 (the negative predictive value).

To summarize the results for our 50-year-old man with anemia, we have revised our pre-test probability of colorectal cancer as follows:

- Without an FOBT, we would assess $p(CRC+) = 0.08$.
- If the FOBT result is positive, we calculate $p(CRC+|FOBT+) = 0.64$.
- If the FOBT result is negative, we calculate $p(CRC+|FOBT-) = 0.015$.
- The probability of a positive FOBT is $p(FOBT+) = 0.1032$.

5.1.6 The effect of pre-test probability in screening

We have seen that the interpretation of a test depended on the test characteristics (sensitivity and specificity) and on the pre-test probability. Let us look at another example of this phenomenon in the context of screening.

EXAMPLE   Your practice has called together a committee to consider screening all adult patients using immunochemical FOBTs. You are concerned about the potential for missing cancers, and also about the anxiety and unnecessary investigation caused by falsely positive tests. Since you do not know how often these may occur, and how their occurrence may vary across different patient groups, you seek more detail about the diagnostic performance and implications of the test.

How should your committee interpret the FOBT in this screening setting? For this task you need to estimate the pre-test probability of colorectal cancer, which in a screening situation is the prevalence in the population. A large trial (3) provided figures from which we can calculate the prevalence of colorectal cancer as approximately one per 1000, two per 1000, and 3.5 per 1000 for persons aged 50–59, 60–69, and 70 + respectively. How does this observation modify the analysis? Let us repeat the steps above, but for the pre-test probability in the 50–59 age group, that is, 1 per 1000. Take a few minutes to try this yourself by filling out a 2×2 table using the four steps above before consulting Table 5.4. To facilitate the calculations it is prudent to start out with a total group of 100 000 subjects, or if you prefer to work with probabilities, be sure to carry at least five digits after the decimal point.

Now the post-test probability after a positive test result is 83/4079 or about 2%. This post-positive-test probability of cancer for a screened person is less than the *pre-test* probability for the 50-year-old anemic patient in our first clinical example, and similar to his *post-negative*-test probability of cancer. Clearly, the post-test probability depends strongly on the pre-test probability of the group we apply the test to, and will strongly influence both how the

Table 5.4 The steps in probability revision for the fecal occult blood test (FOBT) for the diagnosis of colorectal cancer (CRC) in a screening situation with a pre-test probability of CRC of 0.1%

FOBT result	CRC	No CRC	Total by row
Step 1: Use pre-test probability to fix column totals			
Positive			
Negative			
Total by column	100	99 900	100 000
Step 2: Use sensitivity to fill in disease column			
Positive	83		
Negative	17		
Total by column	100	99 900	100 000
Step 3: Use specificity to fill in non-disease column			
Positive	83	3996	
Negative	17	95 904	
Total by column	100	99 900	100 000
Step 4: Compute row totals			
Positive	83	3996	4079
Negative	17	95 904	95 921
Total by column	100	99 900	100 000

person should be managed and what he or she should be told. For example, if we investigate patients with a positive FOBT in this screened group, the patient should know that, of 100 follow-up colonoscopies, only about two will show colorectal cancer.

Figure 5.2 illustrates how the post-FOBT probability varies according to the pre-FOBT probability. Notice that for very low pre-test probabilities the post-test probability is low, irrespective of whether the test result is positive or negative. Similarly, for very high pre-test probabilities the post-test probability is high, again irrespective of whether the test result is positive or negative. The test is particularly useful for intermediate pre-test probabilities, the 'grey zone,' where the test result distinguishes between low- and high post-test probabilities.

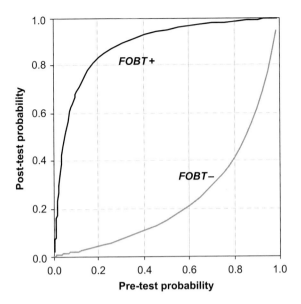

Figure 5.2   Post-test probability after performing a fecal occult blood test (FOBT) depending on the pre-test probability and the test result, either positive (*FOBT+*) or negative (*FOBT−*).

On the book website you will find an Excel worksheet that can help you do probability revision and get insight by playing with the numbers. Similar tools can be found on other websites. In the next section we offer an alternative approach to probability revision, using the mathematics of probability. This device, known as Bayes' formula, is numerically equivalent to the method that uses 2 × 2 tables, although it may be easier to use in some circumstances. While not essential to the remainder of this book, an understanding of the formula and the mathematical basis of probability revision will help the reader with the applications that will be discussed in the next two chapters.

5.2 Bayes' formula

5.2.1 A review of probability notation

The manipulation of a contingency table and probability notation can be combined to yield an important generalization for the revision of pre-test probabilities. Let us review the notation introduced in Chapter 2.

Recall that the expression $p(E)$ indicates the probability of an event or condition E; $p(E \mid F)$ denotes the probability of E contingent upon the presence of F; and $p(E,F)$ stands for the probability of the joint occurrence of both

E and F. The term $p(D+)$, therefore, simply means the probability of disease, or the pre-test probability; $p(T+\,|\,D+)$ denotes the probability that an individual has a positive test result given the presence of disease, which is a relation we expressed earlier in this chapter as the test sensitivity; and $p(T+,D+)$ means the probability of both a positive test result and the presence of disease.

With this notation in mind, let us return to the example of FOBT and colorectal cancer.

5.2.2 Derivation of Bayes' formula

Recall from the laws of probability that we can write the joint probability in terms of conditional probabilities:

$$p(T+, D+) = p(T+\,|\,D+)\,p(D+) \tag{5.1}$$

$$\text{and} \quad p(T+, D+) = p(D+\,|\,T+)\,p(T+) \tag{5.2}$$

Switching the expressions in Equation 5.2 to the other side of the equal sign and dividing both sides of the equation by $p(T+)$ we get:

$$p(D+\,|\,T+) = p(T+,D+)/p(T+) \tag{5.3}$$

that is, the probability of disease among patients with a positive test result equals the proportion of those with a positive result that are also diseased. This equation also follows directly from the definition of the conditional probability $p(D+\,|\,T+)$.

What proportion of patients have a positive test result? Positive results can occur in two ways: true positives among the diseased and false positives among the non-diseased. That is:

$$p(T+) = p(T+,D+) + p(T+,D-)$$

Each term on the right-hand side of this equation can be factored according to the laws of conditional probability, but now we will condition on the presence or absence of disease rather than on the test result:

$$p(T+) = p(T+\,|\,D+)p(D+) + p(T+\,|\,D-)p(D-) \tag{5.4}$$

If we substitute Equations 5.1 and 5.4 into Equation 5.3, we derive the following:

$$p(D+\,|\,T+) = \frac{p(T+\,|\,D+)p(D+)}{p(T+\,|\,D+)p(D+) + p(T+\,|\,D-)p(D-)} \tag{5.5}$$

This equation (Eq. 5.5) is known as Bayes' formula for a dichotomous ($+$ or $-$) test and two disease states. In Chapter 7 we will generalize this expression for multiple test outcomes and multiple diseases. We could also write Equation 5.5 using words rather than probability notation, as follows:

Post-positive-test probability =

$$\frac{\text{Sensitivity} \times \text{pre-test probability}}{(\text{Sensitivity} \times \text{pre-test probability} + (1-\text{specificity}) \times (1-\text{pre-test probability}))}$$

More generally, we can write the above equation for interpreting any test result, R, as,

$$p(D+ \,|\, R) = \frac{p(R \,|\, D+)p(D+)}{p(R \,|\, D+)p(D+) + p(R \,|\, D-)p(D-)} \tag{5.6}$$

The derivation is identical to the derivation in the dichotomous case.

5.2.3 Applying Bayes' formula

Applying Bayes' formula to our first example of a 50-year-old-man with iron-deficiency anemia, we can calculate his post-test probabilities of having colorectal cancer as follows.

If he has a positive FOBT:

$$p(CRC+ \,|\, FOBT+) = (0.83 \times 0.08)/(0.83 \times 0.08 + 0.04 \times 0.92) = 0.64$$

If he has a negative FOBT:

$$p(CRC+ \,|\, FOBT-) = (0.17 \times 0.08)/(0.17 \times 0.08 + 0.96 \times 0.92) = 0.015$$

Both of these results agree with what we obtained in the analysis using 2×2 tables. The above equations are both forms of Bayes' formula (also called Bayes' theorem: Bayes' theorem was developed by the eighteenth-century mathematician Reverend Thomas Bayes). They incorporate two kinds of data: pre-test probabilities of the presence or absence of disease, and information about the characteristics of a given test in individuals with and without disease, or a test's true-positive and false-positive ratios. This information is combined to yield a new probability of the presence of disease in the patient who is the subject of the test. It is in this sense that we refer to test results as revising or modifying our pre-test probabilities of disease.

We began this analysis in response to the question: 'What is the probability of disease in an individual with a positive test result?' The result is given in Bayes' formula by the ratio of the number of individuals who have the disease and whose test results are positive to the number of all those individuals whose test results are positive.

5.3 Bayes' theorem with tree inversion

Thus far we applied Bayes' theorem using a 2 × 2 table and subsequently using a formula. If you look back at the arithmetic you performed while filling in the 2 × 2 table and the arithmetic involved in using the formula you will notice that, in fact, it was exactly the same arithmetic. There is yet another method to do the exact same exercise which may be more appealing to some. Using a chance tree we can visualize the probabilities and then invert the chance tree. Tree inversion is often the most intuitive and error-free method of probability revision with two or more tests.

Figure 5.3 visualizes the probabilities relevant for the first case example. The upper chance tree first divides into colorectal cancer vs. no colorectal cancer with the associated pre-test probability of disease. Subsequently, conditional on the presence or absence of colorectal cancer, the probabilities of a positive vs. negative FOBT result are depicted. This chance tree represents the pre-test probability of disease and the test sensitivity and specificity (Figure 5.4). To calculate the post-test probabilities of disease we need to invert the chance tree so that the tree first models the test result and then the disease status conditional on the test result (Figure 5.4). We calculate the number of cases (or equivalently the probability) for each path through

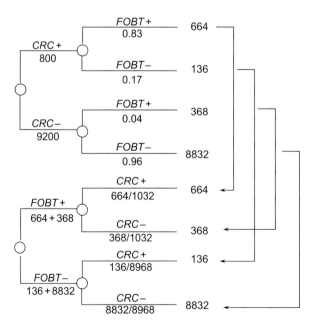

Figure 5.3   Tree inversion to perform probability revision for the fecal occult blood test (FOBT) for the diagnosis of colorectal cancer (CRC) for a patient with a pre-test probability of colorectal cancer of 8%.

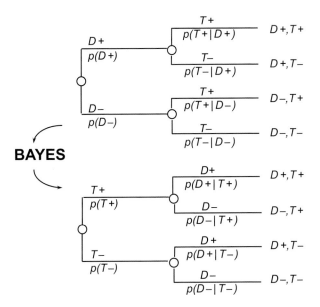

Figure 5.4   Tree inversion to perform probability revision with probability notation.

the tree (Figure 5.3), which is equivalent to filling in the cells of the 2 × 2 table. These numbers are copied to the ends of the branches of the inverted chance tree. The frequency of a positive test result is calculated by summing the true- and false-positive results and the frequency of a negative test result is calculated by summing the true- and false-negative results, which is equivalent to computing the row totals of the 2 × 2 table. Finally, we can calculate the post-test probabilities by dividing the path frequencies by the test result totals. Again, notice the analogy to what we did using the 2 × 2 table.

In Chapter 3 we discussed the importance of sequencing chance nodes in the correct order. Going from left to right, a decision tree should depict the sequence of events as they may occur over time. To model chronologically we would want to model the test result first and then the true disease status. As we can see here, it can sometimes be convenient to model it the other way round: that is, model disease status first followed by the test result. The advantage is that you can use the pre-test probability of disease and sensitivity and specificity in your tree and let the model do the probability revision for you. Because the path probabilities are the same, the end result is the same provided that there are no intervening decisions or events that may influence the course of the disease or affect the probabilities thereafter. The next management decision should always be modeled conditional on the test result, which you observe, and not on the true disease status, which is the underlying truth but unknown to the decision maker as long as a reference test has not (yet) been performed.

5.4 The odds-likelihood-ratio form of Bayes' formula

Bayes' formula, even in the dichotomous (disease vs. non-disease) situation, is too complicated for most people to do as a mental calculation. The 2×2 table also requires calculation aids. For a situation when a quick estimate of revised probabilities is needed, many people find the odds-likelihood-ratio version of Bayes' formula easier to use. This version of Bayes' formula is in fact the mathematical equivalent of clinical diagnostic reasoning: we combine what we believe before doing the test with what we learn from the test to derive what we believe after doing the test. It makes use of the concepts of odds and likelihood ratio, which we define at this point. It also forms the basis for a simple pocket nomogram for rapidly working out post-test probabilities. Finally, we shall find this form of Bayes' theorem invaluable when we turn to the analysis of multiple-valued or continuous-valued test results and the choice of a positivity criterion for such tests, a subject to which we turn in Chapter 7.

5.4.1 Odds

If the probability that an event will occur is p, then the probability that it will not occur is $1 - p$. An event that has a 20% chance of occurring has a corresponding 80% chance of not occurring. Recall from Chapter 2 that the ratio of p to $1 - p$, or $p/(1 - p)$, is called the *odds* favoring the occurrence of an event. The odds against the occurrence of an event can be expressed as $(1 - p)/p$.

If an event has a 0.20 probability of occurrence, the odds favoring the event are 0.2/0.8, or 0.25 (sometimes written 1:4 and read 'one to four'). The odds against are 0.8/0.2, or 4. If an event has a 50% chance of occurrence, then the odds favoring and odds against are both 0.5/0.5, or 1:1, which are called 'even odds.' As probability varies from 0.0 to 1.0, the corresponding odds favoring thus range from 0 to infinity. The relationship of odds and probability may be shown graphically as in Figure 5.5, where each unit on the horizontal axis increases by a multiple of 10 (a logarithmic scale).

DEFINITION   Let p be the probability of an event. Define the following:

    Odds favoring the event

    $Odds = p/(1 - p)$

    Odds against (Odd_A) the event

    $Odd_A = (1 - p)/p$

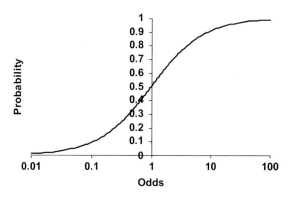

Figure 5.5   Relationship between odds and probability.

We can also reverse the calculation if we know the odds (or odds against) and want to determine the probability by using the equations:

$p = Odds/(1 + Odds)$

and

$p = 1/(1 + Odds_A)$

(In a horse race, the odds given each horse are odds against that horse winning. Thus, if a horse is given odds of 4:1, its probability of winning is 20%, because $0.2 = 1/(1 + 4)$)

5.4.2 Probability revision using odds

The post-test probability of disease is related to the pre-test probability and the test characteristics, through Bayes' formula (Equation 5.6):

$$p(D+|R) = \frac{p(R\,|D+)p(D+)}{p(R\,|D+)p(D+) + p(R\,|D-)p(D-)}$$

Now consider the analog of Bayes' formula for the non-diseased state:

$$p(D-|R) = \frac{p(R\,|D-)p(D-)}{p(R\,|D+)p(D+) + p(R\,|D-)p(D-)}$$

If we divide the first equation by the second equation, we get the simple formula:

$$\frac{p(D+\,|R)}{p(D-|R)} = \frac{p(D+)}{p(D-)}\,\frac{p(R\,|D+)}{p(R\,|D-)} \tag{5.7}$$

This version of Bayes' formula is expressed in terms of odds rather than probabilities. Remember that the odds favoring an event with a probability of

p equals $p/(1 - p)$. The first ratio on the right-hand side of the equation, $p(D+)/p(D-)$, is therefore the pre-test odds favoring disease. The ratio on the far left, $p(D+\,|\,R)/p(D-\,|\,R)$, is the post-test odds given the test result; it is the odds corresponding to the post-test probability $p(D+\,|\,R)$.

To obtain the post-test odds, we multiply the pre-test odds by the ratio $p(R\,|\,D+)/p(R\,|\,D-)$. Let us interpret this ratio. The numerator, $p(R\,|\,D+)$, is the probability of obtaining the test result among individuals who have the disease. The denominator, $p(R\,|\,D-)$, is the probability of obtaining the same test result among persons without the disease. The ratio of the two is a measure of the *relative* likelihood of observing this test result, comparing persons with the disease with persons without the disease. It is called the *likelihood ratio* for the test result R. Evidently, this ratio summarizes all the information we need to know about the test for the purposes of revising the probability of disease.

For a dichotomous test, the likelihood ratio (LR) for a positive test result is denoted $LR+$. It is the true-positive ratio (TPR), which is $p(T+\,|\,D+)$, divided by the false-positive ratio (FPR), which is $p(T+\,|\,D-)$, or:

$$LR+ = \text{sensitivity}/(1 - \text{specificity}) = TPR/FPR$$

The likelihood ratio for a negative test result from a dichotomous test, $LR-$, is the false-negative ratio, $p(T-\,|\,D+)$, divided by the true-negative ratio, $p(T-\,|\,D-)$, or:

$$LR- = (1 - \text{sensitivity})/\text{specificity} = FNR/TNR$$

Now let's apply the odds-likelihood-ratio formula to our FOBT example. The $LR+ = 0.83/(1 - 0.96) = 20.8$; and the $LR- = (1 - 0.83)/0.96 = 0.18$. The pre-test probability for the 50-year-old anemic man was 0.08, and hence the odds were $0.08/(1 - 0.08) = 0.087$. After a positive FOBT, the post-test odds would be $0.087 \times 20.8 = 1.8$. But this is an odds, and we have to convert it to a probability using the relation $p = Odds/(1 + Odds)$. Hence the post-test probability would be $1.8/(1 + 1.8) = 0.64$, which is the answer we had obtained previously.

DEFINITION   The *likelihood ratio* associated with a test result R is the ratio of its probability of occurrence in patients with the disease to its probability of occurrence in patients without the disease. In probability notation,

$$Likelihood\ ratio = \frac{p(R|D+)}{p(R|D-)}$$

Thus, we have four ways of revising probabilities: the 2×2 table, Bayes' formula, tree inversion, and the odds-likelihood-ratio version of Bayes' formula. All give the same answers. All can be calculated with a simple spreadsheet or calculator. Furthermore, web-calculators and smartphone/smart-tablet applications can be found that can conveniently do the calculations.

5.4.3 Using the odds-likelihood-ratio formula to revise probabilities mentally

To show how easy it is to use the odds-likelihood form of Bayes' formula, one of the authors of this book (MCW) recalls the following episode:

When my wife thought she had become pregnant for the first time, about 20 years ago, she went to her gynecologist to have a pregnancy test. Although she felt she was pregnant, the test was negative. She was naturally disappointed and asked her doctor whether the test could be wrong. He told her that about 10% of pregnant women have a negative result on the first pregnancy test. I met her at the doctor's office and found her disheartened by the doctor's report.

I asked her how likely she had thought it that she was pregnant before the test, and she said, 'I was very sure.' I said, 'You mean maybe 95%?' and she answered, 'Yes, about 95%.' I assumed that the false-positive ratio was virtually nil (and thus the true-negative ratio virtually 1), and calculated in my head the post-test probability using the odds-likelihood formulation. Since the pre-test odds favoring pregnancy were about 20:1 and the likelihood ratio for a negative result about 1:10 (that is, false-negative ratio divided by true-negative ratio), I immediately calculated the post-test odds favoring pregnancy as $(20)\cdot(1/10)$, or 2. This was easy for me to convert in my head to a post-test probability of about 2/3. With this conclusion, reached in a matter of seconds, I was able to reassure myself as well as my wife. Rightly so, because she was indeed pregnant.

Even though the pre-test odds used in this illustration were rounded off (from 19:1 to 20:1), this author got a serviceable approximation in a matter of seconds. In a patient-care setting, a pocket calculator, smartphone, smart-tablet, or web-calculator can provide a more exact estimate in as little time.

5.5 Indices of diagnostic test performance for dichotomous tests

The test performance of a diagnostic test with dichotomous test results can be characterized in several ways. The most informative are pairs of indices, such as defined in paragraph 5.1.3, where we defined

sensitivity $(= TP/(TP + FN))$ and

specificity $(= TN/(TN + FP))$,

which together characterize the diagnostic test performance. Not infrequently we will see performance expressed as the

true-positive ratio $(TPR) = TP/(TP + FN) =$ sensitivity and

false-positive ratio $(FPR) = FP/(TN + FP) = 1$-specificity.

The likelihood ratio (LR) of a test result was defined in paragraph 5.4.2. For a dichotomous test two LRs, one for a positive test result $(LR+)$ and one for a negative test result $(LR-)$, are required to fully characterize the test performance:

$$LR+ = p(T+|D+)/p(T+|D-) = \text{sensitivity}/(1 - \text{specificity}) = TPR/FPR$$
$$LR- = p(T-|D+)/p(T-|D-) = (1 - \text{sensitivity})/\text{specificity} = FNR/TNR$$

These LRs are defined to predict presence of disease rather than its absence. Another set of LRs can be defined to predict absence of disease, but that becomes confusing and prone to error and is unnecessary if you recognize that the probability of absence of disease is 1 minus the probability of disease.

An overall measure of diagnostic test performance is the Diagnostic Odds Ratio (DOR):

$$DOR = \frac{TP \cdot TN}{FN \cdot FP} = \frac{TPR \cdot TNR}{FNR \cdot FPR} = \left(\frac{TPR}{1-TPR}\right) \cdot \left(\frac{1-FPR}{FPR}\right)$$

An increase in either the TPR or the TNR will increase the DOR, indicating a better performance of the test. The natural logarithm of the DOR is also commonly used as an overall measure of performance:

$$D = \ln(DOR) = \ln\left(\frac{TPR}{1-TPR}\right) - \ln\left(\frac{FPR}{1-FPR}\right)$$

Finally, Youden's index is defined as:

Youden's index $=$ sensitivity $+$ specificity $- 1$

We will revisit indices of diagnostic test performance in Chapter 7 when we consider multiple test results.

5.6 Subjective estimates of disease probability

This book views diagnostic inference as a problem of revising opinion with imperfect information. Research has shown that the conclusions of unaided opinion revision, the kind physicians do every day, often differs systematically from conclusions they would reach by applying Bayes' formula or other formal aids. Our discussion has focused on post-test probabilities and the cognitive processes involved in getting to a post-test probability. But Bayesian analysis must begin with a pre-test probability. Where do those come from?

In general, as discussed in Chapter 2, we recommend that epidemiological sources and relevant databases be consulted for the starting point of the reasoning process – the pre-test probability. As with finding studies of diagnostic test performance or therapeutic efficacy, this takes some facility with searching computerized databases.

Despite these efforts, published probability data that seem truly relevant and applicable to your particular case may not be available. The data may have been published so long ago that you wonder if the figures are still correct. Or the study was done in a community quite unlike yours, and you wonder if the disease pre-test probability there applies to your locale. For these reasons, and others, clinicians sometimes have to rely upon subjective probabilities – personal opinions formulated as probabilities – to begin to apply Bayes' formula.

Although the mechanics of the calculation with Bayes' formula is the same whether one relies on subjective probabilities or has access to large data sets, there are important possibilities for error and bias in the assessment of subjective probabilities. First and foremost, any individual clinician, or 'probability assessor,' is unlikely to have observed a large enough number of cases to be able to provide a reliable estimate. Furthermore, psychologists have identified three heuristic principles that are commonly employed to generate subjective probability estimates: availability, representativeness, and anchoring and adjustment, which may lead to biased judgment (4).

5.6.1 Availability: reliance on the easily recalled

Availability is employed when the probability of an event (or an underlying disease) is judged by how easy it is to recall instances or occurrences of similar events. When a clinician estimates a probability by remembering a patient very much like the one being evaluated, availability may operate. What is wrong with using this principle to estimate probability? Recall can be affected by factors other than frequency and probability. More recent events ('I just had a patient last week who ...') are often better remembered than more distant ones. On the other hand, memory is also affected by how strange and unusual an event is: commonplace events tend to be forgotten but unusual events are usually remembered very well. We are more likely to remember what we ate at a particularly outstanding banquet years ago than what we had for dinner two weeks ago Monday. Every clinician remembers a very unusual case seen just once, and the result is that the probability of such events is likely to be overestimated. A partial remedy for this bias is to take the precaution of dividing the number of observed cases by the total number of patients one has seen, thereby making reference to the relative frequency of the observed event.

5.6.2 Representativeness: focusing on features at the neglect of pre-test probability

Representativeness is used when the probability of a disease for a particular patient is judged by how closely the clinical picture resembles a larger class of events, such as the 'typical picture' of that disease. Most of the time, this is a rather safe principle to use: physicians commonly diagnose a patient by how closely the clinical picture resembles a classic description. But suppose the clinical picture of a particular case resembles but does not exactly match the typical description of two alternative diseases, or resembles disease A in some respects and disease B in other respects. Let's assume, too, that A is more common than B and that the patient does not have both diseases. In such a situation clinicians may judge A and B to be equally probable, because the observed findings of the case fit both A and B equally well. In doing so, the different pre-test probabilities of the two diseases have been neglected. In other words, the representativeness heuristic is insensitive to pre-test probabilities.

5.6.3 Anchoring and adjustment: under-adjustment for new information

Suppose a clinician consults some epidemiological sources to obtain estimates of the local pre-test probability of various diseases. She decides that none of the published data really fits her community or her patients and that these numbers have to be revised, up or down. The published estimates serve as an anchor, and her subjective probabilities of the pre-test probability in her community are the result of adjustment. The problem is that adjustments are frequently insufficient; the starting point overly influences people. This implies that we could arrive at two different subjective probabilities for a disease, depending on whether we started out with the pre-test probability of 'disease' and adjusted up or if we started with the pre-test probability for 'no disease,' adjusted down, and then converted that subjective probability back to $p(D+)$. Clearly, we should have the same subjective $p(D+)$ regardless of where we started. The anchoring and adjustment heuristic says that frequently these numbers will not be the same.

5.6.4 Value-induced bias

In decision analysis, estimates of probability (the likelihood of an event) and utility (which reflects its value) should be made independently and kept in separate accounts, to be combined during the stage of evaluation. But, in practice, this may be hard to do. Concern about the consequences of a possible disaster makes it more salient and vivid, and these contribute to the workings of availability, so the disaster may seem more likely. Insurance companies use this principle to induce people to buy insurance for very specific, imaginable, but narrowly defined classes of events. In medicine, the probability of serious illness may be overestimated, because the penalties for missing a serious disease are much greater (a malpractice suit?) than the penalties for excessive testing to rule out unlikely possibilities. For example, a patient complains of headache and a medical student concludes the problem is brain cancer. Perhaps the probability of a malignancy is overestimated because of the adverse consequences of missing the case.

5.7 Summary

In this chapter we discussed how information can be interpreted and used to aid decision making. Although we focused on diagnostic (clinical) information that is used to make treatment decisions, the same principles apply to any information that is obtained to guide a decision.

Most information is subject to some degree of error – both false-positive and false-negative results are possible. The accuracy of a test can be summarized with the sensitivity and specificity of the test (or with the true-and false-positive ratios). A sensitive test is very good at detecting patients with the target disease: the high true-positive ratio implies it is sensitive to the presence of disease and the corresponding low false-negative ratio implies it is good at *ruling out* the disease. A specific test is good at screening out patients who do *not* have the disease: the high true-negative ratio and corresponding low false-positive ratio imply that the test is specific to that disease and thus good at *ruling in* the disease.

Our interpretation of the test result, i.e., our estimate of the post-test probability of disease, depends in part on the pre-test probability of disease and in part on the sensitivity and specificity (or true- and false-positive ratios) of the test. Probability revision is the process of converting the pre-test probability of disease to the post-test probability of disease taking the test result into account. Probability revision can be performed with a 2×2 table, Bayes' formula, tree inversion, odds-likelihood-ratio form of Bayes' theorem, or using web-based/smartphone/smart-tablet calculators. In essence all methods do the same thing: the estimate of the probability of disease prior to performing the test (the pre-test probability of disease) is combined with the information from the test result (sensitivity and specificity, or true- and false-positive ratio, or the likelihood ratio) to derive the probability of disease after performing the test (the post-test probability of disease). The process can be used to calculate the post-positive-test probabilities of disease (and no disease) and the post-negative-test probabilities of disease (and no disease). The use of Bayes' formula can help to overcome various biases in estimating probabilities such as the bias due to availability, representativeness, anchoring and adjustment, and value-induced bias.

REFERENCES

1. Weller D, Thomas D, Hiller J, Woodward A, Edwards J. Screening for colorectal cancer using an immunochemical test for faecal occult blood: results of the first 2 years of a South Australian programme. *Aust N Z J Surg*. 1994;64(7):464–9.
2. Whitlock EP, Lin JS, Liles E, Beil TL, Fu R. Screening for colorectal cancer: a targeted, updated systematic review for the U.S. Preventive Services Task Force. *Ann Intern Med*. 2008;149(9):638–58.
3. Mandel JS, Church TR, Ederer F, Bond JH. Colorectal cancer mortality: effectiveness of biennial screening for fecal occult blood. *J Natl Cancer Inst*. 1999;91(5):434–7.
4. Tversky A, Kahneman D. Judgment under uncertainty: Heuristics and biases. *Science*. 1974;185:1124–31.

6

Deciding when to test

Before ordering a test ask: What will you do if the test is positive? What will you do if the test is negative? If the answers are the same, then *don't do the test.*

Poster in an Emergency Department

6.1 Introduction

In the previous chapter we looked at how to interpret diagnostic information such as symptoms, signs, and diagnostic tests. Now we need to consider when such information is helpful in decision making. Even if they reduce uncertainty, tests are not always helpful. If used inappropriately to guide a decision, a test may mislead more than it leads. In general, performing a test to gain additional information is worthwhile only if two conditions hold: (1) at least one decision would change given some test result, and (2) the risk to the patient associated with the test is less than the expected benefit that would be gained from the subsequent change in decision. These conditions are most likely to be fulfilled when we are confronted with intermediate probabilities of the target disease, that is, when we are in a diagnostic 'gray zone.' Tests are least likely to be helpful either when we are so certain a patient has the target disease that the negative result of an imperfect test would not dissuade us from treating, or, conversely, when we are so certain that the patient does not have the target disease that a positive result of an imperfect test would not persuade us to treat. These concepts are illustrated in Figure 6.1, which divides the probability of a disease into three ranges:

(a) do not treat (for the target disease) and do not test, because even a positive test would not persuade us to treat;

(b) test, because the test will help with treatment decisions or with follow-up; and

(c) treat and do not test, because even a negative test would not dissuade us from treating.

Treat implies patient management as if disease is present and may imply initiating medical therapy, performing a therapeutic procedure, advising a lifestyle or other adjuvant intervention, or a combination of these. Do not treat implies patient management as if disease is absent and usually means risk factor management, lifestyle advice, self-care and/or watchful waiting.

145

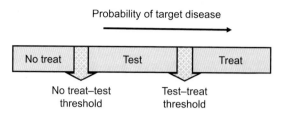

Probability of target disease

No treat | Test | Treat

No treat–test
threshold

Test–treat
threshold

Figure 6.1   Division of the probability of a disease into three ranges: (a) do not treat
(for the target disease) and do not test, because even a positive test result
would not persuade us to treat, (b) test, because the test will help with
treatment decisions; and (c) treat and do not test, because even a negative
test result would not dissuade us from treating.

The aim of diagnostic testing is to improve treatment decisions by reducing
diagnostic uncertainty. Hence, understanding the treatment decision is
important in devising a diagnostic strategy. The treatment threshold (discussed in Chapter 3) is the pivot around which diagnostic testing turns.
Diagnostic testing may be viewed as an attempt to place a patient clearly on
one side or the other of the treatment threshold. Once testing can no longer
change the choice of treatment, it is unhelpful. We must choose despite any
residual uncertainty. Conversely, testing is most helpful when we are near the
treatment threshold, since tests can still change the choice of treatment. Hence
we begin by reviewing the treatment threshold. We then look at how and
when the results of a diagnostic test should alter the treatment chosen by
calculating two threshold probabilities that separate the three zones in
Figure 6.1: the no treat–test threshold and the test–treat threshold (1). (The
supplementary material on the course website illustrates the calculations.)

6.2 The treatment threshold revisited

EXAMPLE   **Chest pain – suspected coronary artery disease (CAD)**

Imagine you are a primary care physician. A 55-year-old well-educated woman
consults you. She recently started having chest pain while running on the beach and
during biking against the wind. The pain is substernal and heavy in nature, is only
present during very strenuous exercise, and disappears immediately with rest. The
chest pain does not bother her in her usual daily activities but she is concerned that
she may be at risk for a myocardial infarction (MI) (heart attack) or another
cardiovascular disease (CVD) event such as sudden cardiac death, stroke, or a
transient ischemic attack (TIA).

She consults you for risk factor assessment and advice on whether to start using
medication (statins, beta-blockers, low-dose aspirin) to reduce the risk of having a
CVD event. She does not smoke, never has. Her blood pressure is 138/80, heart rate

58, total cholesterol is 4.9 mmol/l (190 mg/dl), HDL is 1.3 mmol/l (50 mg/dl), and BMI is 21 kg/m². Her family history is negative for MI and stroke but both parents had essential hypertension. She eats a healthy diet and is physically active.

You enter her risk factors in the European SCORE calculator (for fatal CVD events) and the Framingham risk estimator (for fatal and non-fatal heart attacks) and find that her ten-year risk of having a CVD event (fatal or non-fatal) given her risk factor profile is very low, about 1%. This assumes, however, that her pain is not caused by obstructive coronary artery disease (CAD). If her chest pain is due to CAD the ten-year risk is much higher, about 10%. Optimal medical treatment (OMT) would halve the risk of a CVD event (Relative risk = RR = 50%) irrespective of her baseline risk. Medical treatment, however, carries a ten-year risk of adverse events of about 2% for this patient (serious bleeding due to aspirin use which may be gastrointestinal, epidural/subdural/joint hemorrhage due to (sports) injuries, syncope with serious consequences due to excessive beta-blockade, and myopathy, rhabdomyolysis, or diabetes mellitus due to statins).

For the purpose of this example we will simplify the problem by assuming that CVD events and adverse events from treatment never occur together and that the patient values CVD events and adverse events from treatment as equally undesirable. Furthermore, we assume the patient wants to maximize her ten-year event-free survival.

Let us now tabulate the options in a clinical balance sheet (Table 6.1).

It is clear that neither strategy is dominant: both have advantages and disadvantages and the decision depends on the prior probability p that the patient has the underlying disease (CAD). It will help to calculate the expected value of each option. One way to do this is to draw the decision tree, which will help us structure the sequence of events and probabilities over time. This is shown in Figure 6.2.

To determine the treatment threshold we must compare the benefits and harms of treatment vs. no treatment. As illustrated in Table 6.1 and Figure 6.2, the benefit of OMT if the patient has CAD is that it reduces the ten-year probability of having a CVD event by half (RR = 0.5; 5% absolute ten-year risk reduction if the patient has CAD). There is, however, a 2% probability of adverse events from treatment. Thus, the net benefit is an absolute ten-year risk reduction of 3% (= absolute increase in ten-year event-free survival of 3%) with treatment compared with no treatment if there is underlying CAD (Figure 6.2 and 6.3). What about the harms to those without CAD? The OMT will also halve their risk of an event, reducing it from 1% to 0.5% but that too would come with a 2% risk of an adverse event from treatment. Thus, the net harm of treating patients without CAD when we should not have treated them ('leave the well alone') is 1.5% (= absolute decrease in ten-year event-free survival of 1.5%) (Figure 6.2 and 6.3)

Table 6.1 Clinical balance sheet for alternative management strategies for a patient with suspected coronary artery disease (CAD)

Underlying diagnostic truth	Ten-year outcome	Do not treat	Treat (RR = 0.5)
No CAD	CVD events	0.01	$0.5 \times 0.01 = 0.005$
	Adverse events OMT	0	0.02
	Total events	0.01	0.025
	Event-free survival	**0.990**	**0.975**
CAD	CVD events	0.10	$0.5 \times 0.10 = 0.05$
	Adverse events OMT	0	0.02
	Total events	0.10	0.07
	Event-free survival	**0.900**	**0.930**

RR: relative risk

CAD: coronary artery disease

CVD: cardiovascular disease

OMT: optimal medical treatment

As we have done previously, to determine the no treat–treat threshold probability of disease analytically we use a variable for the prior probability p, calculate the expected value for each strategy (both are expressions with unknown value for p), set the two expressions equal to each other, rearrange the terms, and solve for p. For our example, this can be done using either the ten-year probability of events or using the ten-year event-free survival – the result will be the same. (It is a good idea to check this for yourself. See the Chapter 3 assignment 'Chest pain Suspected CAD' on the book website.)

Recall in Chapter 3 we derived the general equation for the treatment threshold (from the graph) as:

$$Treatment\ threshold = \frac{Harm}{Harm + Benefit} \tag{6.1}$$

Using this equation for the example here gives us a treatment threshold for the probability of coronary artery disease (CAD) of:

$$Threshold\ p(CAD) = 0.015/(0.015 + 0.030) = 0.33 \tag{6.2}$$

Hence, assuming that we can do no further tests, we would prefer not to treat if the chance of CAD were less than 33% and we would prefer treatment if it

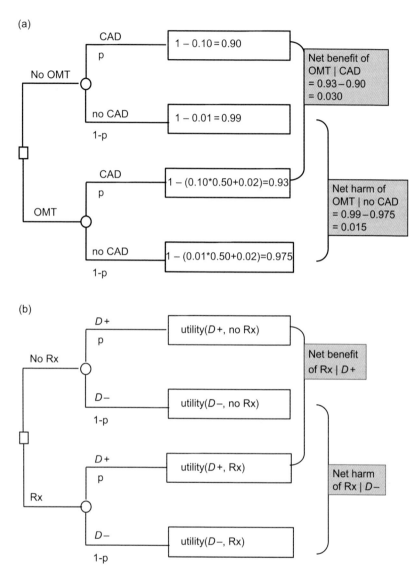

Figure 6.2　　　Decision tree comparing two strategies for (a) suspected coronary artery disease (CAD): optimal medical treatment (OMT) vs. no treatment (no OMT) using ten-year event-free survival as outcome measure and (b) the generic form of the decision tree for a disease (D) comparing treatment (Rx) with no treatment (no Rx). Abbreviations: p prior probability of disease, $D+$ disease present, $D-$ disease absent, u utility/outcome measure. In both (a) and (b) the benefit of treatment conditional on presence of underlying disease and harm of treatment conditional on absence of underlying disease are indicated.

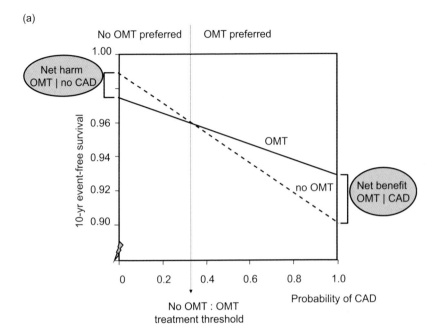

(a)

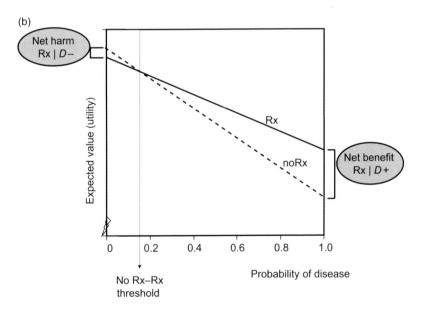

(b)

Figure 6.3   (a) The ten-year event-free survival of preventive treatment (OMT) compared to no treatment (no OMT) as a function of the probability of coronary artery disease (CAD). (b) The corresponding generic graph for expected utility of treatment (Rx) and no treatment (no Rx) as a function of the probability of disease (D). The net benefit and net harm of treatment compared to no treatment for patients with (D+) and without (D−) the disease, respectively, have been indicated. No treatment has the highest expected value for low probabilities of disease, whereas treatment has the highest expected value for high probabilities of disease. The expected value of treatment and no treatment are equal at the treatment threshold. Note how the treatment threshold shifts depending on the harm to benefit ratio. If the harm to benefit ratio decreases (compare Figure 6.3 (b) to (a)), the treatment threshold is lower, broadening the indication for treatment.

were greater than 33%.We can estimate the probability of CAD by consulting a web-based prediction model (2): based on age, gender, and the type of chest pain ('typical' in the example) the probability of CAD is 19%; taking into account that she has no risk factors the probability is 11%. Thus, the probability of CAD is well below the treatment threshold and we would be able to reassure our patient that she should not start medication. A prudent physician would add 'if you experience persistent or worsening chest pain interfering with your daily activities and reducing your quality of life, you should return for non-invasive diagnostic testing. And keep up the healthy lifestyle!'

6.3 Test thresholds: defining the 'gray zone'

In general, a test will only be helpful if a positive result can shift our decision from a tentative decision of 'no treat' to 'treat' or a negative result can shift our decision from 'treat' to 'no treat.' That is, the test result must be able to shift the disease probability across the treatment threshold. Similarly, if after performing the test under consideration further diagnostic testing is still possible, a negative result should shift our decision from 'further diagnostic testing' to 'no treat, no test' and a positive result should shift our decision from 'further diagnostic testing' to 'treat' (Figure 6.4). If a test cannot cause one of these changes in the management plan, then its result has no direct value.

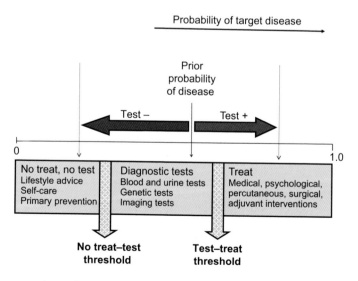

Figure 6.4   A test has value if a positive result shifts our decision to the 'treat' zone and/or a negative result shifts the decision to the 'no treat' zone.

There will be a range of probabilities around the treatment threshold for which the diagnostic test is capable of changing the choice of treatment. The boundaries defining this 'gray zone' of uncertainty are known as the *test thresholds*.

Now let us return to the question of whether to perform further testing on our patient.

EXAMPLE (*cont.*)   **Testing for suspected coronary artery disease**

After a few months the patient returns with persistent symptoms. A friend her age was recently admitted emergently to hospital with a heart attack. She is worried about her own chest pain and would like to undergo a diagnostic workup.

Will testing be useful? And which test would we recommend? Traditionally, the most commonly used test for suspected CAD is exercise ECG which, in women, has a sensitivity of 61% and specificity of 70% (3). There is an alternative test: over the last two decades CT coronary angiography (CTCA) has been developed and has a sensitivity of 90% and specificity of 96% (4). Let us first calculate the post-test probabilities for all possible pre-test probabilities. This was done using the methods explained in Chapter 5 and is shown in Figure 6.5.

When should the results change the treatment decision? In Figure 6.5 the treatment threshold (33%) has been marked on the post-test probability axis, and the zones where testing can change the decision have been indicated. The ability of the test result to change the treatment choice depends not only on its sensitivity and specificity but also on the pre-test probability. For example, at a pre-test probability of 30%, a negative test result (both for exercise ECG and for CTCA), would lower the probability of disease, indicating that the decision not to treat is best, whereas a positive test result would increase the probability (to over 33%), suggesting treatment is best.

DEFINITION   The *test–treat threshold* is the probability at which we are indifferent between testing and immediate treatment. It is the probability for which the expected utility of testing and treating is equal.

At pre-test probabilities above 47%, however, both a negative and positive exercise ECG result would leave us above the treatment threshold, implying that we would choose to treat no matter what the test result, and hence the test does not contribute to the decision. This occurs where the curve of negative test results crosses the treatment threshold. This is the *test–treat threshold*.

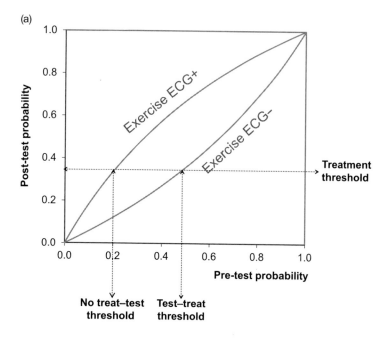

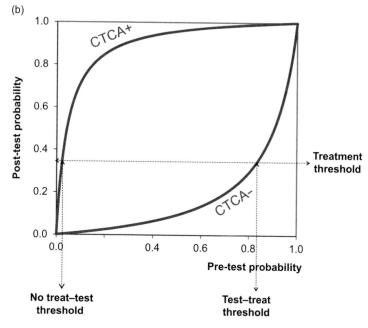

Figure 6.5   Graph of the relationship between pre-test and post-test probabilities for the positive and negative test result of (a) exercise electrocardiography (ECG) and (b) CT coronary angiography (CTCA) for suspected coronary artery disease. Superimposing the treatment threshold on the post-test probability (vertical axis) yields the consequent zone of the pre-test probability (horizontal axis) where (a) exercise ECG and (b) CTCA can change the decision. Using a test with higher sensitivity and/or specificity (CTCA rather than ECG) widens the range over which testing is useful.

By a similar process we can find a lower threshold below which the best treatment is 'no treat,' irrespective of whether the test is positive or negative. The lower threshold is where the positive result curve crosses the treatment threshold, which is at a pre-test probability of 20% for ECG and 2% for CTCA. At all probabilities lower than this threshold, both the post-positive-test and post-negative-test probabilities are below the treatment threshold, implying that we would choose no treatment, no matter what the test result. This is the *no treat–test threshold*.

DEFINITION

The *no treat–test threshold* is the probability at which we are indifferent between testing and not treating. It is the probability for which the expected utility of testing and not treating is equal.

Figure 6.5 shows both of these test thresholds. Within the shaded 'gray zone,' the test is capable of changing the treatment decision, whereas outside this zone it does not. That is, if you test outside the gray zone and base your treatment decision on the test result, then you would do worse than not testing at all. This is an important point, so we shall repeat it. *Imperfect tests performed inappropriately may do more harm than good because of the subsequent inappropriate treatment decisions.* At low probabilities the risk is believing false-positive results, whereas at high probabilities the risk is believing false-negative results. In fact, if the pre-test probability is outside the 'gray zone,' and the test has already been performed, a wise decision maker would be better off ignoring the result than be lulled into acting on it (medical–legal considerations notwithstanding)! In the example, the gray zone for exercise ECG is 20–47% whereas for CTCA it is 2–83%. Note how the range for testing widens with higher sensitivity and specificity of the test.

A general solution to finding any threshold is to draw the decision tree (Figure 6.6) and then perform an appropriate threshold or sensitivity analysis. This is preferably done using decision analytical software. Here we will illustrate an equivalent graphical approach that provides several insights about the effects of individual components of the problem. Let us first modify the benefit vs. harm graph (Figure 6.3) by adding an additional line to represent the test. Figure 6.7 presents the expected value of the do not treat, test, and treat options for the range of probabilities of disease. Notice that the option with the highest utility is optimal: do not treat for low probabilities of disease, treat for high probabilities of disease, and test for intermediate probabilities (the gray zone). Note that at this stage we have not yet introduced any 'toll' from the test itself.

As before, the net harm from treating those without the target disease is represented by the difference of the 'no treat' vs. 'treat' lines on the left-hand

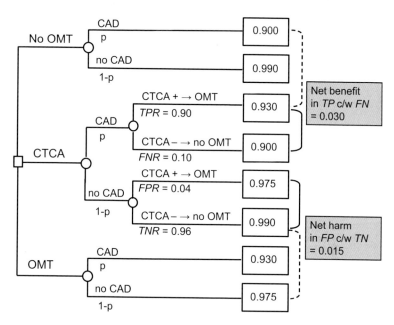

Figure 6.6   Decision tree for the choice between no treat–no test (no OMT), test (CTCA), and treat (OMT) options for the case example. Indicated are the net benefit gained in diseased patients correctly identified by the test and treated (*TPR*: true-positive test results) compared with those missed (*FNR*: false-negative test results, equivalent to diseased patients not tested–not treated), and also the net harm incurred in non-diseased individuals incorrectly labeled as diseased by the test and treated inappropriately (*FPR*: false-positive test results, equivalent to non-diseased individuals not tested but treated) compared with those correctly identified as non-diseased (*TNR*: true-negative test results).

vertical axis (where $p(D) = 0$). The net benefit from treating those with the target disease is represented by the difference of the 'treat' vs. 'no treat' lines on the right-hand vertical axis (where $p(D) = 1$).

Now consider what happens with testing at the extreme probabilities of 0 and 1. When the pre-test probability of disease is 0, no one has the target disease, and all patients with false-positive results would undergo the net harm of treatment (in the example: 0.015 loss of ten-year event-free survival). Hence the expected harm from performing the test instead of not treating is net harm $\times$ false-positive ratio (for exercise ECG in the example: Harm $\times$ $FPR = 0.015 \times 0.30$). This is the difference (vertical distance) between the 'no treat' and 'test' lines along the vertical axis in Figure 6.6 (if the graph had been drawn to scale). However, if we perform the test in those without the disease, patients with true-negative test results are spared the harm of treatment. Hence, the expected harm avoided by performing the test instead of treating equals harm $\times$ true-negative ratio (for exercise ECG in the example: Harm $\times$ $TNR = 0.015 \times 0.70$). This is shown in Figure 6.6 as the difference between

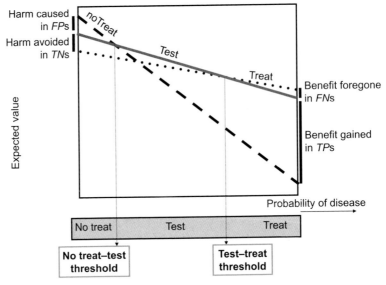

Figure 6.7 Expected value vs. probability of disease showing how a single test influences the treat vs. do not treat decision. For low probabilities of the disease, do not treat has the highest expected value. For high probabilities of the disease, treat has the highest expected value. In between there is a gray zone in which testing has the highest expected value. (Not drawn to scale, for illustrative purposes.)

the 'test' and 'treat' lines along the vertical axis. Similarly, when the pre-test probability of disease is 1, then everyone has the target disease. In that case, all patients with false-negative test results would miss out on the net benefit of treatment (in the example: 0.030 gain in ten-year event-free survival). Hence the expected loss of utility from doing the test instead of treating is benefit × false-negative ratio ($Benefit \times FNR = 0.03 \times 0.39$). This is shown in Figure 6.6 as the difference between the 'treat' and 'test' lines on the right-hand side of the graph where probability of disease equals 1.0. Also, by doing the test, patients with true-positive test results are given the benefit of treatment. Hence, the expected benefit gained by performing the test instead of not treating equals benefit × true-positive ratio ($Benefit \times TPR = 0.03 \times 0.61$). This is shown in Figure 6.6 as the difference between the 'test' and 'do not treat' lines on the right-hand side of the graph where probability of disease equals 1.0.

If the graph is drawn to scale, the test thresholds may be read directly from the graph. If the false-positive ratio increases, the 'test' line drops particularly on the left-hand side of the graph, increasing the no treat–test threshold. Similarly, if the false-negative ratio increases, the 'test' line drops particularly on the right-hand side, decreasing the test–treat threshold. In both cases the range of prior probabilities across which testing is optimal narrows, implying that there is a more limited indication area for testing. Notice that if the false-positive ratio is very high and/or the false-negative ratio is very high, testing can even become suboptimal over the entire range of prior probabilities of disease, that is, either 'no treat' or 'treat' yield a higher expected value, in which case the testing thresholds become meaningless.

We can obtain a more exact and general result for the thresholds using a geometric method. To find the no treat–test threshold (the left-hand test threshold), focus on the triangles made by the 'test' and 'do not treat' lines, together with the vertical axes. At the no treat–test threshold, the ratio of the pre-test probability of disease, $p(D)$, to its complement, $1 - p(D)$, is the same as the ratio of the vertical distance on the axes that form the bases of these triangles. If you have trouble seeing this, look back at Chapter 3, where we explained the geometric proof. (To simplify the equations we use *Harm* to mean 'Net Harm | no disease' and *'Benefit'* to mean *Net Benefit* | disease.)

Therefore, we derive:

$$\frac{p(D)}{1-p(D)} = \frac{Harm \times FPR}{Benefit \times TPR} \tag{6.3}$$

And hence, adding the numerator to the denominator on both sides to convert from odds to probability (i.e., from $x/y = w/z$ follows $x/(x + y) = w/(w + z)$), the threshold is:

$$No\ treat-test\ threshold = \frac{Harm \times FPR}{Harm \times FPR + Benefit \times TPR} \tag{6.4}$$

Similarly, focusing on the triangles made by the 'test' and the 'treat' lines together with the vertical axes, the test–treat threshold can be derived as:

$$Test-test\ threshold = \frac{Harm \times TNR}{Harm \times TNR + Benefit \times FNR} \tag{6.5}$$

These formulae are for tests without a toll, and would enable us to find the exact test thresholds.

Using the benefit and harm for our case example and sensitivity and specificity for the exercise ECG, we can calculate the no treat–test threshold using the above formulae as 20%, and the test–treat threshold as 47%. For CTCA the thresholds are 2% and 83%. Note that the thresholds cannot be read directly from Figure 6.6 because the graph representing the test has not been drawn to scale for illustrative purposes. The actual calculations can easily be performed in a spreadsheet program (see assignment Chapter 6 'Chest pain Suspected CAD' and corresponding solution on the website).

Alternatively, we could have drawn a full decision tree which includes the option of the test as in Figure 6.6. Using a decision tree is the most general and comprehensive method to analyze the value of testing strategies and to calculate testing thresholds. With a decision tree it is fairly straightforward to add additional concerns such as uninterpretable test results, or morbidity and mortality from an invasive test. The latter issues can be added to the graph, but this is not always straightforward. Let us examine such 'tolls' now. Again we will illustrate this with the graph because it provides helpful insights.

6.4 Thresholds for tests with a 'toll'

How would the test thresholds change if the test had some risk, adverse effect, disutility (that is, utility loss), or other 'toll'? The most straightforward examples of 'tolls' from tests are (a) direct health consequences such as direct harms or risks from the invasive nature of the test, e.g., mortality risk (usually small), permanent complications such as stroke, acute adverse events such as infections or allergic reactions to contrast, radiation-induced cancer, or discomfort. We shall show how these types of consequences can be incorporated into the utilities and reflected in the analysis of the test thresholds. A more subtle type of effect of a test would be (b) to delay treatment while awaiting test results. Delay may aggravate the disease and require another treatment, or the test result may become useless if the treatment decision is time-sensitive. For example, a delay in the diagnosis of acute appendicitis increases the risk of perforation of the appendix. Tests may also impose (c) psychological harm, such as anxiety while waiting for results. For example, women with false-positive mammograms may wait several days or weeks before getting definitive negative results and during this time they may experience considerable anxiety. A final negative consequence of tests is (d) the economic costs of the test, including both the direct health-care costs and the patient time costs to undergo the test. Here we will use the term 'toll' to include only the first three of these: the economic costs will be considered separately (Chapter 9).

EXAMPLE (cont.) In the example thus far, we assumed that the exercise ECG and CTCA were available and did not have a risk or cost associated with it. For a first estimate of the usefulness of the test, that is reasonable. In reality exercising a patient who has CAD entails a small risk of inducing a heart attack. Similarly, CTCA is associated with a risk of a contrast reaction, nephrotoxicity, and radiation-induced cancer.

Although the risks of most currently used tests are small, they nevertheless reduce the benefit of testing and need to be considered. Such 'harms' of testing narrow the range in which the test is useful; the test thresholds move in towards the treatment threshold. Let us suppose there is a 'toll' for testing in

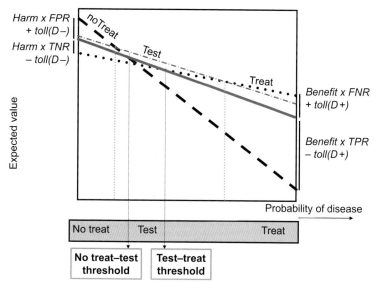

Figure 6.8   Utility graph showing the treat vs. do not treat decision when the test includes a 'toll' (solid line) compared to a toll-free test (dashed line). $D+$, in the presence of disease; $D-$, in the absence of disease; TNR, true-negative ratio; FPR, false-positive ratio; TPR, true-positive ratio; FNR, false-negative ratio. (Not drawn to scale, for illustrative purposes.)

those with disease of $toll_{D+}$, and for testing in those without the disease of $toll_{D-}$. In Figure 6.8 these two tolls lower the intersection of the test line with the right and left axes respectively. Using the same geometric approach as previously we may derive the test threshold with tolls as follows:

$$No\ treat\text{–}test\ threshold = \frac{Harm \times FPR + toll_{D-}}{Harm \times FPR + Benefit \times TPR + toll_{D-} - toll_{D+}}$$

(6.6)

$$Test\text{–}treat\ threshold = \frac{Harm \times TNR - toll_{D-}}{Harm \times TNR + Benefit \times FNR + toll_{D+} - toll_{D-}}$$

(6.7)

These formulae are simpler if the 'tolls' are equal for testing in the diseased and non-diseased groups, as the 'toll' term drops out of the denominator. However, the tolls are often unequal, patients with the disease often being at greater risk of adverse events. For example, when doing a lumbar puncture for suspected meningitis there is a risk of 'coning' in those with meningitis that does not occur in those without meningitis; similarly, endoscopic and angiographic procedures are often more difficult and hence more hazardous in those with the target disease.

Again, these thresholds may be calculated using either a decision tree with a threshold or sensitivity analysis or via these formulae, using for example a spreadsheet. Whichever method is used, it is valuable to obtain the sensitivity graph over the pre-test probability range (Figure 6.8), because this gives a visual representation of where and how the test is useful.

6.5 The expected value of diagnostic information

The test thresholds define when a test is useful, but *how useful* is the test in different parts of this range? Particularly near the test thresholds, the incremental gain from testing may be relatively small. The graphs in the previous section enable us to quantify precisely the value of the test.

6.5.1 Expected value of perfect information

Imagine if we had a perfect and toll-free test. This would enable us to treat all patients with the target disease, and none without. There would be no errors, delays, side effects, or costs! While such tests do not exist, they do give us an upper limit to the potential benefit from any test. The gain from such an imaginary perfect test is the expected value of perfect (diagnostic) information (EVPI).

The EVPI can be read from Figure 6.9a as the distance between the 'test' line and 'do not treat' line for probabilities less than the treatment threshold, and the 'test' line and 'treat' line for probabilities greater than the treatment threshold. The EVPI reaches a maximum at the treatment threshold where we are most uncertain whether to treat or not. As we move away from the treatment threshold, the EVPI diminishes, and it is zero at pre-test probabilities of 0 or 1.

> **DEFINITION** The *expected value of perfect information* (EVPI) in the context of diagnostic testing is the difference between the expected value with a diagnostic test and the expected value without the test when the test reveals the true disease state with certainty and is assumed to have no toll.

6.5.2 Expected value of clinical information

Very few tests in clinical medicine are perfect. For example, the exercise ECG and CTCA in our example both had false-positive and false-negative results. An imperfect test can remove only some of our uncertainty, and hence testing gains only a portion of the EVPI. This lesser value is known as the expected value of (imperfect) clinical information.

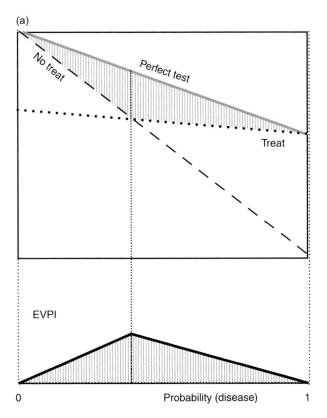

Figure 6.9   Utility graph showing the expected value of (a) perfect information (EVPI)
               obtained with a toll-free diagnostic test that provides perfect information and
               (b) clinical information (EVCI) obtained with a diagnostic test that provides
               imperfect information. If the test line takes into account the toll of the test,
               (*b*) represents the net EVCI. Note that the EVPI and EVCI reach their maximum
               value at the treatment threshold probability of disease.

DEFINITION	The *expected value of clinical information* (EVCI) obtained from a diagnostic test is the difference between the expected value with the test and the expected value without the test, assuming that the test has no toll.

As with the EVPI, the EVCI can be read from Figure 6.9b as the distance
between the 'test' line and the 'do not treat' line for probabilities less than
the treatment threshold, and between the 'test' line and the 'treat' line for
probabilities greater than the treatment threshold. Again, the EVCI reaches
a maximum at the treatment threshold where we are most uncertain
whether to treat or not. As we move away from the treatment threshold,
the EVCI diminishes, and is zero at each of the test thresholds. It is

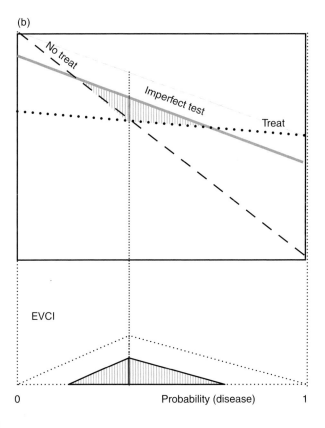

(b)

Figure 6.9 (*cont.*)

negative outside the test thresholds, reminding us that using and selecting treatment based on a test outside the test threshold leads to more harm than good.

Finally, we need to take into account the toll of the test which gives us the net EVCI. Again this can be read from our utility graph if we have plotted the 'test' line taking into account the toll.

DEFINITION	The *net expected value of clinical information* (net EVCI), obtained from a test, is the difference between the expected value with the test and the expected value without the test when the risks of the test itself (the toll) are taken into consideration.

What about the economic costs of the test? We could take the ratio of the financial cost of the test to the net EVCI and obtain an approximate cost-effectiveness ratio. However, this ignores any downstream costs incurred and cost-savings as a consequence of performing the test. For example, if there are further diagnostic testing and treatment costs for the false-positive results, this needs to be incorporated in the economic analysis of the test. Also, if events may occur due to false-negative results, this needs to be included. Without doing this, all we can say is that the cost-effectiveness ratio can only be favorable when the net EVCI is positive and is likely to be best near the treatment threshold. We will deal with cost-effectiveness more thoroughly in Chapter 9.

6.6 Number-needed-to-test

If the scale for the expected value is in natural units, such as events averted, then we can also express the EVCI as its inverse – the number-needed-to-test. This is simply an alternative expression of the same information. For example, for an exercise ECG in patients with stable chest pain, the maximum EVCI at the treatment threshold $(p(CAD) = 0.33)$ is 31 events per 10 000 patients tested, if the test is positive treated, and followed for ten years. For CTCA this is 86 events per 10 000 patients. Inverting the events averted gives a number-needed-to-test of 323 and 116 respectively, that is, we need to test 323 patients with an exercise ECG or 116 patients with CTCA to prevent one event over the course of ten years.

The EVCI (and hence the number-needed-to-test) will vary with the pre-test probability. As we move away from the threshold, the EVCI decreases (and hence the number-needed-to-test increases). The EVCI becomes 0 at both the test thresholds, in which case the number-needed-to-test becomes infinite.

6.7 Summary

Whether or not you explicitly calculate the test thresholds, the important concept in this chapter is that diagnosis is focused around the treatment threshold, and that there is a 'gray zone' around the treatment threshold where testing is worthwhile. There are several different ways of calculating the test thresholds.

Method 1. Use the pre-test post-test graph and the treatment threshold.

Method 2. Draw the decision tree, then analytically or numerically do a threshold analysis or sensitivity analysis on the probability of disease to find the two thresholds. This is the most general method.

Method 3. Use the utility graph, which is useful for visualizing the effects of changes in the parameters. You can add a 'toll' to allow for test morbidity and mortality conditional on whether the patient has the disease or not.

Method 4. Use an extended version of the threshold formula. This can give exact values for the thresholds and be readily incorporated in spreadsheet programs.

Whichever method is used, the central concern is to recognize the existence of the gray zone where testing is useful.

REFERENCES

1. Pauker SG, Kassirer JP. The threshold approach to clinical decision making. *N Engl J Med.* 1980;302(20):1109–17.
2. Genders TS, Steyerberg EW, Hunink MG, et al. Prediction model to estimate presence of coronary artery disease: retrospective pooled analysis of existing cohorts. *BMJ.* 2012;344:e3485.
3. Kwok Y, Kim C, Grady D, Segal M, Redberg R. Meta-analysis of exercise testing to detect coronary artery disease in women. *Am J Cardiol.* 1999;83(5):660–6.
4. Pontone G, Andreini D, Bartorelli AL, et al. Radiation dose and diagnostic accuracy of multidetector computed tomography for the detection of significant coronary artery stenoses: a meta-analysis. *Int J Cardiol.* 2012;160(3):155–64.

Multiple test results

Even though the diagnostic radiologist examines black-and-white images, the
information that is derived from the images is hardly ever black-and-white.

M.G. Myriam Hunink

7.1 Introduction

In the previous chapters we focused on dichotomous test results, e.g., fecal
occult blood is either present or absent. Test results can conveniently be
dichotomized, and thinking in terms of dichotomous test results is generally
helpful. Distinguishing patients with and without the target disease is useful
for the purpose of subsequent decision making because most medical actions
are dichotomous. In reality, however, most test results have more than two
possible outcomes. Test results can be categorical, ordinal, or continuous. For
example, categories of a diagnostic imaging test may be defined by key
findings on the images. These categories may be ordered (intuitively)
according to the observer's confidence in the diagnosis, based on the findings.
As an example, abnormalities seen on mammography are commonly reported
as definitely malignant, probably malignant, possibly malignant, probably
benign, or definitely benign. As we shall see later in this chapter, it makes
sense to order the categories (explicitly) according to increasing likelihood
ratio (LR). Some test results are inherently ordinal, e.g., the five categories of a
Papanicolaou smear (test for cervical cancer) are ordinal. Results of biochem-
ical tests are usually given on a continuous scale, which may be reduced to an
ordinal scale by grouping the test results. Thus, a test result on a continuous
scale can be considered a result on an ordinal scale with an infinite number of
very narrow categories. Scores from prediction models are on an ordinal scale
if there are a finite number of possible scores, and on a continuous scale if
there are an infinite number of scores. When test results are categorical,
ordinal, or continuous, we have to consider many test results R_i, where i
can be any value from two (the case we have considered in Chapter 5 and
Chapter 6, $T+$ and $T-$) up to any number of categories. Interpretation of a
test result on an ordinal scale can be considered a generalization of the
situation of dichotomous test results.

In this chapter, we first generalize the ideas discussed in the context of dichotomous test results and apply them to interpreting diagnostic test information from tests with multiple results. We then discuss the trade-off between true-positive and false-positive ratios. We show the relationship between diagnostic and prognostic information. Subsequently, we extend the ideas to combining multiple results from multiple tests. Summary indices for comparing tests and the choice of an optimal positivity criterion for proceeding to a treatment decision are discussed. Finally, we address the incremental value of new tests and other issues that are important in evaluating and interpreting multiple test results. The discussion will focus on the clinical example introduced in Chapter 6.

Example from Chapter 6 continued: suspected coronary artery disease (CAD)

Our 55-year-old female patient requests a minimally invasive test. She would prefer not having contrast injected and avoiding radiation as much as possible. Performing a plain CT to identify coronary artery calcification (CAC) has been suggested as a triage test. It requires no contrast and is associated with very little radiation (<1 mSv). The presence of calcification is associated with the presence of plaque, indicating CAD. The degree of CAC is generally measured with the Agatston score. The more calcification, the higher the CAC score, the more likely there is disease.

We start by addressing the following question: if we decide to perform the test, how do we combine the pre-test probability with the CAC score?

7.2 Post-test probabilities using multicategory test results

In Chapter 5 we encountered the odds-likelihood ratio version of Bayes' formula. We also saw that Bayes' formula can be generalized from the case of a dichotomous test $(T+, T-)$ to any type of test result (R). This yielded the following generalized formulation of Bayes' formula, in odds-likelihood ratio format:

$$\frac{p(D+\mid R)}{p(D-\mid R)} = \frac{p(D+)}{p(D-)}\frac{p(R\mid D+)}{p(R\mid D-)} \tag{7.1}$$

This formula, which relates the posterior odds of disease to the prior odds of disease, holds whether R is a result from a two-category or multicategory test. For a dichotomous test result, we replace R with either $R + $ or $R -$. For a test with multicategory results $i = 1 \ldots I$, R becomes R_i. For a continuous test, we simply let R be a representative result from among the (possibly infinite) set of possible results $\{\mathbf{R}\}$.

The above expression can also be written as:

Post-test odds = pre-test odds x likelihood ratio of result R (7.2)

Expressed in plain English, this means that the information after doing the test (post-test odds) equals the information before doing the test (pre-test odds) combined with the information obtained from the test (LR). We will apply this generalized formulation of Bayes' formula to our clinical example of the *CAC score*.

7.2.1 Pre-test probability

To determine the potential value of performing a CT and measuring the *CAC score* in this setting, you need to consider the pre-test probability of CAD and the *LRs* of the possible test results. To estimate the pre-test probability of CAD we would ideally like to have information from a setting-specific database that contains information about patients with similar clinical characteristics, i.e., age, sex, type of chest pain, cardiovascular risk factors, and prior history. Rarely do we have such a database available.

The next best would be to search for this information in the literature. For example, we could look for a clinical algorithm, a clinical prediction rule, or a meta-analysis estimate of the probability of CAD (1–3). Our choice of reference depends on which described patient population is the most representative of the patient in front of us, and which study we think provides the best available evidence for the problem (Chapter 8). For example, the Diagnostic Imaging for Coronary Artery Disease (DICAD) consortium demonstrated that the Diamond and Forrester algorithm and the Duke clinical score both overestimate the probability of CAD, especially in women. Subsequently, the consortium developed a new prediction rule which was then cross-validated (2). Using their web-based risk calculator, the prior probability of CAD in our patient is 19% based on age, gender, and the type of chest pain ('typical' in the example) and 11% if we also take into account that she has no risk factors.

7.2.2 Likelihood ratios of the test categories

To decide whether a CT *CAC score* could provide useful information we need to know how good this test is in distinguishing patients with CAD from patients without CAD. The diagnostic performance of the *CAC score* was evaluated by the DICAD consortium (2) and the results are presented in

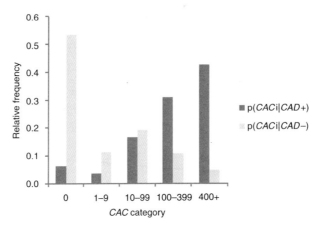

Figure 7.1   Histogram of the DICAD consortium data (2).

Figure 7.1. For illustrative purposes, we have divided the *CAC score* into five categories. The heights of the dark bars (Figure 7.1) represent the frequency distribution of the *CAC* results among patients who *have CAD*. These five proportions sum to 100%. The heights of the light bars represent the frequency distribution of the *CAC* results among patients who *do not have CAD*. These five proportions also sum to 100%.

It is evident from the figure that the *ratio* of the frequency of a particular test result among patients with CAD to the frequency among patients without CAD steadily increases as we move to higher *CAC scores*. This relative frequency, the ratio of the heights of the bars, is the *LR* for each of the five test results. Using the tabulated information (Table 7.1) we can calculate the *LRs* for each of the *CAC* categories. For example, the frequency of a *CAC score* = 10–99 equals 235/1406 = 0.167 among patients with CAD, and 667/3456 = 0.193 among patients without CAD. Hence, the *LR* for the 10 to 99 category equals 0.167/0.193 = 0.866.

If you recall the lessons from Chapter 5, you might be asking whether these *LRs* would apply to a population in which the prior probability of CAD is different from that in the DICAD study. That would be a good question: but the answer is generally that they would apply. Like the sensitivity and specificity of a test, it is generally reasonable to assume that the distribution of test results conditional upon disease status does *not* depend on the prevalence of disease. In fact, because of the conditionality, the true- and false-positive ratios and the *LRs* do not depend on the prevalence of disease. Sometimes, however, both the observed prevalence and the distribution of test results are influenced by underlying variables, in epidemiological terms confounders. For example, the observed prevalence of CAD will depend on the detectability of

Table 7.1 Data on the *CAC score* measured on a plain CT scan in suspected coronary artery disease (CAD)

CAC score	CAD+	CAD−	p(CAC_i|CAD+)	p(CAC_i|CAD−)	LR
0	87	1844	0.062	0.534	0.116
1–9	50	395	0.036	0.114	0.311
10–99	235	667	0.167	0.193	0.866
100–399	436	378	0.310	0.109	2.835
400+	598	172	0.425	0.050	8.546
	1406	3456			

Data from the DICAD consortium (2)

CAC: coronary artery calcification

coronary artery obstructive lesions. The distribution of test results (such as the CT *CAC score*) conditional on disease status, including sensitivity and specificity, may then appear to depend on prevalence but in fact it depends on the location, extent, and disease severity in the examined patient population. These factors may influence both the observed prevalence and test characteristics. Such situations are best handled with multivariate prediction rules, discussed later in this chapter.

7.2.3 Post-test probability

Using the *LR*s corresponding to each specific category, we can calculate the post-test probability of disease conditional on the pre-test probability of CAD and the test result. Thus, given a pre-test probability of 11% and $CAC = 1$–9 result, the post-test probability equals 3.7%. This is obtained from Equation 7.1 as follows. First we convert the pre-test probability of 0.11 to a pre-test odds of $0.11/0.89 = 0.124$. We multiply this prior odds by the *LR* for the $CAC = 1$–9 result ($LR = 0.311$) to obtain the post-test odds of $0.124 \cdot 0.311 = 0.0385$. Finally, we convert this odds back to a probability and obtain the post-test probability $0.0385/(1 + 0.0385) = 0.037$. We can repeat this exercise for varying pre-test probabilities and different *LR*s. (The supplementary material on the book website illustrates these calculations.)

Figure 7.2 presents the relationship between the post-test probability of disease and the pre-test probability of disease for the five different *CAC* categories. As expected, the graph for the $CAC = 10$–99 category is close to the diagonal. Why do we expect this? Notice that if the *LR* for a test result

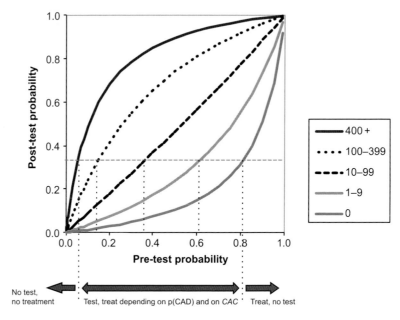

Figure 7.2   The post-test probability of disease as a function of the pre-test probability of disease for the five possible categories of the *CAC score*. The treat–no treat threshold of 33% obtained in Chapter 6 (Eq. 6.2) is indicated by the horizontal dashed line.

equals 1.0 (i.e., it is equally frequent among diseased and non-diseased patients), then the posterior odds equals the prior odds. The test result contributes no information in that case, and the relationship in Figure 7.2 would be a diagonal line. For the $CAC = 10$–99 category in Figure 7.2, the curve is slightly lower than the diagonal, because the LR is slightly less than 1.0, namely 0.866. Hence the post-test probability is little different from the pre-test probability. The graphs for the $CAC = 400+$ and $CAC = 100$–399 results lie to the upper left because of their high LRs (8.546 and 2.835, respectively), and the graphs for the $CAC = 0$ and $CAC = 1$–9 results lie to the lower right because of their low LRs (0.116 and 0.311, respectively). For very low pre-test probabilities, the post-test probability is also low, irrespective of the test result. Similarly, for very high pre-test probabilities, the post-test probability is also high, irrespective of the test result.

Performing a test is, in general, most useful in the gray zone where one is uncertain of the presence or absence of disease. For example, if the pre-test probability of disease is somewhere between, say, 10% and 80%, we would probably be ambivalent about the best management strategy. In such situations the test can have a large impact on the estimated probability of disease. For our patient, with an estimated pre-test probability of 11%, the post-test probability ranges from 1.4% if the $CAC = 0$ to 51% if the $CAC = 400$ or higher.

As we saw in Chapter 6, for a dichotomous test the usefulness of a test in a specific setting is determined by the effect it has on the decision to treat or not. Even if a test result induces a big change in the probability of disease, it is not going to change a decision unless the post-test and pre-test probabilities are on opposite sides of some decision threshold. In our patient, the decision is whether or not to initiate medical therapy for cardiovascular disease. In Chapter 6 we estimated that the threshold probability of disease for treating the patient is 33%. Then by superimposing the treat–no treat threshold probability of disease on the vertical-axis of the graph (Figure 7.2), we can determine how this threshold cuts the pre-test probability into different regions:

- Pre-test probability less than 0.055: don't perform the CT, don't treat.
- Pre-test probability between 0.055 and 0.15: perform the CT and treat if the *CAC score* is 400 or higher.
- Pre-test probability between 0.15 and 0.37: perform the CT and treat if the *CAC score* is 100 or higher.
- Pre-test probability between 0.37 and 0.62: perform the CT and treat if the *CAC score* is 10 or higher.
- Pre-test probability between 0.62 and 0.81: perform the CT and treat if the *CAC score* is 1 or higher.
- Pre-test probability more than 0.81: treat, don't perform the CT.

These pre-test probability thresholds can be calculated by recognizing that the thresholds of interest represent the points where the posterior probability equals the treat–no treat threshold. Thus, at these thresholds p_i the posterior odds (which is the prior odds · likelihood ratio LR_i, according to Bayesian revision) equals the harm/benefit ratio, expressed in an equation:

$$posterior\ odds = \frac{p_i}{1 - p_i} \cdot LR_i = \frac{harm}{benefit} \tag{7.3}$$

$$p_i = \frac{harm}{harm + benefit \cdot LR_i} \tag{7.4}$$

Thus, in this particular setting, the *CAC score* measured on CT is valuable for pre-test probabilities between 0.055 and 0.81, and it has no decisional value if the pre-test probability is outside this range. Inside this range, its expected value of clinical information (EVCI) for the *CAC score* is greater than zero; outside this range, it has no value in decision making.

7.3 Trade-offs between true-positive and false-positive ratios

Tests with continuous or ordinal multiple results typically have two features: (1) a measurable *test variable*, i.e., a measurable property on a categorical, ordinal, or continuous scale that relates to a particular disease, and (2) a *positivity criterion*, which is a particular value of the measured variable that distinguishes patients with the target disease from those without the target disease. If we are interested in hypertension, for example, one possible variable would be the average diastolic blood pressure at three successive readings, and we might choose as our positivity criterion a diastolic blood pressure of 90 mmHg. In the diagnosis of tuberculosis, the variable might be the size (in mm) of the indurated papule induced by injection of a small quantity of antigen into the skin, and the positivity criterion might be a particular size, e.g., 10 mm.

Biologic variables often show a substantial spread in values for populations with and without the target disease. Furthermore, the values in the two groups usually overlap. This overlap makes it impossible to define a positivity criterion that distinguishes perfectly all those with a disease from all those without it. Most clinical tests share this imperfection, but it does not render them useless. Our task is to discover the positivity criterion that makes the best possible separation of those in the population who have the target disease from those who do not have it. Although in reality we commonly have to deal with a variety of diseases and varying degrees of severity of disease, it is useful to dichotomize a continuous test variable into 'positive' and 'negative' regions. This is because most medical action is dichotomous: we decide to operate or not to operate, to initiate treatment or not to initiate it. Even if more than two actions are possible, the problem can generally be redefined as a staged process consisting of successive dichotomous actions. As we shall see later in this chapter, the choice of an optimal positivity criterion depends on the context in which the test is to be used to reach a clinical decision.

For example, we need to decide whether to initiate medical therapy in our 55-year-old female patient with suspected CAD based on the *CAC* result. In this situation we would prefer to avoid further testing because of the patient's explicit preference. Which patients in this situation would you treat? Only those with a *CAC* of 400 or higher? Or would you also treat those with a *CAC score* of 100? In other words, where would we draw our threshold for the choice between treating vs. not treating the patient? First, we need to know how changing the threshold influences the test characteristics, i.e., the true-positive and false-positive ratios.

7.3.1 Graphical representation of the trade-off: ROC curves

Consider the data presented in Table 7.1 and as a histogram in Figure 7.1. If we choose to set the threshold at a value of 400, for example, we would correctly decide to treat 598 patients with CAD (true-positives) but at the same time incorrectly withhold treatment from 808 ($= 87 + 50 + 235 + 436$)

Table 7.2 Data on the *CAC score* measured on CT for suspected coronary artery disease (CAD): calculating cumulative true-positive and false-positive ratios from the absolute numbers, going from a strict criterion to more-and-more lenient criteria (2)

CAC scores considered positive	CAD+	CAD−	True-positive	False-positive
None	0	0	0	0
≥ 400	598	172	0.43	0.05
≥ 100	598 + 436	172 + 378	0.74	0.16
≥ 10	598 + 436 + 235	172 + 378 + 667	0.90	0.35
≥ 1	598 + 436 + 235 + 50	172 + 378 + 667 + 395	0.94	0.47
All	598 + 436 + 235 + 50 + 87	172 + 378 + 667 + 395 + 1844	1.00	1.00
Total	1406	3456		

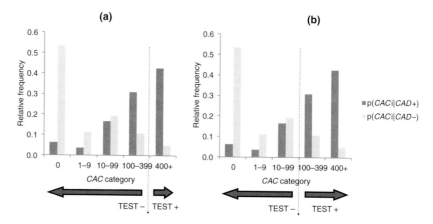

Figure 7.3   Varying the positivity criterium of the *CAC score* for making the diagnosis of CAD and treating accordingly.

patients with CAD (false-negatives) (Figure 7.3A; Table 7.2). If we relax the positivity criterion (i.e., move it up in the table or to the left in the histogram; Figure 7.3B; Table 7.2), we will increase the fraction of patients with CAD who are correctly identified as such (true-positive results). Alas, at the same time we will also increase the number of subjects without CAD who are incorrectly labeled as having the disease (false-positive results). If we tighten the positivity criterion (move the threshold up in the table or to the right in the histogram), the proportion of patients without CAD whose test results are positive will decrease (false-positive results). But, we will also

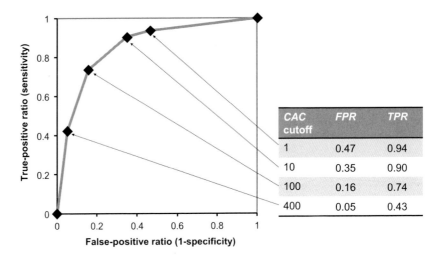

CAC cutoff	FPR	TPR
1	0.47	0.94
10	0.35	0.90
100	0.16	0.74
400	0.05	0.43

Figure 7.4   Receiver operating characteristic (ROC) curve for the *CAC score*.

decrease the proportion of patients with CAD whose positive test results correctly identify the disease (true-positives). Moving the positivity criterion thus entails a trade-off between true-positive and false-positive ratios (Table 7.2). A receiver operating characteristic (ROC) curve demonstrates these trade-offs graphically (Figure 7.4).

An ROC curve thereby evaluates overall test performance independently of the ultimately chosen decision criterion. The points (0,0) and (1,1) are inherent to all ROC curves. The point (0,0) represents the most stringent possible positivity criterion: no patients in any of the test categories are labeled as having the target disease. The point (1,1) represents the most lenient positivity criterion: all patients are labeled as having the target disease. Points on the curve closer to the lower-left corner (Figure 7.4) represent situations in which strict criteria (cutoff at a high *CAC score*) are used to make the diagnosis. In that part of the curve there will be few false-positive test results (low false-positive ratio) but at the expense of missing the diagnosis in a considerable number of patients (low true-positive ratio). Points on the curve closer to the upper right-hand corner represent situations in which lenient criteria (cutoff at a low *CAC score*) are used to make the diagnosis. In that part of the curve many patients are identified as having the target disease (high true-positive ratio), but many non-diseased subjects are also labeled as having the target disease (high false-positive ratio).

DEFINITION   A *receiver operating characteristic (ROC) curve* is a plot of all pairs of possible combinations of true-positive and false-positive ratios achievable with a test as the positivity criterion is varied.

If the diagnostic test has results with numerical values, such as with the *CAC score*, the positivity criterion will be a particular value, above which (or below which, depending on the test) a test will be called positive or negative. With diagnostic imaging this is only possible if some biomarker can be measured. Sometimes no numerical value indicating the presence or absence of disease is produced but instead specific characteristics on the image, such as an ill-defined nodule and microcalcifications on a mammogram, can be used to categorize the results. Alternatively, the reader of the image can (and in the clinical routine usually does) express his or her confidence in the diagnosis based on various criteria.

ROC analysis (in the past also known as relative operating characteristic analysis) was developed by signal detection theorists who needed to distinguish signal from noise, for example in analyzing radar data. The technique is also used in psychology, polygraph lie detection, and weather forecasting. Since the 1970s the technique has been applied to diagnostic tests in medicine.

7.3.2 Likelihood ratios and the ROC curve

In using the term 'likelihood ratio' one needs to distinguish the result-specific *LR* from the cumulative *LR* of a dichotomized test result. For the *CAC*, Table 7.1 shows the result-specific *LRs* for each of the five possible results. Once a positivity criterion has been selected (such as $CAC \geq 100$), a cumulative *LR* can be defined for the group of 'positive' results ($CAC \geq 100$) and for the group of 'negative' results ($CAC < 100$). These cumulative *LRs* are, however, less relevant in the context of multiple test results.

DEFINITION The *result-specific likelihood ratio* for a particular test result is the ratio of the probability of observing that result conditional on the presence of the target disease, to the probability of observing that result conditional on the absence of the target disease. When the results are grouped into categories, we refer to this quantity as the *category-specific likelihood ratio*.

The result-specific likelihood ratio is generally implied when using the term 'likelihood ratio.' It is the most useful ratio because it contains the most information. In probability notation, the result-specific (or category-specific) likelihood ratio (LR_i) of the test result R_i is:

$$LR_i = \frac{p(R_i \mid D+)}{p(R_i \mid D-)} \tag{7.5}$$

where $p(R_i \mid D+)$ is the probability of the test result R_i given presence of the target disease, and $p(R_i \mid D-)$ is the probability of the test result R_i given

Table 7.3 Data on the *CAC score* measured on CT for suspected coronary artery disease (CAD): calculating cumulative true-positive and false-positive ratios based on the category-specific conditional probabilities, going from a strict criterion to more-and-more lenient criteria (3)

CAC scores considered positive	CAD+	CAD−	True-positive	False-positive
None	0	0	0	0
≥ 400	0.425	0.050	0.43	0.05
≥ 100	0.425 + 0.310	0.050 + 0.109	0.74	0.16
≥ 10	0.425 + 0.310 + 0.167	0.050 + 0.109 + 0.193	0.90	0.35
≥ 1	0.425 + 0.310 + 0.167 + 0.036	0.050 + 0.109 + 0.193 + 0.114	0.94	0.47
All	0.425 + 0.310 + 0.167 + 0.036 + 0.062	0.050 + 0.109 + 0.193 + 0.114 + 0.534	1.00	1.00

absence of the target disease. Note that for dichotomous test results the above equation is equivalent to the ratio introduced in Chapter 5.

Notice that we can generate the operating points on the ROC curve by starting at the origin (0,0), and then, beginning with the category-specific probabilities of the high *CAC* result, adding one-by-one the category-specific conditional probabilities (Table 7.3) to the cumulative true-positive and false-positive ratios. Going from one (strict) operating point to the next (less strict) point, we add the category-specific probability given disease to the cumulative true-positive ratio (the vertical-axis in ROC space), and we simultaneously add the category-specific probability given no disease to the cumulative false-positive ratio (the horizontal-axis in ROC space). Thus, the slope of the line joining two operating points of the ROC curve is equivalent to the ratio of the category-specific probabilities given disease and given no disease, which, as we defined above, equals the category-specific *LR*. Using strict positivity criteria in the left-lower corner, the slope of the ROC curve (and the corresponding category-specific *LR*) is high. Walking up the ROC curve the slope of the curve, and the category-specific *LR*, decrease (Figure 7.5*a*). For continuous data the categories are infinitesimally small and the *LR* equals the tangent of the curve (Figure 7.5*b*).

7.3.3 Likelihood ratios and uninterpretable test results

The fact that the slope of the ROC curve, and the category-specific *LR*, decrease as we go from strict to lenient criteria can be helpful in determining

7.3 Trade-offs between true- and false-positive ratios

Table 7.4 Ultrasound for appendiceal disease

Ultrasound result (US$_i$)	AppDis +	AppDis −	p(US$_i$/ AppDis +)	p(US$_i$/ AppDis −)	LR
Positive	39	0	0.75	0.00	Infinity
Dubious	3	3	0.06	0.10	0.60
Appendix not visualized	10	28	0.19	0.90	0.21

AppDis, appendiceal disease; US, ultrasound; US$_i$, specific ultrasound findings as indicated by row: positive, dubious, or appendix not visualized; LR, likelihood ratio. Modified from (4).

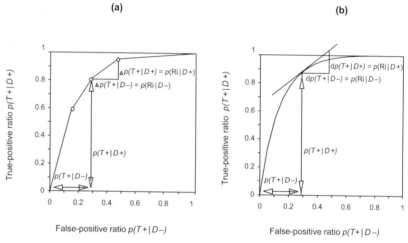

Figure 7.5 Likelihood ratios and the receiver operating characteristic curve (*a*) for categorical data and (*b*) for continuous data.

the value of uninterpretable test results. If uninterpretability is unrelated to the presence or absence of the target disease, we would expect to find an equivalent proportion of uninterpretable test results among those with and without the disease, i.e., the *LR* would equal one, and the uninterpretable test result would convey no meaningful information. If, on the other hand, uninterpretable test results are seen relatively more often in patients without the target disease than in those with the disease, then an uninterpretable result would contain information (low *LR*) and would reduce the probability of disease. This was the case in a study evaluating the use of ultrasound in the diagnosis of appendicitis (Table 7.4; (4)), in which a low *LR* was found for appendices not visualized with ultrasound. Pathophysiologically, the findings can be explained in that a normal appendix is not swollen and thus about 2–5 mm in diameter, which can be very difficult to identify among the bowel loops using ultrasound.

7.4 Diagnostic prediction vs. prognostic prediction

In diagnosis the goal is to predict current ('prevalent') disease, that is, to determine the probability that the target condition is present. The index test result and true disease status are determined at the same point in time, or within a reasonable time window during which neither remission nor progression can take place. The reference standard is defined as the underlying diagnostic truth within that time window. Sometimes follow up is used as part of the reference standard test and as a proxy for what was the diagnostic truth at the time the index test was performed. For example, a thromboembolic event during three-month follow up after an initial suspected thromboembolic event may be considered a sign that disease was present at baseline.

In prognosis events that may or may not happen during follow-up are the focus of attention. The time to a possible event in the future is explicitly taken into account in modeling prognosis. Both the future event and the time-to-event are considered in the outcome (5).

Diagnosis and prognosis are closely related. The aim of diagnosis is to classify patients into meaningful categories that are relevant to therapeutic and preventive decision making. Diagnostic classification should reflect differences in subsequent management which logically depends on prognosis. Thus, diagnostic categories should be chosen to reflect differences in prognosis in order to be meaningful for decision making.

Many methods are common to both modeling diagnosis and modeling prognosis. The concepts discussed above apply to both, as do the methods for combining multiple test results and the summary indices below. The only real difference is that in prognostic prediction models the time-to-event is taken into account whereas in diagnostic prediction this is irrelevant. In practice this implies that diagnostic prediction is commonly performed with logistic regression whereas prognostic prediction of longer term outcome is usually done with Cox proportional hazards models.

In keeping with this generalization, we use the term 'disease' ($D+$) to mean either patients with prevalent disease in the context of diagnosis or patients with an incident event in the context of prognosis, and the term 'non-disease' ($D-$) to mean absence of disease or no event.

7.5 Combining results from multiple tests

In many decision-making situations, it is possible to obtain more than a single test. In using the tests to make treatment decisions, the results from multiple tests are combined. Clinical information, such as age, gender, symptoms, risk factors can be considered 'test results' which need to be integrated with lab results and imaging findings. Decisions must be made about which tests to perform, in what sequence to perform them with each test decision contingent on the results of previous tests, and how to treat based on the composite information from all the chosen tests. Here we focus on the task of estimating the post-test probabilities of the disease of interest, in the presence of multiple test data. The choice of sequential testing strategies is best handled with decision trees, although the probabilities required in the trees will be obtained using the methods described here.

Each test may yield dichotomous results, or results in multiple categories, or results along a continuum. Consider, for example, two tests that can be used in evaluating CAD: a clinical 'test result' from the history, namely the type of chest pain (*CP*: typical, atypical, or non-specific) and the CT coronary artery calcification score (*CAC score*: ranging from 0 to well over 400 and here divided into five commonly used categories). Table 7.5 presents the DICAD data on these two tests. The categories typical, atypical, and non-specific have been ordered according to decreasing *LR*. Note, however, that the data show that atypical and non-specific chest pain have more or less equal *LRs*, implying that these categories could alternatively have been combined into one category. The generalized form of Bayes' formula still applies, but now instead of a single result R we have the combination of results from multiple (in this example, two) tests. In our example, each combination of the two tests may be denoted as $R = (CP, CAC)$. Combining the results from these two tests yields the following formulation of Bayes' formula:

$$\frac{p(CAD+ \mid CP, CAC)}{p(CAD- \mid CP, CAC)} = \frac{p(CAD+)}{p(CAD-)} \cdot \frac{p(CP, CAC \mid CAD+)}{p(CP, CAC \mid CAD-)} \quad (7.6)$$

7.5.1 Conditional dependence and independence of multiple tests

Combining the results of the *CP* and *CAC* requires information of the test characteristics p(*CP*, *CAC* | *CAD*+) and p(*CP*, *CAC* | *CAD*−) for each possible combination of the test results, i.e., the joint distribution of the test results conditional on disease status.

Often it is not possible to find data on the joint distribution of two or more tests conditional upon the disease we are interested in. If we have the test

Table 7.5 Observed data of the tests CP (type of chest pain) and CAC (coronary artery calcification score). The likelihood ratios for the combination test have been calculated from the actual observed data (LR(obs)) of the combined results and from the likelihood ratios of the individual test results combined, assuming conditional independence ($LR_{CP}*LR_{CAC}$). Data from (2)

CP	CAC	CAD+	CAD−	p(R/CAD+)	p(R/CAD−)	LR(obs)	$LR_{CP} \cdot LR_{CAC}$
Typical		652	485	0.464	0.140	3.30	
Non-specific		205	801	0.146	0.232	0.63	
Atypical		549	2170	0.390	0.628	0.62	
	400+	598	172	0.425	0.050	8.55	
	100–399	436	378	0.310	0.109	2.84	
	10–99	235	667	0.167	0.193	0.87	
	1–9	50	395	0.036	0.114	0.31	
	0	87	1844	0.062	0.534	0.12	
Typical	400+	306	33	0.218	0.010	22.79	28.24
Typical	100–399	191	58	0.136	0.017	8.09	9.37
Typical	10–99	109	106	0.078	0.031	2.53	2.86
Typical	1–9	18	53	0.013	0.015	0.83	1.03
Typical	0	28	235	0.020	0.068	0.29	0.38
Non-specific	400+	96	54	0.068	0.016	4.37	5.38
Non-specific	100–399	72	102	0.051	0.030	1.74	1.78
Non-specific	10–99	17	153	0.012	0.044	0.27	0.54
Non-specific	1–9	6	87	0.004	0.025	0.17	0.20
Non-specific	0	14	405	0.010	0.117	0.08	0.07
Atypical	400+	196	85	0.139	0.025	5.67	5.31
Atypical	100–399	173	218	0.123	0.063	1.95	1.76
Atypical	10–99	109	408	0.078	0.118	0.66	0.54
Atypical	1–9	26	255	0.018	0.074	0.25	0.19
Atypical	0	45	1204	0.032	0.348	0.09	0.07

CP, type of chest pain: the categories typical, atypical, and non-specific have been ordered according to decreasing LR; the data show that atypical and non-specific chest pain have more or less equal LRs, implying that these categories could alternatively have been combined into one category. CAC, coronary artery calcification on CT; CAD, coronary artery disease; R_i, category-specific test result, with i the category number; LR_{obs}, likelihood ratio based on the observed results of the combined tests CP and CAC; $LR_{CP} \cdot LR_{CAC}$, product of the likelihood ratios of CP and CAC category, i.e., assuming conditional independence; data from (2).

characteristics per test separately (e.g., from different studies), it would be helpful to be able to derive the joint distributions conditional on disease status from the individual test distributions.

Suppose that the two tests were *independent*, conditionally upon the presence or absence of disease. Recall that two events E and F are independent if their joint probability equals the product of their individual probabilities: p $(E, F) = p(E) \cdot p(F)$. But in the setting of testing, the relevant probabilities of test results are conditional upon disease status, $D+$ or $D-$. Independence conditional upon a common third event, such as the presence of a disease, is called *conditional independence*.

DEFINITION

Two tests, T and U, are said to be *conditionally independent, given disease status D* if, for all possible pairs of results (T, U):

$$p(T, U \mid D) = p(T \mid D) \cdot p(U \mid D) \qquad (7.7)$$

Note that the qualifier 'given disease status D' is part of the definition of conditional independence. It is possible that two tests are conditionally independent given disease status $D+$, but conditionally *dependent* given $D-$, or vice versa.

Also take heed that two tests which are conditionally independent given $D+$ and $D-$ are not usually *unconditionally* independent. If both tests are associated with the presence or absence of disease D, then they will generally be dependent, through the association with D. In other words, if tests T and U are both good tests for D, a highly positive result on T will tend to be associated with a positive result on U, because D is more likely to be present. As the following example illustrates, this can happen even if the tests are conditionally independent.

If we are able to assume conditional independence of the test results given disease status, then the post-test odds of disease for the combination of CP and CAC becomes:

$$\frac{p(CAD+ \mid CP, CAC)}{p(CAD- \mid CP, CAC)} = \frac{p(CAD+)}{p(CAD-)} \cdot \frac{p(CP \mid CAD+)}{p(CP \mid CAD-)} \cdot \frac{p(CAC \mid CAD+)}{p(CAC \mid CAD-)} \qquad (7.8)$$

Post-test odds = pre-test odds $\cdot LR_{CP} \cdot LR_{CAC}$ $\qquad (7.9)$

Note that this equation assumes conditional independence of CP and CAC results in the presence of CAD and conditional independence of CP and CAC results in the absence of CAD. If conditional independence holds in both disease statuses, then the LRs for the combined results equal the products of the LRs for the individual results.

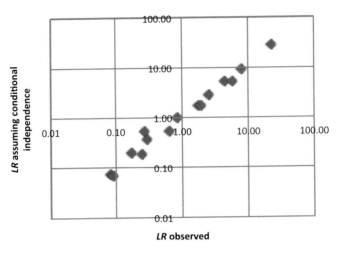

Figure 7.6

Relationship between the *LR*s calculated from the actual observed data on the combination results and the *LR*s calculated from the individual test results when combined assuming conditional independence, plotted on a logarithmic scale. The results confirm that assuming conditional independence is justified in this particular example.

The data collected by the DICAD consortium give us the opportunity to test the conditional independence assumption for the *CP* and the *CAC* category for the diagnosis of CAD. Table 7.5 presents the *LR*s calculated from the actual observed data on the combination results and the *LR*s calculated from the individual test results when combined, assuming conditional independence, and Figure 7.6 presents the relationship between the two *LR*s on a logarithmic scale. The results demonstrate that the two sets of *LR*s are very similar, indicating that assuming conditional independence is justified in this particular example. Often we will find that the *LR*s from the observed data are generally closer to 1.0 than the *LR*s calculated from the marginal probabilities of each test assuming conditional independence, in which case the assumption of conditional independence is not fully correct. In such cases the actual combination categories contain slightly less information than we would expect based on the conditional independence assumption. If we need to use the conditional independence assumption in order to synthesize information from disparate sources, we may therefore overestimate the true value of the combination of tests. More often than not, we will be unable to check empirically whether the conditional independence assumption holds, in which case we need to decide on pathophysiological grounds and our knowledge of the tests whether the assumption is justified.

The combination test categories are by definition categorical and not ordinal. There is no inherent ordering of combinations of test results if

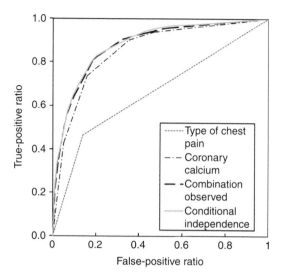

Figure 7.7   ROC curves of the clinical information 'type of chest pain' (*CP*), the coronary artery calcification (*CAC*) measured on *CT*, the combination of the two using the actual observed data on the combination results and the combination assuming conditional independence. The results confirm that assuming conditional independence produces the same ROC curve as the observed data in this particular example.

ordered by their category names as done in Table 7.5. To order the combinations of test results correctly we have to refer to their composite LRs. If we order the combination categories according to decreasing *LR*, i.e., by the information contained in the combination result, we can then construct a ROC curve for the combination test (Figure 7.7). (See the supplementary material 'CAD example ROC curves.xlsx' on the book website for the calculations and for assignments.)

7.5.2 Multivariable Bayes' and multivariable prediction models

If instead of one test we have multiple tests, Bayes' formula applies in a generalized formulation. In the multivariable case, the test result R becomes a set of variables $X = (X_1, X_2, X_3, X_4 \dots X_i \dots)$ with each X_i being either a dichotomous or multicategory variable and i indicating the category number. The set of variables X may be a combination of clinical variables, genetic information, diagnostic test variables, imaging biomarkers, and even response variables to previous treatment. The variables (or covariates) are combined with regression coefficients using logistic regression analysis to derive a score, which may be considered the diagnostic test variable of the combination test. For example, for the CAD example:

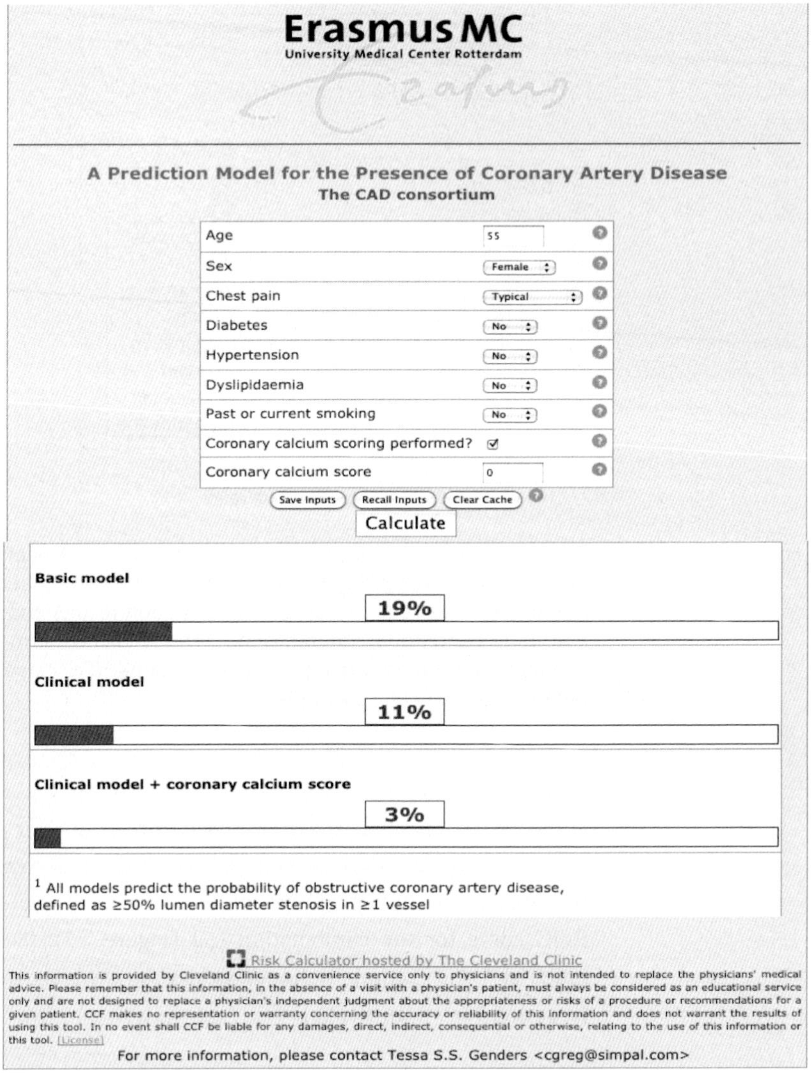

Figure 7.8

Web-based risk calculator for the probability of CAD depending on age, gender, type of chest pain (basic model); including diabetes, hypertension, dyslipidemia, smoking (clinical model); and including the coronary artery calcification score (clinical model + coronary calcium score) (2).

$$Score = \beta_0 + \beta_1 \cdot age + \beta_2 \cdot gender + \beta_3 \cdot typical\ CP + \ldots + \beta_i \cdot CAC$$

$$(7.10)$$

The DICAD risk calculator referred to at the beginning of the chapter is such a prediction rule which combines age, gender, type of chest pain, CVD risk factors, and the coronary artery calcification score (2) (Figure 7.8).

Logistic regression analysis in this context has favorable properties and has been used to derive diagnostic prediction models for various combination tests. The probability of disease given the set of variables (or vector) X can be expressed as:

$$p(D+\,|\,X) = \frac{1}{1 + e^{-score}} \qquad (7.11)$$

The post-test odds of disease given the set of variables X can be expressed as:

$$\frac{p(D+\,|\,X)}{1-p(D+\,|\,X)} = e^{score} = e^{\beta_0 + \beta_1 \cdot X_1 + \beta_2 \cdot X_2 + \beta_3 \cdot X_3 + \ldots + \beta_i \cdot X_i + \ldots} \qquad (7.12)$$

Substituting $e^{\beta_0} = p(D+)/(1-p(D+))$ the above expression can also be written as:

$$\frac{p(D+\,|\,X)}{1-p(D+\,|\,X)} = \frac{p(D+)}{1-p(D+)} \cdot e^{\beta_1 \cdot X_1 + \beta_2 \cdot X_2 + \beta_3 \cdot X_3 + \ldots + \beta_i \cdot X_i + \ldots} \qquad (7.13)$$

in which case $p(D+)$ is the pre-test probability of disease in the reference group. The above expression emphasizes that prediction rules based on the combination of test results are an extension from the univariable formulation of Bayes' formula to a multivariable formulation, i.e.:

$$\textit{Post-test odds} = \textit{Pre-test odds} \cdot LR_X \qquad (7.14)$$

where LR_X is the likelihood ratio of the set of variables (vector) X. If the variables are conditionally independent, LR_X is the product of the individual LR_is of each variable:

$$LR_X = e^{\beta_1 \cdot X_1 + \beta_2 \cdot X_2 + \beta_3 \cdot X_3 + \ldots + \beta_i \cdot X_i + \ldots} = \prod_i LR_i \qquad (7.15)$$

In this formulation X is expressed in comparison to the reference group and the pre-test odds is the odds in the reference group. Conceptually it is easiest to think of the reference group as individuals without the risk factor, in which case the pre-test odds is low in the reference group. The odds ratio (OR) for each group equals the LR in the group with the variable present ($X_i = 1$, $T+$) divided by the LR in the reference group without the variable ($X_i = 0$, $T-$). The OR in the logistic regression analysis is in fact the diagnostic odds ratio:

$$DOR = \frac{LR_{T+}}{LR_{T-}} = \frac{TPR \cdot TNR}{FPR \cdot FNR} = \frac{TP \cdot TN}{FP \cdot FN} \qquad (7.16)$$

Alternatively, the equations may be expressed in comparison to a reference group consisting of individuals with mean values on all variables and the pre-test odds being the odds in this group of hypothetical individuals, which is estimated with the prevalence in the entire group.

If the test variables are conditionally independent, then the LR_X can be derived from studies evaluating each test individually and multiplying the LRs. To account for conditional dependence requires data from a group of patients among whom all the test variables are known. Such a dataset allows for derivation of the LRs adjusted for the effect of other variables. In some situations one may want to combine information on the conditional dependence from one multivariable data set with estimates of more accurate univariable LRs of each of the individual tests from the literature. This can be achieved by adjusting the combined univariable LRs obtained from the literature $(LR_{\text{Test,lit}})$ with an adjustment factor derived from the multivariable dataset (5). This is conveniently done on the logarithmic scale as follows:

$ln(LR_{\text{multi.adjusted}})$

$= combined\ univariable\ LRs$ from the literature$-$

$adjustment\ factor$ from the multivariable dataset

$= (ln(LR_{\text{Test1,lit}}) + ln(LR_{\text{Test2,lit}}) + ln(LR_{\text{Test3,lit}})) -$

$(ln(LR_{\text{Test1,data}}) + ln(LR_{\text{Test2,data}}) + ln(LR_{\text{Test3,data}}) - ln(LR_{\text{multi,data}}))$ (7.17)

7.6 Summary indices of validity

Should we use a clinical prediction model, exercise ECG, CAC, CT coronary angiography (CTCA), SPECT, MRI, or a prediction model combining clinical information and multiple test results for the diagnosis and prognosis of a patient with suspected CAD? Clinicians, local purchasers, and policy makers often need to decide which are the best diagnostic and prognostic biomarkers to use. In summarizing and comparing test performance and prediction models, we need indices that measure the information content of such predictions and the added value of additional test results. This is particularly important with the current proliferation of multiple novel biomarkers.

Important components of this decision should be the validity and the utility of the tests and prediction models and rules. Here we consider the validity: how well does the test or prediction model perform in estimating the risk of disease or an event? In Section 7.8 we consider the utility: how useful is the test or prediction rule in improving outcome? In Chapter 5 we discussed the LR, diagnostic odds ratio, and Youden's index (J statistic) in the context of dichotomous test results, all indices of validity of the test. In this chapter we have already used LRs in the context of multicategory test results. Here we discuss measures of discrimination and calibration. Section 7.8 discusses reclassification, net benefit, and relative utility.

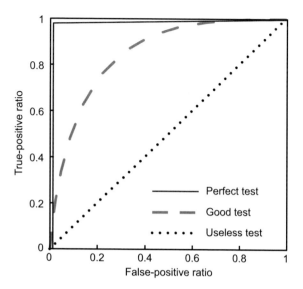

Figure 7.9   Receiver operating characteristic (ROC) curves of perfect (continuous line),
                  good (dashed line), and useless (dotted line) tests, illustrating how the area
                  under the ROC curve is an overall measure of the diagnostic performance of
                  a test.

All these measures can be calculated for the dataset in which the test or
prediction model was developed (internal validation) and, better still, in a new
validation dataset (external validation). If no validation dataset is available
one can split the data into development and test datasets, develop and cross-
validate in subsets of the data, or bootstrap the original dataset (5, 6).

7.6.1 Discrimination: the area under the ROC curve

The ROC curves that go up steeply from (0, 0) and reach near (0, 1) describe a
test that is nearly perfect in discriminating subjects with and without the
target disease. Curves close to the diagonal have little or no discriminatory
power (Figure 7.9), the *LR* being near 1.0 for every point on the curve. Most
tests have an ROC curve somewhere between these two extremes. Thus, the
area under the ROC curve (also referred to as the concordance statistic, the *c*-
statistic) is a summary measure of test performance. An area of 1 represents a
perfect test, whereas an area of 0.5 indicates a test with no discriminatory
power. Note that the area under the curve is a measure of test performance
independent of the chosen operating point on the curve and thus independent
of the probability of disease and the benefits and harms associated with test
outcomes. The area under the ROC curve also has an intrinsic meaning: it
equals the probability that a randomly chosen pair of non-diseased and

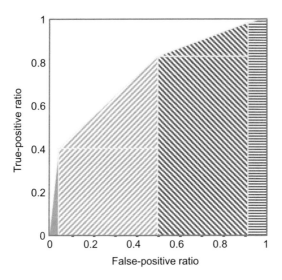

Figure 7.10   Calculating the area under an empirical, non-parametric receiver operating characteristic (ROC) curve.

diseased individuals will be correctly categorized. Statistically the area under the ROC curve is equivalent to the Mann–Whitney U statistic and the rank-order statistic. Most statistical software packages have routines to calculate the area under the ROC curve, either non-parametrically or parametrically. It is prudent to understand the basic underlying methods of how the packages do this, which is explained in the next sections.

7.6.2 Non-parametric estimates of the area under the ROC curve[1]

The most convenient way of calculating the area under the ROC curve is by connecting the calculated points and adding the areas of the trapezoids underneath each part of the curve (Figure 7.10). This is a non-parametric method, that is, no assumptions are made regarding the underlying probability distributions of test results. The method is equivalent to the Mann–Whitney–Wilcoxon U statistic from non-parametric statistics. The U statistic is normally used to test whether the value of a quantitative variable is generally larger in one population compared to another population. Its value in this context is that, in addition to providing a formula for calculating the area, we can also easily determine its standard error according to the Hanley–McNeil algorithm or using a bootstrap algorithm (7, 8). The non-parametric method is adequate, provided that enough data points are present

---

[1] This is advanced material and can be skipped without loss of continuity.

7.6 Summary indices of validity

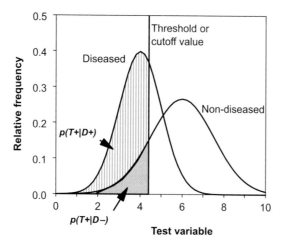

Figure 7.11

The binormal distribution of the results of a test. An arbitrary threshold has been indicated. Areas under the distributions to the left of the threshold represent the true- and false-positive ratios associated with that threshold.

and the points are spread along the curve. The area under the ROC curve is slightly underestimated with this method compared to a parametric estimate, but if comparing tests is the major issue, the underestimation of the area is of little concern.

7.6.3 Parametric estimates of the area under the ROC curve*

Parametric methods are based on the assumption that the test results conform to some well-defined underlying probability distribution (Figure 7.11). The most commonly used parametric method is the one introduced by Dorfman and Alf, which assumes that the underlying distributions of the test results are Gaussian, or normal. Although the distributions of test results are often not Gaussian, it has been shown that the binormal ROC model gives accurate results for many non-Gaussian distributions (9). Other underlying distributions include chi-squared, log-normal, and the negative exponential (9).

When using the binormal ROC model the basic procedure is to convert the true- and false-positive ratios to their corresponding normal deviate values. The ROC curve plotted on binormal deviate axes is a straight line (10). A maximum likelihood estimation algorithm is subsequently used to calculate the slope and intercept of the line (11). Finally, the predicted values are transformed back to ROC space.

---

* This is advanced material and can be skipped without loss of continuity.

7.6.4 Comparing the areas under two or more ROC curves

A plot of the competing ROCs is helpful to visualize the range of values and relative accuracy of the two tests. In particular, it should be noted whether or not the two curves cross, suggesting that each may be better in different areas. To compare the overall performance we need a statistical method. In comparing the area under two ROC curves a two-sided paired t-test is used. If the test results were derived from the same set of patients, one should take into account the correlation between test results (7). The z-statistic is calculated using the formula:

$$z = \frac{A_1 - A_2}{\sqrt{SE_1{}^2 + SE_2{}^2 - 2rSE_1SE_2}} \tag{7.18}$$

where A_1 and A_2 are the areas under the ROC curves of the two tests, SE_1 and SE_2 are the standard errors of the areas, and r is the correlation coefficient between the areas under two ROC curves derived from the same individuals (7). To determine the parameter r we need to calculate the Kendall tau (for categorical scales) or Pearson product moment correlation (for continuous scales) between the two test results for non-diseased and diseased patients. Bootstrapping can also be used for a non-parametric test of the difference between paired ROC areas. These calculations can be readily done with most current statistical software packages.

7.6.5 Calibration

When assessing the validity of a prediction model, either univariable or multivariable, an important step is to check whether the predictions approximate the observed outcomes (5, 6). Calibration refers to the agreement between observed outcomes and predictions. In the context of binary outcomes, calibration can be visualized with calibration plots that present the observed frequency of the disease (or event) on the vertical axis as a function of the predicted probability on the horizontal axis for defined subgroups of the study population (Figure 7.12). The subgroups may be defined by, for example, demographics or clinical presentation. If the subgroups are defined by quantiles of predictions, the calibration plot is a graphical representation of the Hosmer–Lemeshow goodness-of-fit test.

Calibration-in-the-large
Perfect predictions would fall on the diagonal of the calibration plot. Calibration graphs parallel to the diagonal but shifted to the right indicate overestimation of the probability and those shifted to the left indicate underestimation of the probability. This concept is referred to as 'calibration-in-the-large.' The intercept

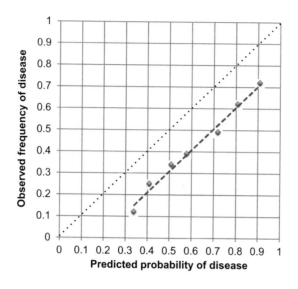

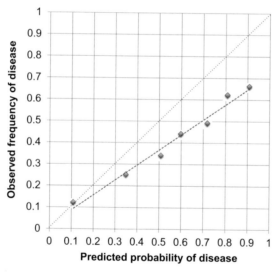

Figure 7.12   Calibration plot: observed frequency of the disease (or event) on the vertical axis as a function of the predicted probability on the horizontal axis for defined subgroups of the study population. Perfect predictions would fall on the diagonal. (a) Calibration-in-the-large shows predictions shifted parallel to the diagonal. Shifts to the right (as shown) indicate overestimation of the predictions. (b) The calibration slope estimates the overall effect of the predictors. A slope less than one (as shown) indicates over-fitting of the model in the development phase. (Made-up data for illustrative purposes only.)

of the calibration plot is a numerical summary of the extent that predictions are systematically over- or underestimating the observed outcomes. A positive intercept indicates that the mean observed proportion in the validation data is higher than the mean predicted probability – that is, the model underestimates the probability. Conversely, a negative intercept would imply that the mean observed proportion in the validation data is lower than the mean predicted probability – that is, the model overestimates the probability. A statistically significant result indicates significant miscalibration, whereas a non-significant result supports validity of the prediction model.

Calibration slope
The calibration slope refers to the overall effect of the model predictors in the validation data. A calibration slope less than one would imply that the overall effects of the predictors in the validation data were lower than those in the prediction model and is generally a sign of over-fitting of the model in the development dataset. Conversely, a positive value would indicate that the overall effects of the predictors in the validation data were stronger than those in the prediction model. A significant result would indicate significant miscalibration of the predictor effects, whereas a non-significant result would indicate no difference in predictor effects, supporting the validity of the model.

Recalibration and re-estimation
One can adjust an existing prediction model to a new setting in a stepwise approach. Each next step is taken only if the previous steps have not led to sufficiently valid results.

Step 1. Recalibration: adjust the intercept to adjust for miscalibration-in-the-large. This step is very often needed to correct for unexplained differences in prevalence in a different patient population.

Step 2. Re-estimation of the overall predictor effects. Typically this would mean shrinkage of regression coefficients, that is, adjusting the overall effect of the linear predictor by shrinking the coefficients when the calibration slope indicates over-fitting of the model.

Step 3. Re-estimation of the individual predictor effects. The regression coefficients for the individual variables are re-estimated.

Step 4: Extension of the prediction model with other variables, for example new biomarkers that have become available since the previous model was developed.

7.7 Choosing a positivity criterion

In using diagnostic tests with multiple results, we need to identify the optimal positivity criterion, i.e., the best threshold value or cutoff point of the test variable to use in making the next management decision. Not all positivity criteria of the test variable, and thus the associated operating points on an ROC curve, will result in equally good patient outcomes. The optimal positivity criterion represents the combination of true- and false-positive ratios that yield the greatest expected utility when applied to a particular decision problem. Utility, as we have seen, can be defined in terms of survival, life expectancy, quality-adjusted life expectancy, or any other metric suitable for the problem at hand. The choice of an optimal positivity criterion is equivalent to choosing a point on the ROC curve – an optimal 'operating point' on the curve. It represents the optimal risk threshold for classifying individuals in diseased vs. non-diseased, taking into account the consequences of that decision. Determining this threshold for a prediction model creates a prediction rule: if the predicted probability > threshold then treat, if the predicted probability < threshold then do not treat. Recall that treat in this context implies patient management as if disease is present and may imply initiating medical therapy, performing a therapeutic procedure, advising a lifestyle or other adjuvant intervention, or a combination of these. Do not treat implies patient management as if disease is absent and usually means risk factor management, lifestyle advice, self-care and/or watchful waiting.

As we shall demonstrate using decision analysis, the optimal operating point (optimal threshold value) depends upon the pre-test probability of disease, the expected net benefit of correctly diagnosing the disease (true-positives), and the expected net harms associated with false-positive results (12). These factors are combined in an expression that equals the slope of the ROC curve, and thus the *LR* of the test result, at the optimal operating point. We will show that the optimal operating point will shift to a less stringent positivity criterion (i.e., higher sensitivity and lower specificity, lower *LR*, and less steep slope) if the probability of disease is higher, the net benefit of diagnosing the disease is larger, or the net harm associated with false-positive results is smaller.

Consider the case example of the 55-year-old woman with which we started our discussion. There is a fairly low pre-test probability of CAD of 11%. If she has CAD, treatment with optimal medical therapy improves her prognosis by reducing the event rate but with a substantial complication rate. These circumstances make it desirable to set a relatively stringent cutoff point, which is to the bottom left on the ROC curve (Figure 7.4) in an effort to minimize the number of false-positive test results. On the other hand, if CAD is likely – as would be the case in an older man with multiple CVD risk factors and typical chest pain – or if CAD has serious consequences if left untreated (which is the case in extensive and severe CAD), then we would prefer to shift our positivity criterion to a more lenient criterion. In that situation we would want to shift the operating point more to the upper right on the ROC curve, in order to increase test sensitivity, in spite of the increased number of false-positive results.

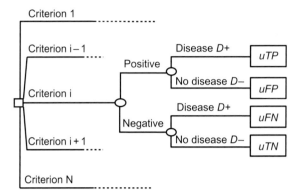

Figure 7.13   A generic decision model to determine the optimal positivity criterion of a test variable. '*u*' is used to indicate the net health benefit or utility associated with an outcome: *uFP* for false positives, *uFN* for false negatives, *uTP* for true positives, and *uTN* for true negatives.

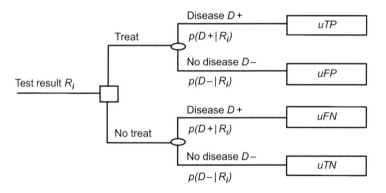

Figure 7.14   Generic decision tree for the decision to treat versus not treat conditional on test result R_i. Thus, $D+$ and $D-$ in our case example indicate presence and absence of CAD, R_i indicates the *CAC* result, and '*u*' is used to indicate the net health benefit or utility associated with an outcome: *uFP* for false positives, *uFN* for false negatives, *uTP* for true positives, and *uTN* for true negatives.

Balancing the risks and benefits to determine the optimal positivity criterion can be done explicitly using decision models (Figure 7.13) in which every possible positivity criterion is considered a choice option. Here we shall instead use an analytical approach based on a decision tree (Figure 7.14) to derive a general equation for calculating the optimal positivity criterion. This approach is especially useful when a test has a large number of categories or for continuous data. We will apply it to our example with the *CAC* that can be considered both on a continuous scale or in categories.

Averaging out the decision tree we get:

$$EU(treat) = p(D+\,|\,R_i)uTP + p(D-\,|\,R_i)uFP \qquad (7.19)$$

$$EU(no\ treat) = p(D+\,|\,R_i)uFN + p(D-\,|\,R_i)uTN \qquad (7.20)$$

To optimize the expected outcome we would use the decision rule:

Treat if: $EU(treat) > EU(no\ treat)$ (7.21)

Thus, substituting the above expressions:

$$p(D+|R_i)uTP + p(D-|R_i)uFP > p(D+|R_i)uFN + p(D-|R_i)uTN \qquad (7.22)$$

This can be rearranged algebraically as follows:

$$p(D+|R_i)(uTP - uFN) > p(D-|R_i)(uTN - uFP) \qquad (7.23)$$

which simplifies to the following comparison of ratios:

$$\frac{p(D+|R_i)}{p(D-|R_i)} > \frac{(uTN - uFP)}{(uTP - uFN)} \qquad (7.24)$$

Recognize that the left side of this inequality is the post-test odds given the test result R_i. The post-test odds can be rewritten as the product of the pre-test odds and the LR of R_i. Thus, the criterion becomes:

$$\frac{p(D+)}{p(D-)}\frac{p(R_i|D+)}{p(R_i|D-)} > \frac{(uTN - uFP)}{(uTP - uFN)} \qquad (7.25)$$

Dividing by the pre-test odds ratio on both sides yields the decision rule:

$$\frac{p(R_i|D+)}{p(R_i|D-)} > \frac{p(D-)}{p(D+)}\frac{(uTN - uFP)}{(uTP - uFN)} \qquad (7.26)$$

Recognize that the left-hand side of the inequality is now the LR of test result R_i. Furthermore, the first term on the right-hand side is the inverse of the prior (pre-test) odds. Also, recognize that $uTN - uFP$ is the net loss due to a false-positive compared with a true-negative which is the Net Harm caused by treating a non-diseased individual, incorrectly labeled as diseased (previously discussed in Chapters 3 and 6). Similarly, $uTP - uFN$ is the net gain due to a true-positive compared with a false-negative which is the Net Benefit of treating a diseased patient correctly identified. Thus, the optimal operating point on the ROC curve is defined by its LR which should fulfill the criterion:

Treat if:

$$LR_i > \frac{1}{prior\ odds} \cdot \frac{Harm}{Benefit} \qquad (7.27)$$

The second term in the inequality is therefore the harm-to-benefit ratio that we first introduced in Chapter 3 and also used in Chapter 6, which is the prior odds at the treatment threshold. Thus, the decision rule is to treat if the LR of the prediction is larger than the ratio of the prior odds at the treatment threshold divided by the prior odds of disease.

Here we have considered utility in a very generic sense. We can optimize the criterion for whatever outcome we choose. For example, this may be life expectancy, quality-adjusted life years, monetary costs, or a measure that combines effectiveness and costs. We will return to the concept of a multi-attribute outcome combining effectiveness and costs in Chapter 12.

Now let us once more consider our patient with suspected CAD. If the patient has CAD and is left untreated, she has a ten-year event risk of 10%. If she does not have CAD the risk is only 1%. Optimal medical treatment can reduce these risks by 50%. The risk of complications, however, is considerable and estimated at 2% during a ten-year period. Using the quoted data, we saw in Chapter 6 that the harm-to-benefit ratio was 0.015 / 0.030, which yielded a treatment threshold probability of 0.33. We could use the *CAC score* as a risk marker to decide whether or not to treat. Assuming the patient has a pre-test probability of 0.11 as determined by the web-based clinical risk calculator and using the derived equation, we would maximize the ten-year event-free survival chances of this patient by treating her if the test result has a *LR* of more than $(0.89/0.11) \cdot (0.015/0.030) = 4.05$. This implies that we should treat her only if the *CAC score* is high, corresponding to a strict criterion on the ROC curve. If we can only choose from the categories as listed in Table 7.1, we would choose a cutoff score of 400 since this is the first category with a *LR* higher than the optimal *LR*. Alternatively, we could interpolate between the *CAC scores* in which case we can define the *CAC* threshold more precisely. (See supplementary material on the website for the calculation.)

Analogous to the calculation of the optimal positivity criterion of a test variable, we can also calculate the optimal positivity criterion for a combination test or for a multivariable prediction model. We can use, for example, the predicted probability of disease (or event) or the score function from a multivariable prediction model which may include signs, symptoms, laboratory tests, genetic information, imaging biomarkers, and response to treatment. The 'test' is now a combination test and the 'test variable' is the predicted probability or score function from the regression model. True-positive and false-positive ratios are calculated by determining the probability of the score being larger than a particular (shifting) value, x, conditional on true disease status, i.e., $p((score > x) \mid D+)$ and $p((score > x) \mid D-)$.

For example, combining the type of chest pain and the *CAC* categories from the DICAD data led to 15 combination categories (Table 7.5). Similar to the calculation we performed to determine the optimal positivity criterion of the *CAC* result, we can determine the optimal positivity criterion of the reordered combination categories, which would lead to a prediction rule for further workup based on the type of chest pain combined with the *CAC* result. Note, however, that the type of chest pain was incorporated in the web-based

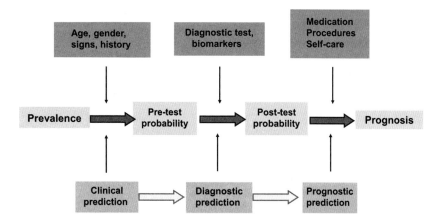

Figure 7.15   The concept of precision medicine: the steps in patient management are based on clinical, diagnostic, and prognostic prediction modeling, determined by patient-specific probability estimates of disease and combined with individual values and preferences.

risk calculator for the clinical probability of CAD, which would imply that we should only use the data from the combination categories in Table 7.5 if our prior probability is based on another source without consideration of type of chest pain, otherwise we would be using 'type of chest pain' twice. Similarly, the web-based calculator also provides the probability of CAD incorporating clinical factors and the *CAC score*, which in fact does the same as we did in Table 7.5 but then including all the clinical information and using logistic regression (Figure 7.8). Thus, it is important to ensure that the right prediction model and corresponding decision rule are used at the right time in the workup of the right patient and used in conjunction with the right prior probability (Figure 7.15). Prediction modeling and Bayesian thinking form the basis of precision medicine, that is, a personalized quantitative approach to medicine that combines diagnostic and prognostic predictions with patient-centered outcomes and individual values and preferences.

7.8 Summary: indices of clinical utility

Test results, biomarkers, and prediction models become prediction or decision rules once a threshold of risk has been defined above which the next step in patient management is justified. For example, above a threshold *CAC score* of 400 we would initiate medical therapy to prevent CVD events. As we saw in Section 7.7, choosing a threshold risk is best done by determining the optimal operating point on the ROC curve which depends on the prior odds and harm-to-benefit ratio. The next important step is to determine the clinical usefulness and patient outcomes when using this threshold risk to reclassify

New classification

Old classification		-	+	++
	-	156	22	10
	+	2	43	8
	++	0	1	25

Figure 7.16   Reclassification table of diseased individuals. Changes in classification in risk categories going from an old model to a new model are indicated. In this example only three individuals are incorrectly 'down reclassified' (lower risk category with the new classification) whereas 40 individuals are correctly 'up reclassified' (higher risk category with the new classification). (Made-up data for illustrative purposes only.)

patients. In this section we consider the utility of using such a test result or a prediction rule: how useful is the test or prediction rule in improving patient outcome? As with the summary indices of validity, the indices of utility are relevant for both diagnostic predictions of disease and prognostic predictions of events. As before, we will use the term 'disease' ($D+$) to mean presence of disease in the context of diagnosis or individuals with the event in the context of prognosis, and the term 'non-disease' ($D-$) to mean absence of disease or individuals without the event.

7.8.1 Reclassification

Reclassification tables (Figure 7.16) demonstrate how classification in risk categories changes when going from an old model to a new model. Typically the new model is an extension of the old model with a novel biomarker that is being evaluated. For example, the *CAC score* is a new imaging marker which has added value in predicting CVD beyond that of the traditional risk factors. The higher the proportion of individuals that change their category going from the old to the new model, in other words that are reclassified, the larger the impact of using the new model. The proportion reclassified, however, can be misleading since not all reclassifications are correct. Thus, the reclassification of diseased and non-diseased individuals should be considered separately (13).

Any 'upward' shift in risk categories for diseased individuals indicates improved classification of risk and any 'downward' shift indicates worsened classification of risk while the reverse is true for the non-diseased. In other words, a useful new marker would reclassify diseased individuals to higher risk groups ('up' reclassification) whereas it would reclassify non-diseased individuals to lower risk groups ('down' reclassification). The net reclassification improvement is a summary index derived from reclassification tables that are constructed for diseased and non-diseased individuals separately (13).

DEFINITION	The *net reclassification improvement (NRI)* is the net change in the correct direction, that is, the sum of differences in proportions of subjects moving up minus the proportion moving down for diseased individuals, and the proportion of subjects moving down minus the proportion moving up for non-diseased individuals. In formula form:

$$NRI = p(up \mid D+) - p(down \mid D+) + p(down \mid D-) - p(up \mid D-) \qquad (7.28)$$

The *NRI* is unreliable when the reclassification table has small cell frequencies. Furthermore, the *NRI* depends on the number of categories and the cutoff values, that is the defined risk thresholds. Finally, although the chosen risk threshold should reflect the harm-to-benefit ratio, this ratio is not explicitly considered in the calculation of the *NRI*. Expressed differently, the *NRI* gives equal weight to improvements in classification for diseased individuals and non-diseased individuals.

Several extensions of the *NRI* have been proposed that address some of these disadvantages (14). *Disease NRI and non-disease NRI* in diagnostic models and *event NRI and non-event NRI* in prognostic models are two subcomponents of the total *NRI* which are useful for a better interpretation of the total obtained reclassification. These are defined and reformulated using conditional probability theory as follows:

$$NRI_{D+} = p(up \mid D+) - p(down \mid D+) = \frac{p(D+ \mid up)p(up) - p(D+ \mid down)p(down)}{p(D+)}$$

$$(7.29)$$

$$NRI_{D-} = p(down \mid D-) - p(up \mid D-) = \frac{p(D- \mid down)p(down) - p(D- \mid up)p(up)}{p(D-)}$$

$$(7.30)$$

A *prospective formulation of the NRI*, relevant to survival data, is the event rate increase among those who are reclassified upwards plus the event rate decrease among those who are reclassified downwards.

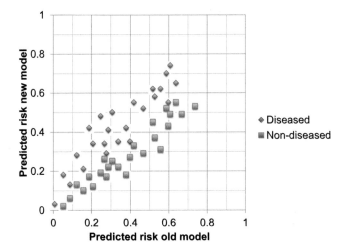

Figure 7.17   Reclassification plot: the predicted risk with the new model on the vertical axis
                     as function of the predicted risk with the old model on the horizontal axis. The
                     diseased and non-diseased individuals are indicated with different markers to
                     separate them. (Made-up data for illustrative purposes only.)

The *weighted NRI (wNRI)* allows for weighting with gains in patient
outcomes or cost savings from improved reclassification. The weighting is
different for diseased $D+$ and non-diseased $D-$ individuals, thus accounting
for the difference in Net Harm and Net Benefit discussed previously.

The *continuous NRI* is category-free and can be applied in the absence of
established risk category definitions. The only constraint is that we need to
define what upward and downward reclassification is. This could be any
change in predicted probability (notated as *NRI(>0)*) or a change larger than
say 1% (notated as *NRI(>1%)*). Subsequently, the above definitions and
equations can be applied. Analogous to the reclassification table, we can make
a *reclassification plot* for prediction on a continuous scale (Figure 7.17) which
presents the predicted risk with the new model on the vertical axis as a
function of the predicted risk with the old model on the horizontal axis for
the diseased and non-diseased individuals separately. A scatterplot with many
reclassifications among diseased individuals above the diagonal and many
reclassifications among non-diseased individuals below the diagonal indicates
that the new marker is clinically useful.

The *clinical NRI* quantifies the improvement obtained by measuring the
new biomarker only in individuals in an intermediate risk group; in other
words, it is the *NRI* conditional on being at intermediate risk according to the
old classification.

A related index is the *integrated discrimination improvement (IDI)*, which
is the sum of the increase in mean predicted probabilities among diseased and

the decrease in mean predicted probabilities among non-diseased. The *IDI* can also be seen as the improvement in average true-positive ratio (sensitivity) and any potential increase in average false-positive ratio (1- specificity).

For a single risk threshold, reclassification indices have a direct relationship with the sensitivity and specificity, the change in area under the ROC curve, and Youden's index. The *NRI* is the sum of the improvement (new vs. old model) in sensitivity and specificity and it is 2x the change in the area under the ROC curve for the single-point ROC curve. The *NRI* also equals the improvement in the Youden index (new vs. old model) and the *IDI* is equivalent to the integrated difference in Youden's indices (13, 15).

7.8.2 Net proportional benefit and decision curves

<table>
<tr><td>**DEFINITION**</td><td>The *net proportional benefit* at the reclassification threshold is a composite index of the corresponding proportion of true-positives and false-positives in a population of size *n*, the latter weighted by the relative harm (or cost) of a false-positive expressed as a loss (that is, with a minus sign):

$$Net\ Proportional\ Benefit = \frac{TP}{n} - w\frac{FP}{n} \qquad (7.31)$$</td></tr>
</table>

Thus, the net proportional benefit is the proportion of true-positives (*TP/n*) in the study population with size *n*, penalized by the weighted proportion of false-positives (*w·FP/n*) (15–18). In this formulation, the net benefit of a true-positive is considered equivalent to the harm of *w* false-positives. The weight *w* expresses the relative harm caused by a false-positive test result. An appropriate weight is the harm-to-benefit ratio that we first calculated in Chapter 3 (and which keeps showing up in our equations!):

$$Net\ Proportional\ Benefit = \frac{TP}{n} - \frac{harm}{benefit}\frac{FP}{n} \qquad (7.32)$$

We can express this in probabilities but keep in mind that we need to distinguish the prior probability of disease in the study population $p(Study\ D+)$ from the prior probability of disease in the target population $p(D+)$, i.e., the patients under consideration. Ideally these are the same but often they are not:

$$Net\ Proportional\ Benefit = TPR \cdot p(Study\ D+) - \frac{harm}{benefit} FPR \cdot p(Study\ D-)$$

$$(7.33)$$

Note that the concept 'net proportional benefit' was originally introduced in the literature as 'net benefit' (16). We have renamed it here to 'net

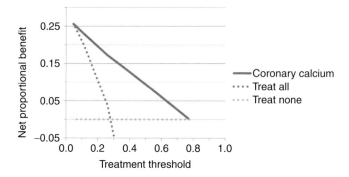

Figure 7.18   Decision curves for the *CAC score* in suspected coronary artery disease. The 'treat all' and 'treat none' strategies have been added as comparison. We present the decision curve for a prior probability in the target population equal to that in the study population. Note that the treat all and treat none lines intersect at the prior probability of 29%. (See Excel sheet on the website.)

proportional benefit' in order to distinguish this concept from the 'net benefit' introduced in Chapter 3, which refers to the gain in outcome, such as ten-year event-free survival, obtained from a true-positive test result compared with a false-negative test result, and which is the denominator in the harm-to-benefit ratio. Recognize that the harm-to-benefit ratio equals the odds at the treatment threshold p_T, therefore:

$$Net\ Proportional\ Benefit = TPR \cdot p(Study\ D+) - \frac{p_T}{1-p_T} FPR \cdot p(Study\ D-)$$

$$(7.34)$$

In the context of a risk prediction model that dictates whether to treat or not, the odds at the treatment threshold is the posterior odds of the threshold risk prediction, and since *posterior odds = prior odds · LR*, we can rewrite this as:

$$Net\ Proportional\ Benefit = TPR \cdot p(Study\ D+) - \frac{p(D+)}{p(D-)} LR \cdot FPR \cdot p(Study\ D-)$$

$$(7.35)$$

Thus, for every threshold (every cutoff on the ROC) we can calculate the corresponding *TPR, FPR, LR*, the threshold risk prediction, and the net proportional benefit. Net proportional benefit can be plotted as a function of the threshold risk, which yields a decision curve (Figure 7.18). A new test is compared with a 'treat none' strategy (i.e., always predict absence of disease) and a 'treat all' strategy (i.e., always predict presence of disease). The net proportional benefit of 'treat none' is zero since there are no true-positives and no false-positives. In the 'treat all' strategy all individuals with disease are true-positives and all those without disease are false-positives, thus:

$$Net\ Proportional\ Benefit_{Treat\ all} = p(Study\ D+) - \frac{p(D+)}{p(D-)} LR \cdot p(Study\ D-)$$

$$(7.36)$$

Decision curves are a way of presenting the clinical consequences of reclassifications using new tests, biomarkers, or prediction models across the full range of possible treatment thresholds without performing a formal and complex decision analysis.

7.8.3 Relative utility

Relative utility expresses the utility of a test or prediction model as the proportion of the maximum gain possible relative to the best baseline strategy for each treatment threshold p_T (15, 19, 20).

DEFINITION   *Relative utility* is the net proportional benefit in excess of 'treat all' or 'treat none' (whichever is larger) divided by the net proportional benefit of perfect prediction:

$$Relative\ Utility = \frac{EU_{p_T} - EU_{All}}{EU_{Perfect} - EU_{All}}, \qquad if \quad prior > p_T \qquad (7.37)$$

$$Relative\ Utility = \frac{EU_{p_T} - EU_{None}}{EU_{Perfect} - EU_{None}}, \qquad if \quad prior \le p_T \qquad (7.38)$$

Thus, the relative utility is the expected value of clinical information divided by the expected value of perfect information as defined in Chapter 5. If there is negligible harm caused by the test itself, then the above expression can be rewritten as:

$$Relative\ Utility = (1 - FPR) - \frac{1}{LR}(1 - TPR), \qquad if \quad prior > p_T \qquad (7.39)$$

$$Relative\ Utility = TPR - LR \cdot FPR, \qquad if \quad prior \le p_T \qquad (7.40)$$

Similar to decision curves, relative utility can be plotted as a function of the treatment threshold, which yields a relative utility curve (Figure 7.19). Also, just as with net proportional benefit, relative utility does not require precise determination of harms and benefits because it is a relative measure and it is calculated for a range of treatment thresholds.

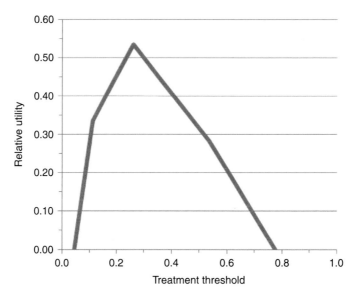

Figure 7.19   Relative utility curve for the *CAC score* in suspected coronary artery disease.

7.9 Other issues

7.9.1 Clustered data

In many situations data can be analyzed at several levels. For example, in the assessment of the coronary arteries, three arteries are distinguished each with multiple segments. Results for the three coronary arteries and for the multiple segments may be correlated, in which case a high sensitivity in one segment would imply that another segment may also have a high sensitivity. In other words, the probability of a positive test result conditional on disease status may increase more-or-less equally across segments, in which case they would be correlated. Similarly, for many organs in the body two exist and many organs have multiple segments or lobes. This is known as clustered data.

When analyzing clustered data, the calculations need to account for the possible correlation. Several methods exist to perform the analysis of clustered data and we refer here to a tutorial on the subject (21). In decision modeling, such clustered data can be unwieldy: modeling each segment of the coronary arteries and the effect on overall patient management is very complex. The key is always to ask oneself how test results may affect further management and at what level decisions are made.

7.9.2 Multiple disease states

Current methods for diagnostic and prognostic test evaluation and interpretation, such as prediction models and ROC analysis, typically focus on discriminating the 'diseased' from the 'non-diseased' population. In reality, multiple diseases generally need to be distinguished. For example, infections, metabolic diseases, malignancy, benign disease, or no disease are diagnoses that need to be distinguished. Furthermore, varying degrees of severity of disease need to be distinguished. Significant carotid artery disease was previously defined as a stenosis of 70% or more, whereas distinguishing a 0–49%, 50–69%, 70–99% stenosis, and an occlusion is more consistent with the results of recent trials of carotid endarterectomy. Different locations of the disease need to be distinguished. For example, diagnosing a stenosis in the tibial artery if the real problem is in the iliac artery can have very serious consequences. Predicting different categorical outcomes can be relevant to the prognosis. For example, in cardiovascular disease myocardial infarction, heart failure, stroke, and death are all outcomes of interest. Also, predicting different ordinal outcomes may be important, such as the five levels on the Glasgow Outcome Scale after head injury.

In diagnostic prediction Bayes' formula can be extended to multiple diseases $(D_1, D_2, D_3, D_4 \ldots D_i \ldots D_n)$ as follows:

$$p(D_i \mid R) = \frac{p(R \mid D_i)\, p(D_i)}{p(R \mid D_1)\, p(D_1) + \ldots + p(R \mid D_i)\, p(D_i) + \ldots + p(R \mid D_n)\, p(D_n)}$$

(7.41)

The problem of differential diagnosis in the presence of multiple tests and multicategory tests (and multiple segments) is complicated. Extensive decision models are needed in order to optimize the use of multiple tests in differential diagnosis and no simple algorithms such as we have seen for single tests exist. Some suggestions have been made in the literature on how to handle multiple disease states (5, 22–27). The most promising of these are polytomous logistic regression, proportional odds logistic regression, and Bayesian hierarchical methods (5, 27). The challenge for the future is to apply these advanced statistical techniques in such a manner that the method and results are understandable for the doctor who will apply the conclusions.

7.9.3 Focusing the development of new diagnostic and prognostic biomarkers

The challenge of evaluating diagnostic and prognostic tests and biomarkers is to do so in a timely fashion. Ideally, one is 'ahead of the game,' i.e., as a novel technology emerges, target values are estimated that this 'new' technology would have to meet to be cost-effective compared to the 'old' technology. One such method exists: challenge ROC regions (12, 28). Challenge ROC curves represent the threshold pairs of true-positive and false-positive ratios that a new test would have to attain to be cost-effective compared to an established test considering all possible operating points on the ROC curve of the established test. All pairs of true-positive and false-positive ratios to the upper left of the challenge ROC curve represent performance parameters for which a new test would be cost-effective compared to the established test. The pairs of true-positive and false-positive ratios can be restricted further to a challenge ROC region by taking into account the slope of the ROC curve at the optimal operating point. Clearly this method can be used to explore new diagnostic technology and focus its development. The limitations of the method lie in the fact that it focuses on replacing one test with another and focuses on discriminating between two disease states instead of multiple states.

7.10 Summary

In this chapter we discussed diagnostic and prognostic prediction using multiple test results. Diagnosis and prognosis are closely related. The aim of diagnosis is to classify patients into meaningful categories that are relevant to subsequent management and which reflect differences in prognosis.

The generalized form of Bayes' formula of test result R is:

Post-test odds = pre-test odds · likelihood ratio of result R

When multiple test results exist, some cutoff of the test variable commonly needs to be chosen to define further management. A trade-off needs to be made between true-positive and false-positive test results. An ROC curve is a plot of pairs of possible combinations of true-positive and false-positive ratios achievable with a test as the positivity criterion is varied. The likelihood ratio at a chosen cutoff of the test variable is the slope of the ROC curve at that point. An ROC curve evaluates overall test performance independently of the ultimately chosen decision criterion.

Combining results from multiple tests can be done assuming conditional independence or, if individual patient-level data are available, with multivariable prediction models. We showed that prediction models based on combination tests are an extension from the univariable formulation of Bayes' formula to a multivariable formulation. Validity of such models is evaluated with the area under the ROC curve as a measure of discrimination and with calibration plots which assess observed frequency of disease vs. predicted risk.

Not all positivity criteria of the test variable, and thus the associated operating points on an ROC curve, result in equivalent outcomes. In using diagnostic tests with multiple results, we need to identify the optimal positivity criterion, i.e., the threshold value or cutoff point of the test variable which yields the highest expected utility. The optimal positivity criterion (operating point on the ROC curve) depends upon the pre-test probability of disease, the expected net benefit of correctly diagnosing the disease (true-positive compared with false-negative results), and the expected net harms associated with false-positive (compared with true-negative) results. The optimal operating point shifts to a less stringent positivity criterion (i.e., higher sensitivity and lower specificity, lower LR) if the probability of disease is higher, the net benefit of diagnosing the disease is larger, or the net harm associated with false-positive results is smaller.

Clinical utility of a new test or a new prediction model can be demonstrated with reclassification tables and plots, with net proportional benefit and decision curves, and with relative utility curves.

REFERENCES

1. Diamond GA, Forrester JS. Analysis of probability as an aid in the clinical diagnosis of coronary artery disease. *N Engl J Med*. 1979;300(24):1350–8.
2. Genders TS, Steyerberg EW, Hunink MG, et al. Prediction model to estimate presence of coronary artery disease: retrospective pooled analysis of existing cohorts. *BMJ*. 2012;344:e3485.
3. Pryor DB, Harrell FE, Jr., Lee KL, Califf RM, Rosati RA. Estimating the likelihood of significant coronary artery disease. *Am J Med*. 1983;75(5):771–80.
4. Puylaert JB, Rutgers PH, Lalisang RI, et al. A prospective study of ultrasonography in the diagnosis of appendicitis. *N Engl J Med*. 1987;317(11):666–9.
5. Steyerberg EW. *Clinical Prediction Models: A practical approach to development, validation, and updating*. Springer: 2009.
6. Steyerberg EW, Vickers AJ, Cook NR, et al. Assessing the performance of prediction models: a framework for traditional and novel measures. *Epidemiology*. 2010;21(1):128–38.
7. Hanley JA, McNeil BJ. A method of comparing the areas under receiver operating characteristic curves derived from the same cases. *Radiology*. 1983;148(3):839–43.
8. Efron B, Tibshirani RJ. *An Introduction To The Bootstrap*. CRC Press; 1998.
9. Hanley JA. The robustness of the 'binormal' assumptions used in fitting ROC curves. *Med Decis Making*. 1988;8(3):197–203.
10. Swets JA. ROC analysis applied to the evaluation of medical imaging techniques. *Invest Radiol*. 1979;14(2):109–21.
11. Dorfman DD, Alf E. Maximum likelihood estimation of parameters of signal detection theory – a direct solution. *Psychometrika* 1968; 117–24.
12. Phelps CE, Mushlin AI. Focusing technology assessment using medical decision theory. *Med Decis Making*. 1988;8:279–89.

13. Pencina MJ, D'Agostino RB, Sr, D'Agostino RB, Jr, Vasan RS. Evaluating the added predictive ability of a new marker: from area under the ROC curve to reclassification and beyond. *Stat Med.* 2008;27(2):157–72; discussion 207–12.

14. Pencina MJ, D'Agostino RB, Sr, Steyerberg EW. Extensions of net reclassification improvement calculations to measure usefulness of new biomarkers. *Stat Med.* 2011;30(1):11–21.

15. Van Calster B, Vickers AJ, Pencina MJ, et al. Evaluation of markers and risk prediction models: overview of relationships between NRI and decision-analytic measures. *Med Decis Making.* 2013;33(4):490–501.

16. Vickers AJ, Elkin EB. Decision curve analysis: a novel method for evaluating prediction models. *Med Decis Making.* 2006;26(6):565–74.

17. Vickers AJ, Cronin AM, Elkin EB, Gonen M. Extensions to decision curve analysis, a novel method for evaluating diagnostic tests, prediction models and molecular markers. *BMC Medical Informatics & Decision Making.* 2008;8:53.

18. Vickers AJ, Elkin EB, Steyerberg E. Net reclassification improvement and decision theory. *Stat Med.* 2009;28(3):525–6; author reply, 6–8.

19. Baker SG. Putting risk prediction in perspective: relative utility curves. *J Natl Cancer Inst.* 2009;101(22):1538–42.

20. Baker SG, Cook NR, Vickers A, Kramer BS. Using relative utility curves to evaluate risk prediction. *J R Stat Soc Ser A Stat Soc.* 2009;172(4):729–48.

21. Genders TS, Spronk S, Stijnen T, et al. Methods for calculating sensitivity and specificity of clustered data: a tutorial. *Radiology.* 2012;265(3):910–16.

22. Steinbach WR, Richter K. Multiple classification and receiver operating characteristic (ROC) analysis. *Med Decis Making.* 1987;7(4):234–7.

23. Chakraborty DP, Winter LHL. Free-response methodology: alternate analysis and a new observer-performance experiment. *Radiology.* 1990;174:873–81.

24. Ananth CV, Kleinbaum DG. Regression models for ordinal responses: a review of methods and applications. *Int J Epidemiol.* 1997;26(6):1323–33.

25. Harrell FE, Jr., Margolis PA, Gove S, et al. Development of a clinical prediction model for an ordinal outcome: the World Health Organization Multicentre Study of Clinical Signs and Etiological Agents of Pneumonia, Sepsis and Meningitis in Young Infants. WHO/ARI Young Infant Multicentre Study Group. *Stat Med.* 1998;17(8):909–44.

26. Dreiseitl S, Ohno-Machado L, Binder M. Comparing three-class diagnostic tests by three-way ROC analysis. *Med Decis Making.* 2000;20(3):323–31.

27. O'Malley AJ, Zou KH. Bayesian multivariate hierarchical transformation models for ROC analysis. *Stat Med.* 2006;25(3):459–79.

28. Hunink MGM, Kuntz KM, Fleischmann KE, Brady TJ. Noninvasive imaging for the diagnosis of coronary artery disease: focusing the development of new diagnostic technology. *Ann Intern Med.* 1999;131(9):673–80.

Finding and summarizing the evidence

It is surely a great criticism of our profession that we have not organized a critical summary, by specialty or subspecialty, adapted periodically, of all relevant randomized controlled trials.

Archie Cochrane

8.1 Introduction

Good decision analyses depend on both the veracity of the decision model and on the validity of the individual data elements. These elements may include probabilities (such as the pre-test probabilities, the sensitivity and specificity of diagnostic tests, the probability of an adverse event, and so on), estimates of effectiveness of interventions (such as the relative risk reduction), and the valuation of outcomes (such as quality of life, utilities, and costs). Often we lack the information needed for a confident assessment of these elements. Decision analysis, by structuring a decision problem, makes these gaps in knowledge apparent. Sensitivity analysis on these 'soft' numbers will also give us insight into which of these knowledge gaps is most likely to affect our decisions. These same gaps exist in less systematic decision making as well, but there is no convenient way to determine how our decisions should be affected. In this chapter we shall cover the basic methods for finding the best estimate for each of the different elements that may be included in a formal decision analysis or in less systematic decision making.

Sometimes, but not as often as one would like, the estimates one is looking for can be inferred from a published study or from a series of cases that someone has reported in the literature or recorded in a data bank. This is generally considered the most satisfactory way of assessing a probability, because it involves the use of quantitative evidence. Often we will have a choice of data sources, so it is useful to have some 'rules' to guide the choice of possible estimates. One helpful concept is the 'hierarchy of evidence' (see www.cebm.net) which explicitly ranks the available evidence; 'perfect' data will rarely be available, but we need to know how to choose the best from the available imperfect data. This choice will also need to be tempered by the practicalities and purpose of each decision analysis: what is feasible will differ with a range from the urgent individual patient decision to a national policy decision to fund an expensive new procedure. The hierarchy we suggest is:

1. *Systematic review of primary studies.* A systematic review aims to identify all relevant primary research, undertake standardized appraisal of study validity, and synthesize the studies of acceptable quality. This is a considerable undertaking, so, if a systematic review is already available, then you will usually want to use it. If not, then you might consider doing a systematic review yourself for the most critical element(s) in the decision analysis – but this may take weeks to months of work.

Meta-analyses are a special type of systematic review that entails using quantitative techniques for combining estimates from different sources. The term is used broadly to encompass methods that simply pool observations across studies, to methods that consider both within-study and between-study variability (including hierarchical models). Meta-analyses can be grounded either in frequentist statistical theory, which restricts inference to the observed data, or in Bayesian methods that incorporate prior beliefs.

2. *'Best' single study.* A simpler alternative to a systematic review is to search for all relevant studies, but choose the largest study that meets some minimum quality criteria. For example, to estimate the effectiveness of an intervention you might choose the largest randomized trial, where 'largest' is not necessarily the largest number of patients, but the largest number of events or person-time.

3. *Subjective estimates.* An estimate should not necessarily be adopted from a study or data set just because it is available. A modified assessment for an individual patient or population, based in part on your own experiences, knowledge of the patient or local population, and the judgments of experts, may be required to adjust a particular estimate. Sometimes no data will be available for the estimate, and you must instead choose the most plausible value.

Finding the best data can be hard work, and sometimes impossible (firmly establishing that no data exist is often a time-consuming task). Sometimes the estimation may be straightforward. For example, suppose that you want to know the probability that a particular surgical procedure will result in perioperative death. A report in the literature states that of a series of 1000 patients who underwent the operation, 23 died in surgery. Thus, an obvious estimate of p[death] is 23/1000, or 0.023. The larger the sample, the more confident we can be that the observed frequency in the sample is a good estimate of the actual probability in the general population. Based on this sample, and assuming that the patient outcomes were independent with a common mortality probability, p[death], a 95% confidence interval for p[death] is: 0.015 to 0.034 – which may then be used in a sensitivity analysis.

Sometimes the estimation will be less straightforward: even when the data are found they may not be in the format required for the model, and may need to be adjusted, either by modeling or subjectively. For example, life expectancy is steadily increasing, and estimates based on historical or even current data will tend to underestimate the likely true value.

There are several caveats in translating the results from a single study or systematic review into an estimate for use in your particular decision problem.

First, the treatments (or diagnostic procedures) may not be entirely comparable to yours. Different personnel, equipment, facilities, or variations in the actual procedure may result in different probabilities. For example, while a study may be based on the experience with a new surgical procedure, the performance of surgeons may have improved considerably since the time of the study's data collection.

Second, the study population may be different in some important respects from your population or patient. Those patients in the study population may have been older or younger, or in better or worse health. They may have volunteered or have been specially selected for the treatment in question. The potential effects of this difference may best be examined by sensitivity analysis. This will enhance the ability of the analyses to be applied and adapted to a variety of situations, populations, and individuals. We will return to this in Section 8.5.

8.2 Finding the 'best' studies

The best study type will depend on the type of estimate required. We may classify most of the decision elements into the following different types of questions, which then guides our search for data:

1. *Proportion or frequency.* How common is a particular feature or disease in a specified group? For example, what is the prevalence of osteoporotic fractures at various ages, or the frequency of a particular gene such as BRCA1 for breast cancer, or the prevalence of risk factors for cardiovascular disease? The appropriate study design here is to perform a standardized measurement in a representative sample of people, which is a cross-sectional study. If we are interested in the trends over time, such as the increase in obesity over time, we would need a repeated cross-sectional study.

2. *Diagnostic performance.* How accurate is a sign, symptom, diagnostic test, or screening test in predicting the true diagnostic status of a patient? This essentially involves a comparison between the test of interest and some reference ('gold') standard test. Note that if we move from an interest in diagnostic performance to an interest in the effects

on patient outcomes, then the question becomes one of intervention – we are interested in whether the test predicts the effects of treatment. Diagnostic performance is an intermediate outcome rather than the final outcome of workup and treatment. The analyst has a choice whether to model the causal chain from diagnostic performance to intervention to outcome, or whether to rely on direct evidence of the effect of testing on outcome. Diagnostic performance is evaluated in cross-sectional studies or, if follow-up is part of the reference standard test, in cohort studies.

3. *Risk factor: etiology and prognosis.* Is a particular factor, such as age, gender, laboratory measurement, or family history, the cause for the occurrence of disease or adverse outcomes? Inferring that a factor is causal requires that the six criteria of Hill be fulfilled: the cause precedes the effect, the cause–effect relationship is biologically plausible, there is a consistent association between the cause and effect, the association is strong, there is a dose–response relationship, and removing the cause reduces the risk. Etiology is initially often studied with case-control studies but confirmation of the findings require a longitudinal cohort study. Prognosis requires a longitudinal cohort study. Often data on the association between risk factors and the occurrence of disease or an event are available in the form of a statistically estimated risk function relating one or more risk factors to a measure of frequency of disease, such as the incidence rate, or to a measure of association, such as relative risk. Commonly encountered statistical models of this type include logistic regression models, proportional hazards (Cox regression) models, and multilevel (mixed) models.

4. *Intervention effectiveness.* What are the effects of an intervention on patients? The intervention may be a pharmaceutical, surgery, a minimally invasive procedure, a dietary supplement, exercise training sessions, psychotherapy, yoga classes, etc. Some interventions are less directly related to patient outcome, such as early detection (screening), patient educational materials, or legislation. The key characteristic is that there is some manipulation of the person or his or her environment. To study the effects of interventions requires a comparable control group without the intervention, and thus a randomized controlled trial (RCT) is the ideal design. Preferably both the patient and the investigator are unaware of which treatment the patient was allocated to (double-blind design) but this is not always possible in which case a pragmatic design is used. Results from RCTs are presented with measures of association such as the relative risk, relative risk reduction, absolute risk reduction, hazard rate ratios, and numbers-needed-to-treat.

5. *Patient preferences and costs.* In all of the previous questions, additional outcomes of interest will commonly be patient preferences and costs. For example, we may be interested in patient outcomes and costs of the intervention, and any potential downstream cost savings caused by improved patient outcomes.

The first four (1–4) of these are probabilities. Appraising studies reporting these probabilities was covered in Chapter 2. If you find several potential studies then the appraisal should guide you to the best single study. If there are several studies which appear of equal quality, then you will need to either choose the largest or, preferably, synthesize the results using meta-analytic methods.

8.2.1 Electronic searching

Most searching will be done electronically using words or phrases relevant to each estimate needed. A useful tactic is to break down the particular question into components: the Population, the Intervention (or test or risk factor), the Comparison (or control), and the Outcome (these may be remembered by the acronym, PICO). The search terms should include identifying potential synonyms for each component. In addition, an appropriate 'methodological filter' may help confine the retrieved set to the most valid primary research studies. For example, if you are interested in whether hemoccult screening reduces mortality from colorectal cancer (an intervention), then we may wish to confine the retrieved studies to the controlled trials evaluating screening.

It is useful to break the study question into its components, and then combine these using the special terms AND and OR. For example, in the Venn diagram of Figure 8.1, 'mortality AND screen*' represents the overlap

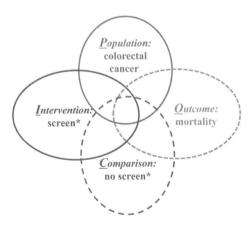

Figure 8.1   Four components (PICO) of a question that might be considered in designing a search strategy, and their overlap of 'hits'. For this example, the 'C' is unnecessary, and 'O' may be optional (dashed circles).

Table 8.1 Using the components of a question to guide the literature search

Component of question	Example of search term	Synonyms and related terms
Population/ setting	Adult, human	
Intervention, test, or risk factor	Screen for colorectal cancer	Fecal occult blood test, early detection
Comparison	No screening	
Outcome	Colorectal cancer mortality	Bowel cancer, colorectal neoplasm and death, survival
Study design[a]	Controlled clinical trial	

[a] Study design is an option needed only when the search results are unmanageable – see Section 8.2.2.

between these two terms, i.e., only those articles that use both terms. 'screen* AND colorectal cancer AND mortality,' the small area where all three circles overlap, will require articles that have all three terms. Complex combinations are possible, e.g., '(mortality AND screen) OR (mortality AND colorectal cancer) OR (screen AND colorectal cancer)' captures all the overlap areas between any of the circles. Note that the Comparison – no screening – is unnecessary for this example; generally the P and I are needed, and the O and C added only if we need to further restrict the results.

Though the overlap of all three parts will generally have the best concentration of relevant articles, the other areas may still contain many relevant articles. Hence, if the population (or disease) AND intervention ('colorectal cancer AND screen') combination (union of the two corresponding circles in the figure) is manageable, it is best to work with this and not restrict the search any further, e.g. using outcomes ('mortality'), or else use very broad terms for the outcome fields.

When the general structure of the question is developed it is then worth looking for synonyms for each of those components. This process is illustrated in Table 8.1.

Thus a search strategy might be: '(screen* OR fecal occult blood test OR early detection) AND (colorectal cancer OR bowel cancer OR colorectal neoplasm) AND (mortality OR death OR survival).' (The term 'screen*' is shorthand for words beginning with screen, e.g., screen, screened, screening, etc.)

In looking for synonyms one should consider both text words and key words in the database. The MEDLINE keyword system, known as the Medical

Subject Headings (MeSH), is worth understanding: the tree structure of MeSH is a useful way of covering a broad set of synonyms very quickly. For example the 'explode' feature allows you to capture an entire subtree of MeSH terms within a single word. Thus for the colorectal cancer term in the above search, the appropriate MeSH term might be:

Colonic neoplasm (exp)

With the 'explode' the search incorporates the whole MeSH tree below colonic neoplasm, viz:

Colorectal neoplasms
    Colonic polyps
    Adenomatous polyposis coli
Colorectal neoplasms
    Colorectal neoplasms, hereditary non-polyposis
Sigmoid neoplasms

While the MeSH system is useful, it should supplement rather than usurp the use of text words, lest incompletely coded articles are missed.

8.2.2 Methodological filters

A search may be made more specific by including terms indicative of the best appropriate study design, and hence filter out inappropriate studies (details and references for filters are given at http://www.ncbi.nlm.nih.gov/pubmed/clinical). For example, if you are interested in studies of an intervention's effectiveness then you may initially try to confine the studies to randomized trials. These filters might use specific methodological terms or compound terms.

What are 'methodological' terms? MEDLINE terms not only cover specific content but also a number of useful terms on study methodology. For example, if we are considering questions of therapy, many randomized trials are tagged in MEDLINE by the specific methodological term randomized-controlled-trials to be found under publication type (pt) or as controlled-clinical trials. Be aware, however, that many studies do not have the appropriate methodological tag.

8.2.3 Electronic databases

Which databases should I use? Most commonly you will use MEDLINE (e.g., through PubMed or OVID or one of the other interfaces to MEDLINE), but other databases to use depends on the content area and the type of question being asked. For example, there are specific databases for nursing and allied health studies (e.g., CINHAL) and for psychological studies (e.g., Psyclit). If it is a question of intervention, then the Controlled Trials Registry within the Cochrane Library is a particularly useful resource, as it contains over half a million references for randomized controlled trials, identified by a systematic search of databases and hand-searching of selected journals.

Given almost half of clinical trials and other study types remain unpublished, reviews should also check registries such as the WHO registry http://www.who.int/ictrp/en/ which allows a search across multiple trials registries.

8.3 Systematic reviews and meta-analyses

The purpose of a systematic review is to evaluate and interpret all available research evidence relevant to a particular question. A systematic review contrasts with a traditional review by its concerted attempt to identify all relevant primary research, by its standardized appraisal of study quality, and its systematic (and sometimes quantitative) synthesis of the studies of acceptable quality. A systematic review generally requires considerably more effort than a traditional review. The processes are described here in brief. For more extensive treatment there are several good textbooks, and the Cochrane Handbook is available for free on the web. For intervention studies go to: http://www.cochrane-handbook.org/. For diagnostic tests performance studies go to: http://srdta.cochrane.org/handbook-dta-reviews.

The two major advantages of systematic reviews and meta-analyses are the increase in power and the improved ability to study the consistency of results. Many studies have insufficient power to detect modest but important effects. Combining all the studies that have attempted to answer the same question considerably improves the statistical power. Furthermore, similar effects across a wide variety of settings and designs provide evidence of robustness and transferability; if the studies are inconsistent, then the sources of variation can be examined. Thus while some people see the mixing of 'apples and oranges' as a problem of systematic reviews, we see it as a distinct advantage because of its ability to enhance generalizability and transferability.

A protocol outlining the question and methods is advisable prior to starting the review; indeed this is required for all Cochrane systematic reviews (1). The term 'systematic review' is preferred to meta-analysis because it suggests this careful review process. While it may provide a summary estimate, this is neither necessary nor sufficient to make a review 'systematic.'

It is useful to think of the process of doing a systematic review in a number of discrete steps:

1. *Defining the review questions.* The process of decision analysis breaks a problem down into many components, many of which will require relevant

data. It is helpful to set up a table of the data items, their definitions, and the potential data sources.

2. *Finding studies.* The aim of a systematic review is to answer a question based on all the best available evidence, published and unpublished. Being comprehensive and systematic is important in this critical, and perhaps most difficult phase of a systematic review. Finding some studies is usually easy. Finding all relevant studies is almost impossible. However, there are a number of methods and resources that can make the process easier and more productive.

3. *Appraisal and selection of studies.* The relevant studies identified will usually vary greatly in their quality. This phase entails undertaking a critical appraisal of each of the identified potentially relevant studies, and then selecting those of appropriate quality. To avoid a selection, which is biased by preconceived ideas, it is important to use a systematic and standardized approach to the appraisal of studies. The appraisal should include a systematic assessment of the risk of bias in the included studies.

4. *Summary and synthesis.* Next, the relevant data from each of the studies needs to be extracted, summarized, and synthesized. The initial focus should be on describing the study's design, conduct, and results in a clear and simple manner – usually in a summary table. Following this, some summary ('forest') plots will be helpful, particularly if there are a large number of studies. Finally, it may be appropriate to provide a quantitative synthesis in a meta-analysis. However, as indicated above, this is neither a sufficient nor necessary part of a systematic review.

5. *Generalizability and heterogeneity.* Following the summary and synthesis of the studies we will need to ask about the overall internal and external validity of any results and conclusions. Is there a large difference in settings, methods, and results across studies? How and to whom are the results of the synthesis applicable? How will the effects vary in different populations and individuals?

It is vital to understand the type of question, and to specify the components of the question clearly before starting. This will define the process in the next three phases of: finding, appraising, and synthesizing the studies.

8.3.1 Finding relevant primary studies

Finding all relevant studies that have addressed a single question is not easy. MEDLINE indexes only about 15–20% of biomedical journals, and even the MEDLINE journals represent several hundreds of thousands of journal articles per year. Beyond sifting through this mass of literature, there are the problems of duplicate publications and with accessing the 'gray literature,' such as conference proceedings, reports, theses, and unpublished studies. A systematic approach to this literature is essential if we are to identify all of the best evidence available that addresses the question. There are various issues to take into account when searching the literature:

8.3.1.1 Is there a good recent systematic review?

Before doing a systematic review yourself though, you should ask 'Has a systematic review already been done?' Published reviews may answer the question, or at least provide a starting point for identifying the studies. Finding such reviews takes little effort, but several good 'filters' have been developed to help make this easier. For example, one 'balanced' filter for PubMed is:

Meta-analysis [Publication Type] OR meta-analysis[Title/Abstract] OR meta-analysis [MeSH Terms] OR review[Publication Type] OR search* [Title/Abstract]

This filter has a sensitivity of 98% and a specificity of 91% (2). Of course, not all reviews will be well done, so you need to check the quality of the review process. A simple appraisal mnemonic is FAST: (i) Find – Did they find all the primary studies, that is, was their search sufficiently thorough? (ii) Appraise – Did they appraise the primary studies, and select only the better ones? (iii) Synthesize – Did they provide a graphic plot of the results, and, if sufficiently homogeneous, pool the results together? (iv) Transferability – Did they consider how robust the findings are and how generalizable they would be to different settings? A more extensive appraisal can be done with the PRISMA checklist for systematic reviews – www.prisma-statement.org/. Finally, you should check how up to date the review is, which is determined by the date of the last search, not the publication date. Even good reviews might need some supplementary searching to identify subsequent important primary studies.

8.3.1.2 Finding published original studies

It is usually easy to find a few relevant articles by a straightforward literature search, but the process becomes progressively more difficult as we try to identify additional articles. Eventually, you may sift through hundreds of articles in order to identify one further relevant study. There are no magic formulae to make this process easy, but there are a few standard tactics, which, together with the assistance of a librarian experienced with the biomedical literature, can make your efforts more rewarding.

In addition to the general methods of electronic searching described above, there are some additional methods that should be considered in a thorough search for all relevant studies.

Snowballing

The process of identifying papers is an iterative one – sometimes referred to as 'snowballing.' The results of the initial search are used to retrieve relevant papers, which can then be used in several ways to identify missed papers:

(a) the bibliographies of relevant papers are checked for articles missed by the initial search,

(b) a citation search, which uses tools such as the *Science Citation Index* or *Scopus* to identify papers that have cited the identified relevant studies, some of which may be subsequent primary research,

(c) use the key words of relevant papers in a new search.

Hand-searching

If the relevant articles appear in a limited range of journals or conference proceedings, it may be feasible and desirable to search these by hand. This is obviously more important for unindexed or very recent journals, but may also pick up relevant studies not easily identified from titles or abstracts.

Is it worth writing to experts?

Experience varies on this question. However, an analysis of a recent review of the value of near-patient diagnostic tests (diagnostic tests which can be done entirely within the clinic, e.g., dipstick urine tests) showed that writing to experts may be quite useful (3). Of 75 papers eventually identified nearly one-third were uniquely identified by writing to experts. The data are shown in Figure 8.2, which also illustrates the general point that it is worth using multiple sources.

Is it worth including non-English literature?

If at all feasible, it may be worth including non-English language literature. Commonly, however, this poses problems in that the papers need to be translated professionally. A published analysis demonstrated that expanding the search to include non-English literature retrieved very few papers that fulfilled the inclusion/exclusion criteria of the review and did not change the overall conclusion of the systematic review and meta-analysis (4).

Updating the search

Immediately prior to submission of the systematic review it is wise to update the search and include any recently published papers. Keep this in mind when starting out on the project so that you can set up the proper procedures to update your database of papers, your analysis, and your report in an efficient and easy manner. Also, it is important to ensure some overlap in time of the original and updated searches since indexing of papers in electronic literature databases lags behind.

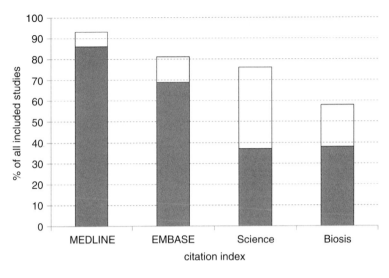

Figure 8.2

Papers identified by different search methods in a systematic review of near-patient ('point of care') diagnostic tests. Shaded area, unique; no shading, non-unique.

8.3.1.3 Publication bias

What is publication bias?

'Positive' studies are more likely to be published than 'negative' or 'inconclusive' studies, which biases any review (traditional or systematic) towards a 'positive' result. This is the essence of publication bias – the positive correlation between the results of the study and our ability to find that study. In 1979 Rosenthal described this as the 'file drawer problem' where 'the journals are filled with the 5% of the studies that show Type I errors, while the file drawers back at the lab are filled with the 95% of the studies that show non-significant (p > 0.05) results' (5). A follow-up of 737 studies approved by the Institutional Review Board at John Hopkins University found that the odds ratio for the likelihood of publication of positive compared with negative studies was 2.5 (6). A recent systematic review of 12 such studies found similar results across countries, times, and disciplines (7).

Does publication bias affect the results of the reviews?

Systematic exclusion of unpublished trials from a systematic review will introduce bias if the unpublished studies differ from the published, e.g., because of the statistical significance or the direction of results. In a seminal review (8) of multiagent versus single-agent chemotherapy for ovarian cancer,

Table 8.2 Comparison of published versus registered studies of multiagent vs. single-agent chemotherapy for ovarian cancer

	Published studies	Registered studies
Number of studies	16	13
Mortality ratio (relative risk)	0.86	0.95
95% confidence interval	0.78–0.94	0.89–1.02
p-value	0.02	0.25

Data from (8).

the authors found statistically and clinically different results between 16 published studies and 13 registered studies – see Table 8.2. Since the registered trials were registered at inception rather than completion, their selection for inclusion in the review was not influenced by the outcome of the study – therefore they constitute an *unbiased* set of studies.

8.3.2 Appraising and selecting studies

All studies have flaws, ranging from the small to the fatal. Assessment of individual studies for such biases is crucial, as the added power of the systematic review will allow even small biases to result in an 'apparent' effect. For example Schulz has shown that studies evaluating treatment effects using unblinded outcome assessment gave on average a 17% greater risk reduction than those using blinded outcome assessment (9).

Providing an explicit and standardized appraisal of the studies identified is often useful for two reasons. First a systematic review should try to base its conclusions on the highest-quality evidence available. To do this requires a procedure to select from the large pool of studies identified so that only the relevant and acceptable quality studies are included. Second, it is important to convey to the reader the quality of the studies included as this tells us about the strength of the evidence for any recommendation made.

Is it important to perform a structured appraisal?

Unfortunately, if unstructured appraisals are made, we tend to look more critically at the studies whose conclusions we dislike. For example, 28 reviewers were asked to assess a single (fabricated) 'study' but were randomly allocated to receive either the 'positive' or 'negative' version (10). The identical Methods sections of this fabricated study were rated significantly worse by the reviewers of the 'negative' study compared with the 'positive' study! Hence, it is essential to appraise all papers equally. This can be accomplished by using a standardized checklist and ideally by quality appraisal while blinded to the results and conclusion of the study.

How many reviewers are required?

Using more than one reviewer is rather like getting a second opinion on a medical diagnosis. When feasible and depending on the importance of the data element being sought, at least two reviewers should be used. Each of these reviewers should independently read and score each of the potentially included studies. They should then meet to resolve any discrepancies between the evaluation of the paper by open discussion. This discussion is a useful educational procedure in itself, which probably increases the consistency and accuracy of the appraisals of the paper.

How should the appraisal be used?

A critical appraisal of the retrieved papers addresses the methodological quality of the studies and the risk that studies overestimate or underestimate the true effect. It can be used in several ways:

1. *Decide which studies merit inclusion in the main analysis.* For example, with a question of treatment, we may confine ourselves to RCTs. But even deciding whether a study is properly randomized or not from the report can be difficult, which emphasizes the need to appraise papers carefully.

2. *Provide a table (or chart) summarizing the risk of bias in the included studies.* Specific features of each study are addressed and a judgment of bias for each is as 'low risk,' 'high risk,' or 'unclear risk.' The 'unclear' category indicates either lack of information or uncertainty over potential bias. For interventions the summary would typically include sequence generation (selection bias), allocation sequence concealment (selection bias), blinding of participants and personnel (performance bias), blinding of outcome assessment (detection bias), incomplete outcome data (attrition bias), and selective outcome reporting (reporting bias) (1). For diagnostic test performance the QUADAS-2 instrument is useful, which includes appraisal of representativeness, an acceptable reference standard, avoidance of differential verification, blinding of test interpretation, reporting of uninterpretable test results, and explanation of withdrawals (11).

3. *Group or sort by study design and/or methodological criteria.* It is useful to consider an exploratory analysis on study design and methodological criteria. Reports may be categorized by study design (e.g., randomized, cohort, case-control) or sorted by quality features and then plotted in rank order, with or without providing summary estimators for each of the groups of studies. One then needs to determine whether this influences the results.

4. *Meta-regression on design/methodological criteria.* An alternative procedure is to look at whether individual items make a difference to the effects seen in the studies. For example do the blinded studies give different results to the unblinded studies? Do the studies with good randomization procedures give different results to those with doubtful randomization procedures? It is possible to extend this further by looking at all the study design and methodological criteria simultaneously in a so-called meta-regression. This does, however, require sufficient original studies.

8.3.3 Summarizing and synthesizing the studies

How should the results of the identified studies be synthesized?

First, it is helpful simply to produce tabular and graphical summaries of the results of each of the individual studies, even if there is no attempt to combine their results. Second, if the studies are considered sufficiently homogeneous in terms of the question and methods, and this is supported by absence of statistical heterogeneity, then it may also be appropriate to combine the results to provide a summary estimate. The method for combining studies will vary depending upon the type of questions asked and the outcome measures used.

8.3.3.1 Graphical presentation of results

The most common and useful presentation of the results of the individual studies will be the plotting of a point estimate together with some measure of uncertainty (confidence interval) for each. This can be done whether we are reporting an effect measure on risk of an event such as the relative risk or hazard rate ratio of a CVD event or a specific outcome measure such as reduction in blood pressure. Studies can be sorted, e.g., by intervention type, by patient population, by study design, by publication year, or by breadth of the confidence interval. In addition, because studies with wide uncertainty draw greater visual attention, it is useful to specifically indicate visually the contribution of the study by the size of the 'dot' at the study's estimator of effect; specifically, the area of the dot could be made proportional to the inverse of the variance of the study's estimator. These principles are illustrated in Figure 8.3, which shows the results of the systematic review of colorectal cancer (12).

8.3.3.2 Summary estimates

Summary estimates may be reported as pooled relative risk (RR), relative risk reduction (RRR), risk difference (RD), absolute risk reduction (ARR), hazard

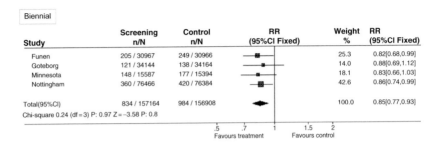

Figure 8.3 Relative risk (RR) of mortality from colorectal cancer in screened vs. unscreened randomized trials evaluating annual and biennial fetal occult blood test screening. CI, confidence interval. From (12) with permission.

rate ratio (HRR), odds ratio (OR), mean difference (MD), standardized mean difference (SMD), the proportion, the summary receiver operating characteristic (SROC) curve, or multivariate pooled outcomes (Table 8.3). Except in rare circumstances, it is not advisable to simply pool the results of the individual studies as if they were one common large study. This can be demonstrated to lead to significant biases because of confounding by the distribution of the intervention groups, particularly if the arms are unequal. Instead the appropriate method is to obtain an estimate of the effect for each individual study, along with the measure of the error (variance or standard error). The individual studies can then be combined by taking a weighted average of the individual effect estimates from each study, with the weighting being based on the inverse of the variance of each study's estimator. For example, Figure 8.3 shows, for colorectal cancer screening, the combined estimate (the center of diamonds on the line marked 'total') and its 95% confidence interval (the ends of the diamonds).

Although this principle is straightforward, there are a number of statistical issues, which make it far from straightforward. For example, the measures of effect have to be on a scale that provides an approximate normal distribution to the error (for example using the log odds ratio rather than just the odds ratio), and allowance must be made for zeros in the cells of 2×2 tables or outliers in continuous measurements. Fortunately most of the available software for doing meta-analysis provides such methods, and readers are referred

Table 8.3 Methods of meta-analysis for different types of questions

Question	Major quality issues	Databases	Usual goal of synthesis	Common analytical methods
Frequency or proportion	1. Random or consecutive sample 2. Adequate ascertainment (>80%) 3. Diagnostic reference standard	MEDLINE, EMBASE	Proportion	Pooled proportion
Diagnostic test performance	1. Random or consecutive sample 2. Independent reading of test and reference standard 3. Adequate verification (>80% or adjustment for sampling) 4. Adequate reference standard	MEDLINE, EMBASE	Pooled sensitivity and specificity Summary ROC	Hierarchical models: bivariate analysis Linear regression on transformed *FPRs*, *TPRs*
Prognosis	1. Random or consecutive sample 2. Patients at first presentation (or other defined time-point) in disease 3. Adequate (>80%) follow-up 4. Adequate measurement of outcomes	MEDLINE, EMBASE	Proportion or duration RR, HRR, OR	Inverse variance method Mixed models
Multivariable prediction rules (prognostic or diagnostic)	As per question (diagnostic or prognostic), plus: Was the rule tested in a validation cohort?	MEDLINE, EMBASE	Multivariable rule	Individual patient-level meta-analysis
Intervention effectiveness	1. Randomization of groups 2. Adequate follow-up (>80%) 3. Blind and/or objective assessment of outcomes	MEDLINE, EMBASE, Cochrane Central Registry, Trial Registries	RR, RRR, RD, ARR, HRR, OR, MD, SMD	Mantel–Haenszel methods Inverse variance method Random-effects meta-analysis. Mixed models

Abbreviations: RR, relative risk; RRR, relative risk reduction; RD, risk difference; ARR, absolute risk reduction; HRR, hazard rate ratio; OR, odds ratio; MD, mean difference; SMD, standardized mean difference; ROC, receiver operating characteristic; *FPR*, false-positive ratio; *TPR*, true-positive ratio.

elsewhere for the details of the properties of the various alternative statistical methods (13–17).

8.3.4 Generalizability and heterogeneity

The variation between studies is often considered a weakness of a systematic review but, if approached correctly, it can be a considerable strength. If the results are consistent across many studies, despite variation in populations and methods, then we may be reassured that the results are robust and transferable. If the results are inconsistent across studies then we must be wary of generalizing the overall results – a conclusion that a single study cannot usually reach. However, any inconsistency between studies also provides an important opportunity to explore the sources of variation and reach a deeper understanding of its causes.

The causes of variation in results may be due to population factors such as gender or genes, disease factors such as severity or stage, variation in the precise methods of the intervention or diagnostic test, or, finally, differences in study design such as randomization vs. cohort design, duration of follow-up, and blinding of outcome measurements. If the meta-analysis can adjust for the variation of these various factors across studies (through meta-regression) and any residual variation is thought to be due to limited sample size of the studies, then some fixed underlying true value is assumed to exist and we refer to such a model as a fixed effects model. When residual variation is due to both limited sample size of studies and due to residual heterogeneity (after adjustment) across study populations, we speak of a random effects model (15).

8.3.5 Question-specific methods

In addition to the general issues that have been described, there are additional issues and methods specific to the different types of questions: frequency, diagnostic test accuracy, risk factors and etiology, prognosis, and intervention. The principles of finding, appraising, and synthesizing apply to each, but specific literature search methods, appraisal issues, and methods of synthesis are needed. Table 8.3 outlines some of these specific issues. For example, column two lists some of the important quality issues relevant to each type of estimate. For further background on the appraisal for each type, we recommend the updated *JAMA* User's Guides series (18) http://jamaevidence.com/resource/520 and the *Cochrane Handbooks*.

There are various software packages available to perform the calculations and plots. None of these is comprehensive and most packages focus on a single question type. Even for addressing a single question more than one package may be required to provide all the needed calculations and plots. Available software includes Revman (from the Cochrane Collaboration), Meta-analyst, Comprehensive Meta-analysis, MIX, and macros in statistical programs such as Stata (for a updated list and URLs see: http://en.wikipedia.org/wiki/Meta-analysis#Software).

8.4 Subjective estimates

Sometimes it is not possible to assess a probability from 'hard' data. Even if we are comfortable in assuming that the patient at hand is representative of some well-defined population, we may not have any data available on what proportion of individuals in that population have experienced the event of interest. For example, the intervention being considered may be too new for any reliable studies to have been published.

While data on other patients might help us to assess each individual situation, since each patient and each circumstance is unique, a physician must often rely on some personal judgment. A probability based on a judgment as to one's strength of belief that an event will occur is called a *subjective probability* (or *personal probability* or *judgmental probability*). Subjective probability is a judgment, belief, or opinion ('the chances are ...') but we do not restrict the use of the word 'probability' to events for which true, underlying frequencies exist. Finally, subjective probabilities, as we have defined them, should obey all of the laws of objective probabilities, such as the summation principle. Subjective probabilities (a) should add to 1 for a mutually exclusive and exhaustive set of possibilities, and (b) are combinable by multiplication using the laws described in Chapter 3. If so, they are logically and mathematically equivalent to objective probabilities, and one can be unhesitatingly substituted for the other in decision trees, expected utility calculations, or Bayes' formula.

8.4.1 A definition of 'subjective probability'

Leaving the medical world temporarily, suppose that you are asked to estimate the probability that the next president of the United States will be a Republican. If the record over the past century is that 13 of the last 25 elections had been won by Republicans, you might estimate the probability as 13/25, or 0.52. Though useful background data, times have changed, and this may now be a poor estimate. An alternative approach would be to first marshal all the information at your disposal, then to answer subjectively questions of the following kind:

'Do you think it more or less likely that a Republican will be elected than that a flip of a coin, whose sides are equally weighted, will come up heads?'

An answer of 'more likely' indicates that: $p*$ [Republican] > 0.5,

where the asterisk reminds us that this is a subjective probability.

An answer of 'less likely' means that: $p*$ [Republican] < 0.5.

Suppose that your subjective answer is 'less likely,' then you might proceed by answering the following question:

'Do you think it more or less likely that a Republican will be elected than that the roll of a six-sided dice will come up with one or two dots?'

An answer of 'more likely' narrows the range further, so that $1/3 < p*$ [Republican] $< 1/2$.

We could continue to narrow the range by analogy to 'known' probabilities until we settle on a point estimate. In many clinical decision problems, it is sufficient to narrow to a range of probability (e.g., $0.3 < p < 0.4$), depending on the results of sensitivity analysis.

DEFINITION	Suppose that a person believes that an event E is just as likely to occur as another event whose probability of occurrence is defined objectively as $p*$. Then $p*$ is this person's *subjective probability* that event E will occur.

8.4.2 Why use subjective probabilities in decision analyses?

When the probabilities used in a decision analysis are based on objective evidence, we may have confidence in using such an analysis to help guide decision making. In effect, the decision analysis provides a structure for the information you want to take into account in reaching a decision. The analysis incorporates this information and the structural assumptions in a systematic fashion so that conclusions may be drawn.

When all of the required probabilities cannot be estimated from objective data, however, and subjective probabilities are used, the decision analysis continues to produce a quantitative conclusion that one strategy is better than another. By the nature of the method, however, the conclusion drawn is no more than a synthesis of the information that enters into the analysis. Therefore, if the probabilities are based on incomplete evidence or unsubstantiated personal judgment, then why bother with a formal analysis? This is a serious question and one that requires a serious answer, because many probabilities that are needed for decision analyses are not available from the medical literature. Here we offer a brief response to this question.

Most important is the observation that decisions must be made with or without decision analysis. Consider the following scenario. Suppose that you structure a decision analysis for a problem you face but find that one key probability cannot be estimated objectively. You agonize over this situation, but in the end you are unwilling to base your decision on an analysis into which is built a 'best guess' of this unknown probability. Since you have to make a decision, you do so based on your best intuitive judgment. In effect, you are discarding the entire analysis because of one weak link, this unknown probability. Now, suppose that you were to use the decision analysis, but instead of inserting your 'guess' for the unknown probability, you perform a threshold analysis that will indicate over what range of this probability your intuitive decision would be optimal. You find that your intuitive decision would be optimal only if the unknown probability is greater than 0.9. Therefore, in effect, your decision is consistent with an implicit belief that this probability is greater than 0.9. Whatever your beliefs about this unknown probability, *you have acted as if the probability were greater than 0.9.* If, in fact, you are quite confident that the probability, while unknown, is less than 0.5, you have acted inconsistently. Would it not have been better to make a subjective assessment of the probability, if only so that you could take advantage of the rest of the analysis? Then, when you find the result, you can always go back and do a sensitivity analysis with respect to that probability.

The point here is that decisions must be made and are implicitly based on judgments about probabilities of uncertain events. Why not be as explicit as possible about your strength of belief if you are going to act implicitly on that strength of belief in any case?

8.4.3 Probability assessments by groups of experts

When a probability is crucial to a policy decision but there is no direct evidence available, one approach to obtaining such probability assessments for policy decisions is to poll a group of experts. The premise in doing so is that, by interacting with each other, the group members will not be as prone to bias. Formal methods for obtaining group assessments are most likely to be useful in situations in which it is desirable to convince others of the validity of the decision analysis, objective estimates are not available, the personal opinions of a single decision maker will not suffice, and sensitivity analysis indicates that the conclusion is especially sensitive to a particular probability assessment.

One method for obtaining an answer is simple: ask each expert independently and take the average. While individuals can be poor at probability

Table 8.4 Delphi estimates of rabies after different types of exposure

Exposure	25th percentile	50th percentile	75th percentile	Range	Recommend PEP (% 'yes')
Skunk (bite)	0.05	0.05	0.05	0.1–0.01	100
Dog (bite)	0.00001	0.00001	0.0001	0.001 –0.00001	95
Dog (lick)	0.000001	0.000001	0.000001	0.00001–0.000001	10
Cat (bite)	0.0001	0.001	0.001	0.01–0.00001	100
Cat (lick)	0.000001	0.000001	0.000001	0.0001–0.000001	5

Data from reference 19; PEP: post-exposure prophylaxis

assessment, their average tends to be closer to the truth. Another more elaborate process is the Delphi method: each member of the group of experts is asked for their assessment, along with the reasons for the assessment, then, the results of this round of assessments are fed back to the members of the group, but in a way that preserves the anonymity of the assessors. Thus, they might be told that five assessors gave a probability between 0.2 and 0.25, ten assessors gave a probability between 0.25 and 0.30, and so forth. Then another round of assessments is solicited, and the process of feedback is repeated. The process continues until some specified level of consensus is reached or until a certain number of rounds have been conducted, whichever happens first. The theory behind the Delphi method is that the interaction of opinions still leads toward a consensus and will help eliminate individual biases. It is also held that the anonymity of responses will prevent the participants from reaching an agreement simply because of peer pressure. The method has been applied in studies of medical decisions and convergence was achieved.

In a recent example, a policy was needed on which people exposed to rabies should receive post-exposure prophylaxis (PEP), but information was lacking on the risk of rabies after different types of exposure. So a panel of 20 experts was used to assess these risks. In each round of the Delphi survey, responses were recorded under a pseudonym. For subsequent rounds, each expert received the aggregate results and was encouraged to provide comments about why they agreed or disagreed with the aggregated results and to explain the thought process behind their estimates.

A possible serious drawback of the Delphi method is that the tendency toward consensus may reinforce, and not eliminate, the biases that underlie some of the participants' probability assessments. Moreover, there is no guarantee that an assessment is accurate just because a group of experts can be made to agree on it. Caution should therefore be exercised in interpreting the probability assessments derived from a Delphi or other group procedures. Sensitivity analysis should always be used, just as for individual assessments, and there should be no misconceptions that a Delphi study of expert opinion is a substitute for a well-designed clinical study. For purposes of a clinician's own decision making, group assessment methods are generally impractical, although they can be used in certain hospital and group practice settings as part of a program of clinical rounds or, in particular, for developing guidelines.

8.4.4 Decision making versus truth

Many physicians and public health professionals object to the use of subjective probabilities and utilities because they are viewed as 'unscientific.' Some might also view subjective adjustments to objectively estimated probabilities, or syntheses of estimates from different data sources, as unscientific. Agreed, if your purpose is to state a scientific conclusion that one treatment is better than another, then subjective probabilities have no role to play. If you want to know the truth, then a 'best guess' is not acceptable, and you are right to insist on unimpeachable evidence, low p-values, and complete objectivity. If, however, you want to prescribe decisions *that have to be made* one way or another, then decision analysis is a tool for incorporating evidence, beliefs, and values in a systematic way. A careful decision analyst couches all conclusions as *conditional upon the assumptions*, and performs extensive sensitivity analyses to back up that outlook. A scientist in search of truth states conclusions as unconditional: $E = mc^2$, the earth is round. If Columbus and his peers had demanded unimpeachable evidence, the discovery of the New World by Europeans might have been delayed until the advent of satellite imagery!

In the following section, we consider some techniques designed to improve a clinician's skill in probability assessment and to permit several clinicians to pool their opinions in a structured way.

8.4.5 Integrating the evidence and subjective probabilities

What do you do when the literature does not quite fit your patient or target population? Over the past decade hundreds, perhaps thousands, of studies have been conducted and published which provide relevant and useful data for decision making. These include scores of studies of clinical outcomes, both randomized and non-randomized clinical trials, studies of new technologies, new drugs, clinical prediction rules, and so forth.

So, all things considered, whether a decision concerns choosing a treatment or assessing the usefulness of a diagnostic procedure, a clinician searching for relevant evidence is far more likely to find published evidence now than

20 years ago. Still, situations do arise when the literature doesn't quite fit and has to be somehow 'adjusted.' For example:

1. Your patient is not precisely the same as those in the sample used in any published study. In many randomized clinical trials, patients with co-morbidities are rigorously excluded, so that the effect of the experimental treatment on the index disease can be assessed with minimal confounding. Hence, patients in RCTs are less likely to have confounding co-morbidities. Your patient, on the other hand, may not match those who were enrolled. Your patient may be younger or older, sicker or healthier, and have more or different co-morbidities. The same problem may arise if you want to extrapolate the findings from a clinical study to the general population.

2. Of the studies bearing on your problem, the study whose sample most closely resembles your patient or target population appears to be the least trustworthy, perhaps due to flaws in the research plan, small sample size, or simply being older and perhaps out of date.

Given what we have said about possible errors in estimating subjective probabilities and the poor fit between your patient and the findings reported in the literature, we seem to have a dilemma: on the one hand, one must treat subjective probabilities cautiously, and on the other hand, one cannot avoid using them if the evidence in the literature really does not apply to your problem.

What can be done in these situations? There are a number of possible routes out of this dilemma:

1. Determine if the clinical situation, as you see it, is sensitive to variations in the plausible range of relevant probabilities. For example, your subjective estimates of the probabilities of various outcomes may be different from the frequencies provided in the literature, but in a simple decision tree, a threshold analysis may show that both estimates are on the same side of the treatment threshold. A related point is that sensitivity analysis and threshold analysis are always available as ways of improving your confidence in the conclusions of a decision analysis. We will return to the role of sensitivity analysis in the context of subjective probabilities shortly.

> (An important advantage of pursuing the analysis, even with subjective probabilities, is that it permits a more focused discussion of a clinical problem among physicians or policy makers. We believe that clinical and policy discussions are much more productive when the source of the disagreement over a decision can be isolated than when the discussion ranges unsystematically from issues of treatment efficacy to issues of valued outcomes to issues of treatment options. It is helpful to be able to focus on a subjective probability (or a utility value) as the source of dispute. The evidence pertaining to this probability can then be marshaled and, if a consensus cannot be reached, at least the parties to the discussion may be able to agree as to the reasons for their disagreement.)

2. If the different estimates lie on opposite sides of the treatment threshold, reflect on possible reasons for the discrepancy between the literature and your views:

    (a) Is your clinical impression based on audit or retrospective analysis of 30 or 50 or 150 local cases? Or is it based on three or fewer memorable cases? Memorable cases are likely to be unusual (due to the availability bias) and may be an unreliable guide to future experience.

    (b) Is your preferred line of action driven by regret minimization rather than by expected utility maximization? Are you really willing to forgo a fairly sizeable gain to avoid a very small chance of causing serious harm? Recall what we said in the opening chapter: the fundamental assumption of decision analysis is that the decision maker wishes to maximize expected utility. The techniques we have discussed in this book are designed to reach that goal. Regret minimization is sometimes a powerful motive, but it is not what decision analysis generally aims to achieve, although methods to include regret could theoretically be developed.

    (c) Ask if your subjective estimates are overly optimistic. If surgery is being considered for your patient and your estimates of the probability of a good outcome are substantially better than what is reported in the literature, consider this: is it probable that local outcome experience is substantially better than the pooled outcome data in a series of published studies? If you believe it is, what kind of data can be reviewed to support this claim? In other words, try to put your subjective estimates to the test of local evidence.

3. Go with a literature-derived composite and ignore personal and local experience. Limited personal clinical experience with the problem at hand, especially compared to the sample sizes reported in the literature, argues for this strategy. Also, this strategy may help you persuade others that your conclusion applies more broadly, an important consideration if you want to get your analysis published.

4. Ignore published literature and go with personal experience. It is tempting to do this because it will circumvent the prescriptive–descriptive issue. But this strategy is unwise if you expect to publish your work or convince others of its merits.

5. Combine estimates. The following approach should help to minimize undesirable effects of anchoring and adjustment:

    (a) Anchor on your personal or local experience and adjust your estimate in the light of the evidence.

    (b) Repeat this process, except now anchor on the evidence and adjust in the light of your clinical experience and beliefs.

(c) Split the difference between these estimates, weighting for the likely differences in the sample sizes behind each.

6. Formally revise a prior probability distribution on the unknown quantity. Formal Bayesian approaches may be helpful here. For example you may assess a subjective prior probability distribution for the quantity of interest. Then, using the evidence, revise your probability distribution using Bayes' theorem.

To illustrate the 'fully Bayesian' approach, suppose that you want to estimate a frequency, p, such as the prevalence of disease in your local clinic. You aren't sure what the value of p is, but you assess a distribution, assigning probabilities to the range of possible values of p from 0 to 1. The family of β distributions is often convenient for this purpose. Next, specify the likelihood of the observed data in the literature, conditional upon each possible true value of p. Data generated from a proportion p are usually modeled according to the binomial distribution, so it is possible to write down the binomial probabilities for the observed data. Finally, use Bayes' theorem to revise your prior distribution on p. This can be done with software designed to perform Bayesian probability revision, such as WIN-BUGS. If your prior distribution was a β distribution, the posterior distribution will also be a β distribution. Useful distributions for continuously valued quantities include the normal (Gaussian) distribution, the lognormal distribution, and the γ distribution. (For details, see a textbook on Bayesian statistics, such as [20]).

8.5 Sensitivity analysis revisited

How precise do our estimates of probability and values need to be? There is no single answer to this question. Rather it depends on whether changing a particular parameter changes the optimal decision. This in turn will depend on three things: how influential the parameter is in the analysis, its range of uncertainty, and how close the decision is to a particular threshold.

The influence of a probability or value depends on its overall contribution to the expected value, or more precisely, its contribution to the *difference* in expected value of different decision options. Some parameters may have little influence on a decision, even if they appear to be a large component. For example, if two drugs have similar toxicity profiles then the choice of drug will be insensitive to the values placed on those toxicities. However, the decision to use a drug at all may be very sensitive to those values. A better understanding of the influence of different probabilities and values may be gained through a series of sensitivity analyses. Ideally, a sensitivity analysis should be done for each parameter over its range of uncertainty. If you have good external relevant data, then the confidence interval may be used for the range of uncertainty. If there is only a subjective estimate then a subjective range may be needed.

If the sensitivity analysis shows that the decision is particularly sensitive to one or two parameters, then you should devote more care to how these were estimated. For example, you may consider doing a systematic review to obtain a combined estimate for a probability that is crucial to the decision. You may even consider that you need to initiate further research to obtain better values for future similar decision problems. Decision analysis is not just a tool for making an individual or policy decision – its real strength is in identifying what information is most needed to improve decision making. As we will see in Chapter 12, we would strongly recommend conducting a decision analysis and extensive sensitivity analysis before undertaking any new research to justify the new study and so that the study can be designed to gather information on the most relevant parameters.

8.6 Summary

The merit of a decision analysis depends on both the overall structuring of the problem and on the accuracy of the individual probabilities and values used. It is therefore important to access the best available information for these parameters. Some probabilities and values will come from external data. When there are several potential sources, we would ideally find or perform a systematic review and meta-analysis. However, performing a systematic review and meta-analysis is considerable work, and hence to make the analysis practical you may need to focus on the best single source available (using appraisal methods such as those described in Chapter 2). In choosing a source there may be a trade-off between the quality of the source (internal validity) and its relevance to your particular situation (external validity). There is no perfect 'objective' data, as there is always some degree of mismatch between the available data and your requirements. Hence expert judgment is required and subjective adjustment may be needed. If there is no external data, we still need to make a decision, and hence we may need to rely on subjective probabilities. Whether the probabilities are objective or subjective, you should undertake sensitivity analysis to check the robustness of any conclusions.

REFERENCES

1. Higgins JPT, Green S. *Cochrane Handbook for Systematic Reviews of Interventions.* (Version 5.1.0, updated March 2011) Oxford: The Cochrane Collaboration; 2011. http://handbook.cochrane.org/. Accessed Jan 14, 2014.
2. Montori VM, Wilczynski NL, Morgan D, Haynes RB. Optimal search strategies for retrieving systematic reviews from Medline: analytical survey. *BMJ.* 2005;330 (7482):68.

3. McManus R, Wilson S, Delaney B, et al. Review of the usefulness of contacting other experts when conducting a literature search for systematic reviews. *BMJ*. 1998;317(7172):1562.

4. Moher D, Pham B, Lawson M, Klassen T. The inclusion of reports of randomised trials published in languages other than English in systematic reviews. *Health Technol Assess*. 2003;7(41):1–90.

5. Rosenthal R. The file drawer problem and tolerance for null results. *Psychological Bulletin*. 1979;86(3):638–41.

6. Dickersin K, Min YI, Meinert CL. Factors influencing publication of research results. Follow-up of applications submitted to two institutional review boards. *JAMA*. 1992;267(3):374–8.

7. Song F, Parekh-Bhurke S, Hooper L, et al. Extent of publication bias in different categories of research cohorts: a meta-analysis of empirical studies. *BMC Medical Research Methodology*. 2009;9(1):79.

8. Simes RJ. Confronting publication bias: A cohort design for meta-analysis. *Stat Med*. 1987;6(1):11–29.

9. Schulz KF, Chalmers I, Hayes RJ, Altman DG. Empirical evidence of bias. *JAMA*. 1995;273(5):408–12.

10. Mahoney MJ. Publication prejudices: An experimental study of confirmatory bias in the peer review system. *Cognitive Therapy and Research*. 1977;1(2):161–75.

11. Whiting P, Rutjes AW, Reitsma JB, Bossuyt PM, Kleijnen J. The development of QUADAS: a tool for the quality assessment of studies of diagnostic accuracy included in systematic reviews. *BMC Medical Research Methodology*. 2003;3:25.

12. Hewitson P, Glasziou P, Irwig L, Towler B, Watson E. Screening for colorectal cancer using the faecal occult blood test, Hemoccult. *Cochrane Database Syst Rev*. 2007;1.

13. Arends LR, Hamza TH, van Houwelingen JC, et al. Bivariate random effects meta-analysis of ROC curves. *Med Decis Making*. 2008;28(5):621–38.

14. Cooper H, Hedges LV, Valentine JC. *Handbook of Research Synthesis and Meta-Analysis*. Russell Sage Foundation; 2009.

15. DerSimonian R, Laird N. Meta-analysis in clinical trials. *Controlled Clinical Trials*. 1986;7(3):177–88.

16. Littenberg B, Moses LE. Estimating diagnostic accuracy from multiple conflicting reports a new meta-analytic method. *Med Decis Making*. 1993;13(4):313–21.

17. Rothman KJ, Greenland S, Lash TL. *Modern Epidemiology*. Philadelphia: Lippincott Williams & Wilkins; 2009.

18. Guyatt GH, Rennie D, Meade MO, Cook DJ. *Users' Guides to the Medical Literature: A Manual for Evidence-Based Clinical Practice*. 2nd edn. American Medical Association, The McGraw-Hill Companies, Inc.; 2008.

19. Vaidya SA, Manning SE, Dhankhar P, et al. Estimating the risk of rabies transmission to humans in the US: a Delphi analysis. *BMC Public Health*. 2010;10(1):278.

20. Gelman A, Carlin JB, Stern HS, Rubin DB. *Bayesian Data Analysis*. 1995.

Constrained resources

There is no question that financial and medical effects will both be considered when making health care decisions at all levels of policymaking; the only question is whether they will be considered well.

Elaine J. Power and John M. Eisenberg

9.1 Introduction

Medical care entails benefits, harms, and costs. Until this chapter our approach has involved weighing benefits against harms for individuals and groups of patients and choosing the actions that provide the greatest expected health benefit. Now we extend our analysis to consider expressly the economic costs of health care and resource allocation decisions for populations.

As with all economic goods and services, the provision of health care consumes resources. Hospital beds, medical office facilities, medical equipment, pharmaceuticals, medical devices, and the time of physicians, nurses, other health-care workers, and family members all contribute to health care. The consumption of these resources constitutes the economic costs of health care.

Sometimes the word *cost* is used to refer to any negative effect of an action; for example, we might refer to the side effects of a drug as a 'cost' of treatment. In this chapter, however, we use *costs* only in the specific economic sense of resources consumed, whether materials or time.

Resources available for health care are limited in supply. This means that whenever resources are used for one activity, they are not available for other activities. An hour of a physician's time spent with one patient is unavailable for another, and an intensive care bed occupied by one patient cannot be used that day for another. Resources devoted to a smoking cessation campaign cannot be spent to increase seat belt use. Society can add to the resources devoted to health care by training more nurses, building more clinics, or launching new outreach programs. But even in the longer term, resources available for health care will be finite. Any medical decision or policy decision that entails the use of resources implicitly excludes those resources from alternative possible uses.

DEFINITION   *The opportunity cost* of a resource consumed in the provision of a good or service is the value of that resource in its next best alternative use.

Health resources are consumed in order to produce health benefits. Given the limited availability of resources, we are led naturally to ask questions about their most efficient use: is this particular expenditure of health resources worthwhile, given the alternative uses to which they might be put?

DEFINITION   *Costs* of health-care services are the economic resources (such as equipment, supplies, professional and non-professional labor, and the use of buildings) consumed in the provision of those services.

Our aim in this chapter is to introduce the conceptual and analytic issues surrounding decisions that involve the allocation of health resources. We will begin by considering a type of decision concerning the allocation of resources that busy clinicians face every day: the allocation of their time. Then we will introduce the principles underlying the efficient allocation of limited resources and discuss the major elements of cost-effectiveness analysis (CEA). Next we will focus on the correct calculation of incremental ratios for comparing the cost-effectiveness of interventions, describe current guidelines for the conduct of CEAs, and review methodological and ethical concerns. By the end of the chapter, you should know the rationale underlying CEAs, be able to assess them critically, and appreciate the potential for different conclusions about preferred interventions and programs when resource costs are ignored versus when they are included.

9.2 The efficient allocation of constrained resources

9.2.1 Time as a constrained resource for the clinician

Physicians and other clinicians know they cannot spend as much time with every patient as might be ideal. The constraints on time, which may have been pressing in years past, are even more pronounced in the current, more competitive health-care environment. Time spent addressing one health concern is time that is not spent in addressing another. Thus, time is a constrained resource that needs to be spent wisely.

Let us say that a primary care physician is considering what forms of preventive services to provide in order to maximize the overall health benefits to patients, given a limit, for example, of 20 minutes of contact time with a patient during an annual physical. Ideally the physician has estimates of the impact of various forms of preventive services in terms of the expected number of days of disability prevented or some other relevant health outcome measure. Note that this 'expected' benefit would not accrue to every patient but would accrue on average over the long run. Armed with this information, the physician would then be able to determine how best to allocate the 20 minutes among the possible preventive services in order to maximize the overall health benefits to the patient. This is done by ranking the possible care (s)he can provide in terms of resource-effectiveness and choosing those that provide the greatest gain in effectiveness for the amount of time spent until the 20 minutes are filled. (If you want to work through an example, see Exercise 9.1 on the book website.)

Other examples of this sort of allocation that physicians regularly perform include triage in an emergency room and the allocation of intensive care unit beds. Although the constrained resources in these examples include skilled nursing care and intensive care unit beds, the same principles of ranking in terms of resource-effectiveness and choosing according to the order of greatest efficiency apply.

9.2.2 Analytic tools for resource allocation: an overview

The analytic methods we present in this chapter are premised on a desire to use available resources to gain the most health benefit. We begin with the proposition that it is not possible to provide all beneficial health services to all people. In many countries, there is a fixed budget for health care; limited resources like hospital beds and specialized medical procedures are allocated by eligibility rules and waiting lists. Patients and clinicians alike are cognizant of the reality of resource limits. In the US, where there is no fixed budget for health care, the pressures of competing demands for tax dollars and employee compensation, and of price competition among insurers and providers, nonetheless constrain health-care spending.

There are several ways to control health-care costs. We can eliminate inefficiency in the delivery of care. Thus, many hospital services that can be provided on an outpatient basis with no loss in quality have been shifted to the lower-cost setting in recent years. We can weed out interventions known to be ineffective, saving the resources devoted to these interventions for productive purposes. We can make scheduling of operating room time more efficient to reduce the capacity required to handle the demand. Some have argued that investing resources in preventive services will save on future costs of chronic illness, although this proposition is not true in many cases. But in the end it is necessary to make choices among potentially beneficial health services.

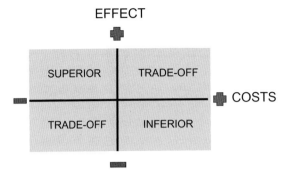

Figure 9.1 The cost-effectiveness plane, with costs on the *x*-axis and effectiveness on the *y*-axis.

Figure 9.1, known as the 'cost-effectiveness plane', categorizes health inter-ventions in terms of their cost (on the *x*-axis) and their health effect (on the *y*-axis) relative to the status quo (the origin in the figure). For interventions that can improve health and save resources at the same time (upper-left quadrant), there is no need for further analysis; they should be adopted. Similarly, there is no question that interventions that decrease health and consume resources (lower-right quadrant) should be discontinued if currently used and not adopted if new. Interventions falling into the other two quadrants, however, require choices if health benefit is to be maximized subject to available resources. These are interventions that improve health yet cost resources – the majority of effective interventions. In addition, actions that save resources, although at some loss of health outcome, should be considered if the resources saved could produce even more benefit if used elsewhere. These decisions apply to effective interventions currently in place that achieve less benefit with the resources they require than would a different use of these resources.

There are several related but distinct approaches to the assessment of health practices, which allow comparisons among interventions so that deci-sion makers can trade off opportunities for health-care investments falling in one of these two quadrants. These are included under the general heading of *economic evaluation*. The first, *cost-minimization analysis*, compares inter-ventions based solely on their net cost. This method applies when alternative options have (or are assumed to have) the same effectiveness. The measure used for comparison is the net difference in resource costs. Because health benefits, which are often difficult to quantify, do not enter into the calculation, cost-minimization analysis is generally simpler to undertake than other methods of economic analysis. But this restriction also limits its applicability.

Cost-effectiveness analysis compares interventions based on a common measure of their costs and a common measure of their health effectiveness.

The measure used for health effectiveness may be cases of a disease prevented, cases cured, lives saved, or years of life saved. It may also be a preference-based measure such as quality-adjusted life years (QALYs) gained, discussed in Chapter 4. Analyses using health measures that are expressed in quality-adjusted units are sometimes referred to as *cost–utility analyses*. Here, we use the term CEA to include this subset of analyses. The CEA can be used when alternative options have different costs and, when a common metric such as the QALY is used, different types of health consequences; by definition, however, all interventions compared must affect health.

Cost–benefit analysis requires that all effects of alternative interventions, as well as all costs, are valued in monetary terms. It can be used to compare very different interventions, including health and non-health investments of resources. Alternatives are considered on the basis of their net monetary benefit: options with a positive net monetary benefit should be implemented while those with a negative net monetary benefit should not. Cost–benefit analysis is used less frequently in health care than CEA, because many people are uncomfortable valuing health effects, such as human lives and the quality of life, in monetary terms. Objections are both technical, concerning the validity of methods used to assign a value to health effects, and ethical.

Because the concerns regarding cost–benefit analysis have led to a preference for CEA in the realm of health care, our focus in this chapter is on CEA. However, cost–benefit analysis is used in a sizeable fraction of economic analyses concerning health, particularly those examining environmental programs and other interventions that have important effects in non-health domains as well as affecting health.

Within the health-care sector, the term 'cost-effectiveness analysis' is often used interchangeably with 'economic evaluation', due to the overwhelming popularity of CEA as a technique. Therefore, when clinicians or analysts refer to 'CEA' they might be referring to the general approach of economic evaluation (including cost-minimization and cost-benefit analysis as well as CEA), or to the specific technique of CEA.

9.2.3 Perspectives for analysis

Resource allocation decisions are often made in the context of diverse views and preferences. Although there is sometimes an identifiable decision maker, such as a patient facing a decision regarding her own choices of therapy, often there is not. Many health and medical policies seem to 'emerge' or follow a tradition. More often than not, decisions made are the result of complex processes involving many protagonists.

Although actual decisions may involve a mix of perspectives and interests, CEA, as a prescriptive decision-making tool, begins with the specification of the decision-making perspective – the perspective of the analysis. The explicit specification of perspective is essential to economic evaluation generally and CEA in particular. An explicit perspective provides a framework for analysts in conducting an analysis and for users of that analysis, in making judgments about its validity. For example, in deciding whether to offer a particular screening program, a health plan would consider more than its costs to run the program and the potential health benefits to current enrollees. Factors such as the attractiveness of the program to desirable enrollees, its attractiveness to the medical staff, and the likelihood of those benefiting remaining enrolled would also be part of the equation. When the perspective of the analysis is clear, it is also clear what properly belongs in the analysis.

It is generally the consideration of resources in health and medical decisions that makes perspective a critical issue. If we consider only benefits and harms of health-care decisions, we usually encounter no conflicts of interest affecting these decisions. A notable exception involves communicable diseases, for which the actions of some individuals may affect the health of others: preventing or curing infection may reduce the risk of transmitting infection to others, and vaccination may reduce community risk through herd immunity. But in most cases, when cost is disregarded, the decision belongs to the patient and family, even when health-care providers and patients have different information about an intervention or different values concerning the outcomes.

Once concerns about health resources are introduced, however, the different perspectives invariably come into play. The owners of these differing perspectives have different goals for the allocation of resources. In addition, they experience different costs and different effects of interventions. For example, the benefit of successful knee surgery may be very different to a surgical practice or hospital, or to the health benefits manager of a professional sports franchise, than to an employer of computer programmers or the benefits manager of a symphony orchestra. The cost of a follow-up visit for a child's ear infection will be different for an uninsured patient facing a billed amount, an insured patient with a per-visit charge or co-pay, or a private pediatrician, whose cost would reflect her own time and her office expenses.

Resource allocation issues arise whenever decision makers face budget constraints. In the health-care arena, a range of decision makers confront these decisions. These include hospitals, clinics, private insurers, government entitlement programs, patients, and managed-care organizations, in addition to clinicians.

The societal perspective

Although some CEAs intended to assist patients, clinicians, and administrators with a specific decision will take the perspective of the individual or institution making the decision, many decisions require a broader analysis conducted from the societal perspective, because the resource consequences extend beyond the individual or institution making the decision. The societal perspective is the most comprehensive perspective for a CEA. It considers all ramifications of a decision: all costs, regardless of who experiences them, and similarly, all health benefits. The societal perspective is that of society at large – the sum of all individuals in society.

The societal perspective is prescribed for analyses that consider programs affecting the distribution of societal resources. In health care, however, many if not most decisions have implications for broader resource allocation. Societal implications are perhaps most obvious in decisions regarding government health policies and public health: programs financed by taxes for disease prevention, food and drug regulation, and publicly financed health care. But decisions in much more local contexts may also have implications for societal resource allocation. Choices concerning medical education and the practice of medicine may have a localized effect in the context of any particular patient but have a significant influence on society when they establish patterns of medical practice.

DEFINITION	*The societal perspective* is the one that considers everyone affected by an intervention and all significant effects and resource uses of the program.

Because a prime benefit of CEA is to allow decision makers to compare and make choices among programs, it is important that there be a bank of comparable CEAs. For this reason, analysts sometimes choose to conduct an analysis from the societal perspective instead of, or in addition to, an analysis from the patient, provider, or organizational perspective. Conducting analyses from different perspectives can also highlight situations where the incentives being faced by the person or party taking the decision are likely to lead them to take a decision that would be inefficient when judged from a broader perspective. For example, the system of funding hospitals might encourage them to retain some cases as inpatients, where it might be more cost-effective overall to treat them as outpatients.

Another perspective often encountered in published CEAs is the 'health care system' perspective, which includes costs that are considered part of the health-care delivery system, but which excludes non-health-care costs such as nutritional supplements and the time of unpaid caregivers. Sometimes the term 'payer perspective' is used to refer to this perspective, but that is not quite correct if some health-care services are not fully covered by the payer.

9.2.4 The cost-effectiveness analysis model

As described earlier, the underlying premise of CEA in health problems is that, for any given level of resources available, the decision maker wishes to maximize the aggregate health benefits conferred to the population of concern. Alternatively, a given health benefit goal may be set, the objective being to minimize the cost of achieving it. In either formulation the analytic methodology is the same. First, health benefits and health resource costs must each be expressed in terms of some unit of measurement. Health resource costs are usually measured in monetary terms but might equivalently be expressed in units of hospital days or hours of clinician time. Health effectiveness (or health benefit) is expressed in terms of some unit of output, such as the number of cases of cancer detected or in terms of a measure of ultimate outcomes, such as the number of lives or years of life saved. The use of QALYs has the advantage of incorporating changes in survival and morbidity in a single measure.

The cost-effectiveness measure is the ratio of costs to benefits and is expressed, for example, as the cost per year of life saved or the cost per QALY saved. Alternative programs or services are ranked from the lowest value of this cost-per-effect ratio to the highest, and then they are selected starting with the highest-ranked program or service until available resources are exhausted. The cost-per-effect ratio at which one is no longer willing or able to pay the price for the benefits achieved becomes the cutoff level of permissible cost per unit of effectiveness. For example, the level of blood pressure at which antihypertensive treatment is recommended might be based on some number of dollars per QALY. The application of this procedure ensures that the maximum possible expected health benefits will be realized, subject to whatever resource constraint is in effect.

The cost-effectiveness formulation

The cost-effectiveness ratio contains the net increase in health-care costs for an intervention *as compared to an alternative* in the numerator, and the net increase in health effect in the denominator. This ratio ($\Delta C/\Delta E$) can be summarized as follows:

$$\Delta C/\Delta E = (\Delta C_{Prog} + \Delta C_{Ind} + \Delta C_{Morb} + \Delta C_{SE} + \Delta C_{Prog\Delta Le})/\Delta E \quad (9.1)$$

where: ΔC_{Prog} = the cost of the program or intervention; ΔC_{Ind} = the cost or savings for procedures induced or avoided as a result of the program;

ΔC_{Morb} = the cost or savings for morbidity averted; ΔC_{SE} = the cost of treating side effects and complications; $\Delta C_{\text{Prog}\Delta\text{LE}}$ = the cost of health care in added years of life; ΔE = the change in QALYs or other measure of health benefit. These components of cost and health benefit are explained further in the sections on costs and effectiveness below.

CEA has been approached from more than one disciplinary direction. Cost-effectiveness research is conducted by economists, psychologists, physicians, and policy analysts. In this book, we present CEA in the context of a broader discussion of decision analysis. Decision-analytic concepts and methods are frequently used to perform CEA. The CEAs often contain important areas of uncertainty; as a result, the calculation of net health benefits[1] and net costs on the basis of a complex set of possible events and the probabilities associated with them is a primary challenge of the analysis. The methods described in this book – the construction of decision trees, Markov modeling, and the valuation of health outcomes – are central to CEA, although these elements may also be found in a variety of other analytical approaches. Other tools, including epidemiological analyses, spreadsheet programming, and simulation modeling, may also be employed to calculate the net costs and net health benefits in the cost-effectiveness ratio.

9.3 Costs

When health-care resources are limited, the consumption of resources by one patient means that somewhere, at some time, resources are unavailable for some other health-care purpose. It is thus the consumption of resources that constitutes the cost of care. As was mentioned earlier, the measure of cost is the value that is forgone when resources are used for one purpose rather than for the next preferred use. This amount – the value of resources in the next best use – is known as the *opportunity cost* of the resource.

The perspective of a CEA plays an important role in determining the opportunity cost of a resource. According to economic theory, the price of

---

[1] Note that here the term *net health benefit* refers to the overall net gain in effectiveness whereas in Chapter 12 the term *net health benefit* is used to express the overall gain in effectiveness minus the weighted monetary costs required to obtain that gain in effectiveness, the weight being the inverse of the threshold willingness-to-pay per unit of effectiveness. Distinguish these meanings from the term *net benefit* introduced in Chapter 3, and used in Chapters 6 and 7, which refers to the net gain in effectiveness from treating patients with the disease compared to not treating them. Yet one more similar term was introduced in Chapter 7, *net proportional benefit* (originally termed net benefit) which is the proportion of true positives in a study population minus the weighted proportion of false positives, the weight being the harm/benefit ratio of the treatment.

goods being sold in a competitive market should equal their opportunity cost. For a health-care insurer that pays this price, the price is indeed the opportunity cost; this is the amount that could be spent on the next best alternative if it were not used in this purchase. From the perspective of an insured patient, however, the cost of a drug may be equal not to its price but to the co-payment the patient pays. From the societal perspective, opportunity cost may also be difficult to ascertain, since impediments to perfect competition may push the price up or down relative to true opportunity cost. In the health care sector, these impediments include the existence of monopoly suppliers for some specialist services and the fact that some consumers (i.e., patients) may not be fully informed about the range of possible treatments and the benefits they may confer. Some practical approaches to the calculation of cost from the societal perspective are discussed in the next section.

It is important to note that real resource consumption is different from the transfer of resources from one party to another. The distribution of costs is an important but separate issue. If the government sends a check to a pharmacist as reimbursement for a prescription, this in itself does not constitute a resource cost from the societal perspective, because the resource pool is in no way depleted. From the societal perspective, the cost occurs when the drug is produced (and delivered to the pharmacy and ultimately to the patient), because resources put to this use cannot be put to another societal use. The cost is assigned to the patient who consumes the drug, because (s)he is the end-user of the resource, and this cost is unaffected by whether the patient, an insurer, the hospital (through unreimbursed care), or the government actually pays for it. Note that if only the government's perspective were considered, the government insurance payment would be a cost, because it would deplete the government's resources – the only resources of relevance in an analysis from this perspective. In CEA, the governmental perspective is different from the societal perspective.

9.3.1 Components of cost in CEA

9.3.1.1 Types of costs

Several types of cost comprise the total resource use to be considered in comparing health-care interventions. The first category, *health-care resources*, is perhaps the most obvious. Health-care resources used to produce a dental appointment, an inpatient admission, an X-ray, a pre-natal class, or other health-care service consist of supplies, pharmaceuticals, equipment and facilities, and tests. The time of health-care personnel – physicians, nurses, dieticians, and others – is often the most important health-care resource.

Non-health-care resources may also be required to produce a health-care service. For example, the transportation a patient needs to reach a clinic is a non-health-care resource, as is the television time used for a substance abuse prevention campaign. Costs associated with dietary changes or exercise routines taken up for health improvement purposes are other examples of non-health-care resources that are inputs to a health-care intervention.

The costs of time for the recipient of services are another resource used in the production of almost every health-care service. These *time costs* reflect the time required for transportation, for waiting in a clinician's office, and for receiving a service. They are distinct from the costs of health-care professionals' time, categorized as health-care costs, as described earlier. From the societal perspective, the value of an hour of the patient's time – the opportunity cost from the point of view of society – is assumed to be equal to the value of that time to the patient, and, for work time, is assumed to be reflected in the patient's wage. From other perspectives, however, the patient's time cost may be very different. The physician or managed-care organization may value the patient's time at zero. The patient herself, receiving paid sick leave, might also assign a cost of zero to time spent in recovering from an illness.

A related category of resource use is *caregiver time*. Caregiver time includes the value of time spent by informal caregivers ministering to a patient, and which would otherwise have been devoted to other activities. These individuals may be volunteers or family members. (If caregivers are paid a market rate for their services, they are generally included in the category of health-care resources, rather than counted as 'caregiver time.') Perspective again plays a role in determining the value of caregiver time. From the perspective of a hospital or managed-care organization, the time of a family caregiver is free. From the societal perspective or the perspective of the patient's family, the caregiver's time has an opportunity cost.

Illness (and death) affect the individual's ability to perform his or her normal activities. The lost or impaired ability to do work results in costs from the societal perspective. These costs are referred to as *productivity costs*. Since individuals trade off leisure and work based on their relative value, according to economic theory, productivity costs include the value of lost leisure as well. Productivity costs are in addition to time costs, which only account for the time the recipient of health care devotes to the health-care program or intervention. Productivity costs reflect the societal value of time spent sick or in reduced health, or of time lost through death.

In cost–benefit analysis, effects on longevity and impaired or improved productivity are translated into their monetary value. These productivity costs are combined with other types of costs and savings to obtain a summary measure of net benefit in monetary terms. In CEA, these same consequences are treated as 'effects' and placed in the denominator of the cost-effectiveness ratio, measured in terms of quality of life and life extension. Technically, we could monetize part or all of these productivity effects and place them in the numerator. In fact, a number of analyses have used this approach. The only caveat is that an effect on productivity must not be double-counted by being placed in the denominator (e.g., as a reduction in QALYs) and in the numerator (as a monetary cost) at the same time. The economic value of productivity gains to individuals *other than* the patient – to employers, to taxpayers, and to the rest of society – should ideally be counted in the numerator, although this is not always done if the so-called 'external benefit' is small.

Whether or not respondents take account of productivity effects in their valuations of health states has been the subject of debate. Some instruments for valuing health states explicitly ask respondents not to take into account the impact on ability to work by asking them to imagine that their income would be protected by unemployment insurance (1). However, many instruments are silent on this matter. Tilling et al. argue that avoiding mentioning income effects in health-state valuations may induce a minority of respondents to include them, but the impacts on the QALY estimates are minor (2). In a further study, where respondents used the time trade-off method to value EQ-5D states, explicit inclusion or exclusion of income effects had little impact on the health-state valuations (3).

In addition to the possibility of double counting, there are two other reasons why productivity costs are often excluded from economic evaluations. First, if an analyst is conducting a CEA from the perspective of a health-care decision maker, it could be argued that the decision maker's main concern is to maximize the health gain from the budget at his or her disposal. This argument is often made in budget-constrained systems, like the UK National Health Service (4). Secondly, if productivity gains are valued, as in a cost-benefit analysis, with reference to the patient's wages, a higher value would be given to providing health-care interventions for those in highly paid jobs. It is sometimes argued that this infringes the equity principle, although the problem can be minimized by using national average wages to value productivity gains, as opposed to the wages of the particular patients receiving a given treatment.

9.3.1.2 Sequence of costs

The costs of health-care resources, non-health-care resources, patient time, and informal caregiver time may be accrued in a single time period or in progressive stages associated with an intervention. Analysts generally calculate the net cost of an intervention by laying out the stream of events occurring with the intervention and the stream of events occurring without the intervention, and then comparing the costs associated with each scenario. This process of 'laying out' the scenarios can be done through a simple itemization of events, a decision tree, a Markov model, or a complex simulation of events.

The costs in the event streams fall into the categories of *initial costs, induced costs*, and *averted costs*. The *initial costs* are those associated with the intervention itself, such as the costs associated with a physician visit and pathology examination for cervical cancer screening. The *induced costs* are those that result from the intervention. In the case of cervical cancer screening, costs for the follow-up of a positive test are induced costs – for the investigation of false-positive as well as true-positive results. The costs of treatment for cases of cancer detected would also be induced costs. *Averted costs* are the costs associated with the stream of events that would have occurred in the absence of the intervention, but because of it did not occur. The cervical cancer screening program would detect some pre-cancerous lesions and early-stage cases of cervical cancer, and by doing so, it would avert some cases that would have been detected in later stages. All costs associated with averted cases – costs associated with their future detection, diagnosis, and treatment and any costs associated with the morbidity they would have imposed – are included in the scenario that would have occurred without the intervention, and thus included in the calculation of *net* cost for a CEA.

9.3.1.3 Costs in added years of life

One of the outcomes that may ultimately result from a successful intervention is an increase in life span. Many health-related programs, including legislation requiring child safety seats and interventions such as antihypertensive medications, have been shown to increase longevity. Although these added years are part of the scenario that occurs with the intervention – and are included in the calculation of net *effectiveness* almost without exception – there is some debate about whether to include all of the *costs* associated with these added years of life.

The costs associated with *health-care interventions* during added years of life are typically included. Thus, if a drug regimen averts a fatal myocardial infarction at age 53, but a fatal stroke occurs at age 83, the costs of medical care for the myocardial infarction and the stroke are included in the respective scenarios. Most decision analysts and health economists include costs for health-care interventions whether these costs are related or unrelated to the specific disease spectrum at issue. For example, in this case, 'unrelated' health-care costs would include those for treating osteoporosis or cancer in later life. One argument sometimes given for not including them in (say) the evaluation of a hypertension treatment program is that they result from later treatment decisions that should be evaluated on their own merits. An argument for including 'unrelated' costs is that it is often difficult to distinguish 'related' from 'unrelated' costs. Further details on this issue may be found in papers by Meltzer (5) and Johannesson (6).

A more vexing question is whether *non-health-related* resource use for years of added life should be included in the treatment scenario. The non-health-related costs, for example for food and clothing, represent real resource use and theoretically should be included as costs associated with added years of life. For example, Meltzer (5) develops a theoretical argument for considering the impacts on all aspects of an individual's consumption and production. However, some have argued that including costs of living as real 'costs' to society runs counter to the social objective of lengthening life. Furthermore, it may lead on to the conclusion that some individuals are more worthwhile keeping alive than others! Other analysts argue on a technical level that the consistent exclusion of these costs would simply result in consistently lower cost-effectiveness ratios, and therefore would not affect decisions made using CEA results (7), although it is likely that their inclusion or exclusion would affect the *relative* cost-effectiveness of programs aimed at young individuals as opposed to those aimed at the elderly (8). In practice, most CEAs have not explicitly included these non-health-related costs of life extension.

9.3.1.4 The scope of costs associated with an intervention

The sequence of initial, induced, and averted costs reflects the timeline of costs that are included in a CEA. However, it is also important that an analysis reflect the breadth of costs associated with an intervention. These include costs associated with side effects and complications of an intervention. The costs may be short-term, such as the costs of acetaminophen for a fever or soreness following a child's vaccination. They may also be long term, such as the costs associated with treatment of chronic mental disorders or of long-term disability associated with stroke.

Events initiated by an intervention may also spill over to individuals other than those directly receiving the intervention. Treating a patient with human immunodeficiency virus (HIV) infection may prevent transmission to a spouse or others in the community. Vaccinations protect others in the community through 'herd immunity,' whereby the vaccinated individual can no longer transmit the infection. A smoking cessation program may prevent morbidity among household members as well as the smoker himself. In general, analysts decide on whether to include costs associated with these chains of events extending from an intervention based on their potential importance in the analysis. Large spillover costs should be included, while relatively small ones can safely be ignored.

9.3.2 Measuring costs – health-care resources

From most analytic perspectives, the measurement of health-care resource costs – their opportunity cost – is relatively straightforward: it is the price the patient or health-care institution pays for a drug, an hour of physician time, or other resource. It is clear in this individual or institutional setting that the price reflects the value of resources that are no longer available for an alternative use. The measurement of such costs from the societal perspective is conceptually and practically more challenging; most of this section will be devoted to costs from this perspective.

Society's opportunity cost for a resource is also, in theory, equal to the market price for those goods or services in a competitive market. In practice, however, opportunity cost may be much more difficult to establish. For one thing, the assumption that market price reflects opportunity costs implies that the marketplace meets the criteria set forth in welfare economics for a perfectly competitive market – or at least, that the market does not diverge too much from these criteria. But the health-care marketplace is non-competitive in many respects. Because medical science is complex, the consumers of health care frequently are not the 'fully informed' buyers that consumers of commodities are assumed to be. In addition, the patient is frequently covered by insurance and therefore does not experience the full cost of a purchase. For these reasons and many others, the economic forces of supply and demand cannot be presumed to function in the same way as in the market for bananas or bicycles.

There are many other reasons why 'prices' in the health-care arena must be viewed with skepticism. Prices are often set administratively by an insurer or government program. In the USA, physicians facing one set of administrative prices from Medicaid, may adjust their prices to recoup earnings from other payers, making it even more difficult to determine the 'real' price. Hospital charges may be inflated above cost by an arbitrary ratio, with the amount depending upon the purchaser. In public clinics and hospitals that have an annual budget, there may be very little accounting of the costs of clinician time and no way to determine costs in relation to specific patient diagnoses. Managed-care organizations, too, do not have prices for specific health-care services.

There are two general methods of developing cost estimates for health-care services that have multiple components, such as a hospital inpatient day, a clinic visit, or complete pre-natal care. The first is to begin with an existing price or set of prices and adjust for known influences. This method, sometimes referred to as *gross-costing*, draws upon fee or payment schedules. In the USA, frequently used sources include the Medicare fee schedules for professional and ambulatory care and the hospital payment schedule based on diagnostic-related groups (DRGs). Hospitals' fee schedules are also used, adjusted using cost-to-charge ratios that may be applied broadly or to specific cost centers. Adjustments for geographic price variations or practice variations may also be used.

The second method, *micro-costing*, involves enumerating the inputs to a service, collecting data on unit prices, and then compiling the cost estimate. For example, an HIV counseling and testing session might be broken down into many components, including the counselor's time, the nurse's time, the test supplies, other medical supplies, telephone time, and written materials (9). Each of these components would be assigned a unit cost, for example, $4 for each ten minutes of the counselor's time. The cost estimate would then be developed using the estimates of resource use and the unit cost estimates.

Some rules of thumb have been developed for pricing resources commonly used in health care. The cost of pharmaceuticals, for example, is often taken from the cost paid by government formularies in countries that have them. In the US, the average wholesale price, which approximates drug prices in discount pharmacies, and the average sales price, which reflects a wider range of purchasers, are frequently used.

9.3.2.1 Long-run versus short-run resource costs

One important consideration in assessing the cost of a service is whether and how to include 'overhead' items such as telephone, rent, or office equipment and other 'fixed' costs. In assessing the cost-effectiveness of an intervention, fixed costs – those that are not affected by the decision under consideration – should not be included in the analysis. Thus, if a clinic is deciding whether or not to add an evening health education class that will use the facility during hours when it would otherwise be closed, the cost of running the class should not include an allocation of the clinic's rent. However, the initial start-up costs, such as for training volunteers or purchasing extra chairs, should be included. And if the class requires the clinic to add hours for their cleaning service, this incremental cost should also be included as a cost of the program. The costs that vary as a result of the program are termed 'variable costs.'

The determination of whether a cost is fixed or variable depends to a great extent on the time frame of the analysis. The costs of implementing a community-based cancer screening program or developing a drug are variable when the decision is whether to undertake the program, but they are fixed once a program has been started, a drug has been developed, or a large capital investment has been made. Costs for rent or for large pieces of equipment are typical examples. The marginal cost for one additional computed tomography (CT) scan examination may be low, and this is the appropriate cost to use in a short-run decision. The marginal cost of letting a patient remain in a hospital bed for an extra day when there is extra capacity on the hospital floor is also relatively low – presumably, it does not affect staffing levels, costs for heat or electricity, administration, or any other of the 'fixed' costs of running the hospital.

However, costs that are fixed in the short run are generally variable over the longer term. Utilization levels over time will determine decisions regarding staffing levels, the purchase of additional equipment, and construction of additional capacity over the long term. As a result, equipment such as the CT scanner, items included in 'overheads,' and other seemingly fixed costs, should be included in any analysis that has general policy implications or implications for health-care practices over the long term. As a general rule, CEA should employ *long-run marginal costs*.

When the decision has been made to include the cost of a relatively long-lasting resource, there are a variety of methods for spreading the cost over the life of the investment – a process known as *depreciation*. The simplest method of depreciation is to divide the purchase cost (less the residual value at the end of useful life) by the number of years the resource will be used. This gives the yearly cost of the capital investment. If a new piece of diagnostic equipment is purchased for $2 million and is fully depreciated over ten years, its cost could then be calculated as $200 000 per year. This method is known as *straight-line depreciation*.

However, straight-line depreciation does not reflect the time value of money – the opportunity cost of resources over time – which is reflected in part by interest rates on bond or loans. In order to capture the time value of money the annual cost can be calculated using an amortization formula. The amortized annual cost is the amount that would have to be paid during each year of the useful life of the capital investment in order to repay the principal plus interest on a loan (e.g., mortgage) to purchase the investment. Since construction and capital equipment are often financed through borrowing, amortization frequently approximates the actual timing of expenditures. If the annual interest rate is i, the term (useful life) is N years, and the purchase price is P, then the amortized annual cost M (i.e., the annual mortgage payment for payments incurred at the beginning of the year) is given by the formula:

$$M = P \cdot i \cdot \frac{(1+i)^{N-1}}{(1+i)^{N}-1} \tag{9.2a}$$

If the mortgage payments are incurred at the end of each year, the formula is:

$$M = P \cdot i \cdot \frac{(1+i)^{N}}{(1+i)^{N}-1} \tag{9.2b}$$

From the societal point of view, the amortized value is more accurate than the straight-line value, because money invested in equipment cannot be used productively elsewhere to yield the normal rate of return. Therefore, the imputed annual cost should reflect not only the purchase price but also the forgone interest.

9.3.2.2 Adjustments to prices

9.3.2.2.1 Inflation

Most of us are accustomed to the idea that $20 today can buy less than $20 years ago, say in the 1950s. These differences in purchasing power result from inflation. Because of inflation, expenditures or savings occurring in different years cannot simply be added together. They must first be converted to a common year by adjusting for inflation.

Inflation-adjusted amounts represent real resource costs in the chosen year. Dollar amounts that are inflation-adjusted are said to be in *constant dollars* or *real dollars*.

Analysts in the US generally adjust for inflation using the Consumer Price Index (CPI). (In other countries, and also sometimes in the US, analysts may use an index of inflation called the gross domestic product [GDP] deflator.) The CPI, published annually by the Bureau of Labor Statistics, is derived by evaluating the changes in price for a given market basket of goods. Although this index may be subject to error if the composition of the market basket is not reflective of purchases generally, the CPI is an accepted standard for price adjustment.

DEFINITION	*Inflation* is a fluctuation in the value of a currency resulting in an increase in prices unrelated to changes in the value of commodities.

The CPI is available for all items and for various categories of goods and services, such as medical care, medical care commodities, and dental services. The component indices are more accurate than the general CPI for categories of goods or services, experiencing a different rate of inflation than the overall economy. Health economists do not agree on whether the overall CPI or the Medical Care CPI should be used in health-related CEA. While it would seem silly to factor in price inflation for items having little to do with the production of health care, there are inevitable limitations in the way price inflation is measured for health care that render it questionable. For example, the quantity and quality of health services, such as a hospital day, are hopelessly intermingled, leaving open to question whether the Medical Care CPI really measures the relative prices of a fixed market basket of health-related items.

9.3.2.2.2 Cross-national conversions

To compare cost-effectiveness results across national boundaries or to use cost estimates from different countries, currencies must be converted to the same metric, for example Canadian dollars or Japanese yen. This can be done simply by applying current currency conversion rates – or rates for another base year. A superior approach would be to use purchasing power parities where these exist, since these eliminate the impact of short-term fluctuations in exchange rates. However, those conducting cross-national comparisons must use caution, because analyses from different countries may contain many assumptions that affect cost-effectiveness results. For example, the relative rates for physician labor and prices for pharmaceuticals often differ sharply, depending on the country. More significantly, the actual quantities of resources used for a service may differ widely from country to country. In a CEA of hypertension treatment, for example, it would be incorrect to apply the averted costs for stroke and heart disease in the USA and simply convert the currencies, if the practice patterns and interventions for treating cardio-vascular disease differ markedly across countries. (The issues of transferring economic data or analyses from one setting to another are discussed in more detail in Section 9.9.)

9.3.3 Measuring time and other resource costs

9.3.3.1 Time

According to economic theory, the value of patient and caregiver time, like the value of health-care commodities, is equal to the opportunity cost of these resources. Although the opportunity cost of medical supplies, drugs, and other direct health-care resources may be indicated by its market price, this measure does not exist for patient and caregiver time.

To assign a value to patient and caregiver time from the societal perspective, analysts generally look to the market price – wage – for an hour of time of employed people with similar characteristics. Thus, the opportunity cost for the value of the time of a 45-year-old, college-educated woman caring for an elderly parent at home would be estimated using the average hourly wage of similar women in her geographic area.

However, strictly speaking, the value of time should depend on what is being sacrificed in terms of paid work, unpaid work, or leisure. Koopmanschap et al. (10) review several methods for valuing caregiver time. Van den Berg and Ferrer-I-Carbonell (11) estimate the value by assessing the level of compensation caregivers would require to maintain the same level of well-being after providing informal care.

One dilemma in using wages is how narrowly to define the group for which the wage is assessed. For example, if a patient is a 20-year-old Hispanic woman, should her time cost be approximated using an average wage for all 20-year-olds? All 20-year-old women? All Hispanic 20-year-old women? Narrower definitions can produce more accurate estimates of the individual's true opportunity cost. However, a broader definition may be preferred if it captures relevant characteristics and omits spurious ones. Broader categories may also be preferred on equity grounds, to avoid systematically valuing the time of some groups more than others.

9.3.3.2 Measuring productivity costs

As noted earlier, productivity costs may be included as monetary costs in the numerator of a CEA or subsumed in the QALY measure in the denominator. Even when the patient's valuations of productivity changes are subsumed in the QALYs, there is still a need to value the productivity-related benefits to others, such as employers and taxpayers.

As stated earlier, the economic theory of competitive labor markets suggests that gross earnings (i.e., the full costs of employing the worker, including pensions and related benefits) reflect the value of an individual's productivity. (This is known as the *human capital* approach to the valuation of workers' time.) Economic theory holds that this valuation also applies to leisure time, as long as the individual has the opportunity to adjust hours worked in response to opportunities. Physicians call it moonlighting, professors call it consulting, laborers call it overtime, but these are all examples of this phenomenon. The implication for CEA is that, if one chooses to measure the value of productivity in monetary terms, the wage is a good place to start.

However, some special issues arise when considering the value of productivity to parties other than the patient. Employers who have to replace workers in the short run incur replacement costs. These costs may already be reflected in the 'sick pay' and 'vacation pay' they consider part of the full cost of retaining an employee. But if an employee is lost for the long term, there are costs of recruitment, training, and waiting for the new employee to reach the same place on the 'learning curve' as the former employee. In addition, workers who continue to work at a lower level of productivity after an illness impose costs on their employers.

This approach to estimating production losses, known as the *friction cost* method, was first proposed by Koopmanschap et al. (12). The essence of the approach is that the loss in productivity when a person is sick depends on the *friction period*, the time it takes for the employer to restore production to its original level. The friction period will depend on the industry, the type of job, and the nature of the illness (e.g., short-term or long-term). Koopmanschap et al. argue that this is a superior approach to the human capital approach, since the latter assumes that the full value of the worker's production is lost in all instances, whereas in reality adjustments are often made to minimize the impact of a worker's illness.

One potential downside of the friction cost approach is that the estimates are harder to generate, given their dependence on the specific job situation. However, Koopmanschap et al. (12) were able to generate estimates of the production losses from absence from work, disability, and mortality for the Netherlands. Estimates obtained by the friction cost method were around 11.5% of those calculated using the human capital approach.

9.3.3.3 Valuing outcomes in cost–benefit analysis

In cost–benefit analysis, all resource use and all health benefits are monetized, so that effects on both health and productivity are always expressed in monetary terms. The classic approach to valuing these outcomes in cost–benefit analysis is called the *human capital* method. The human capital approach equates the value of health to earnings. Thus, the value of lost years of life is estimated as the value of projected future earnings, taking into account such factors as the age, gender, and education of the individual. Some who have taken this approach use the *net* value of earnings, subtracting the individual's anticipated consumption from expected earnings. This approach implies that the individual's value is only what he or she contributes to the rest of society, excluding himself or herself. Others use the *gross* present value of earnings, effectively counting the individual as one of the intended beneficiaries of his work.

The other main monetary method for valuing added years of life and improved functioning is the calculation of the amount an individual is willing to pay for these improvements. The *willingness-to-pay* method takes into account subjective values associated with health and life. We introduced the willingness-to-pay method in the context of valuing health states, and in this regard it functions much like a utility scale. When the values from a population are aggregated, willingness to pay provides a measure of the societal value attached to a given health benefit.

Estimates of willingness to pay can be obtained either by looking at revealed willingness to pay – actual purchases or risk trade-offs – or by eliciting willingness to pay from individuals. For in vitro fertilization, for example, revealed willingness to pay could be determined by looking at the amounts paid by couples not covered by health insurance. (This would provide an upper-bound estimate, as couples who are willing to pay a lower amount would be unable to purchase the service.) Willingness to pay could also be elicited by presenting couples with various scenarios concerning their probability of becoming pregnant with and without in vitro fertilization, and asking their willingness to pay for the intervention.

Like the human capital approach, willingness to pay has important limitations as a measure. A person's willingness to pay varies according to the baseline probability of death or illness and by the amount the intervention reduces the risk. However, since these variations do not have a linear relation to risk changes, willingness to pay cannot easily be inferred across a range of initial probabilities, posing a daunting task for a researcher requiring willingness-to-pay information for a broad range of possible risk scenarios. Furthermore, willingness to pay can assign higher values to life-saving interventions and quality-of-life improvements for the affluent, since willingness to pay increases with wealth. On a practical level, it may also be difficult for subjects to contemplate how much they would be willing to pay for changes in low-probability risks. Despite the challenges it presents for valuing health outcomes, cost–benefit analysis is preferred by many economists, and by some regulatory agencies in the US. The Environmental Protection Agency (EPA) uses an explicit value per statistical life saved (not per life year saved), based on willingness to pay.

9.4 Effectiveness

As discussed earlier, health benefits in CEA are described using non-monetary measures. A wide variety of measures has been used. These include both single measures and combined measures of health benefit.

9.4.1 Single measures of health outcome

The outcomes of programs and interventions are frequently multidimensional, but in some instances an analyst may be interested in only one dimension of a health outcome. Single measures of health effect include, for example, the number of cases of polio prevented, number of cases of breast cancer detected, or a reduction in average number of cigarettes smoked per day. These measures are appropriate for very targeted analyses, where an immediate goal has been identified and the objective of the analysis is to determine efficient ways of reaching this goal. Because the outcome measure is an initial or intermediate outcome, the analysis will not be able to contribute to assessing longer-term goals of health care, quality-of-life improvement or longevity. Another limitation is that cost-effectiveness ratios that use such outcomes can be used only to compare programs whose only important health effect is on this single measure.

Data collected for a CEA very often will focus on a short-term outcome. For example, a study of a smoking cessation program would collect data on outcomes reflecting the amount of smoking and the length of time smoking cessation or reduction is maintained. The study would be unlikely to collect data on morbidity or longevity long term. However, the CEA, if it is to contribute to broad resource-allocation decisions, can and should link these initial outcomes to long-term outcomes, using data from other studies to model length and quality-of-life effects. A careful ascertainment of the links between initial and longer-term outcomes is essential to insure that the initial outcome is in fact meaningful in terms of its real implications for health.

Single measures of health effect can also be measures of long-term outcomes. Number of lives saved and number of life years saved are measures of health benefit that are frequently used alone. Their drawback is that they are usually incomplete measures of the effect of interventions, which generally influence quality of life over a span of time as well as length of life. Furthermore, the notion of 'saving a life' is really meaningless, since lives cannot be saved, only extended. It is possible for a single intervention in an individual patient to 'save' the same life many times over! For interventions that primarily extend life, however, the measure of life years gained may be adequate.

9.4.2 Combined measures of health outcome

For interventions where both effects on quality of life and length of life are important – or where the timing of quality-of-life effects is important – the preferred outcome measure is the QALY, which combines measures of length and quality of life. As described in Chapter 4, QALYs are calculated by using a scale to value the quality of life in a particular health state, multiplying by the amount of time in the health state, and then summing these weighted values.

Two important methodological concerns in developing QALY estimates for CEA concern the appropriate type of weight to be used for adjusting life-years and the appropriate source of the weight.

9.4.2.1 Preference-based measures vs. health status measures

The measures of quality of life used in CEA are preference-based. *Preference-based measures* are those that reflect the value an individual attaches to a health state. Thus, these measures do not simply characterize a state of health but demonstrate people's preferences for these states. Preference weighting gives meaning to QALY measures in that results can be interpreted to reflect the relative desirability of health outcomes (Chapter 4).

Preference-weighted measures are distinct from the health status measures that currently abound in the field of health services research. *Health status measures* are systems for defining and describing health states. These measures define a set of domains of health, such as physical health, mental health, and role functioning, and describe health status based on an instrument that assesses health in each domain. The result is a numerical score, such as obtained by the Medical Outcomes Study SF-36 (13). Numerical disease-specific scales are also used to summarize health status for many chronic conditions such as arthritis and depression.

Health status measures can be used as part of the process of estimating QALYs, describing the health states to which preferences are applied. However, they are not in themselves preference-weighted measures – in fact, they are not weighted at all, either using preferences or other weights. Their preferred use is in assessing health status in population surveys or clinical trials, rather than in CEA. So, for example, the SF-36 has been used in studies monitoring health status for patients with diabetes, cancer, and other conditions, and examining the outcomes of medical and surgical interventions.

Preference-based measures fall into two categories: those derived from utility theory, such as the standard gamble and time trade-off, and psychological scaling methods such as the rating scale. As pointed out in Chapter 4, however, there is no justification for using the numerical values from a rating scale in calculating quality-adjusted life expectancy, because there is no indication that these reflect either preferences under uncertainty, or trade-offs between longevity and quality of life, let alone both. For this reason, many analysts prefer utility-based methods for assigning weights to be used in CEA.

Utility-based methods include the standard gamble and time trade-off. These methods involve comparisons of hypothetical choices between the certainty of time in a health state and a gamble between a better and a worse option. Respondents' preferences are used to reveal their utility for a health outcome, a preference that satisfies the axioms of utility theory. These preferences are theoretically suitable for computation of expected utilities to represent preferences among alternatives with uncertain outcomes. The main disadvantage of utility-based measures is that they can be conceptually difficult for respondents, as discussed in Chapter 4.

9.4.2.2 Sources of preferences for CEA: community vs. patient preferences

An important consideration in determining QALYs is the source of preferences to be used in an analysis. In an analysis from the patient's perspective, the patient is clearly the appropriate source. In an analysis from the societal perspective, the choice is less evident. Patients and their families have the most experience with a given health state and are most familiar with implications for quality of life. However, people's views about illness and disability change based on their experience, and from an *ex ante* perspective, it is perhaps the general population that has claim to the more 'objective' point of view.

Use of patient preferences is often preferred when an analysis is designed to compare different interventions for the same patient group. For example, in a CEA comparing two drug therapies for coronary artery disease, preferences could be solicited from cardiac patients without introducing concerns regarding the relative valuation of health states that are cardiac disease-related vs. those that are not. The advantages of using patient preferences in this type of analysis include convenience – the patient population is likely to be more available and more interested in a survey of preferences than a general population sample – and the feasibility of obtaining a more sensitive outcome measure, because of the patients' ability to discriminate among a variety of states they have experienced. The main disadvantage to using the patients' preferences is that this analysis would not be as comparable to analyses using general population preferences.

General population preferences (often referred to as *community prefer-ences*) are preferred for CEA designed to inform broader resource-allocation decisions. From the societal perspective, which is intended to represent the public interest rather than the interests of any particular group, these prefer-ences are the most defensible choice. The ideal source of preferences would be an unbiased, broad community sample of people who are well informed about the health states in question. This sample would probably include people who had some experience with the illness or condition under study, in proportion to its occurrence in society. Those with no experience would be giving their views about the health state without knowing whether they would, in the future, experience the condition. From behind this so-called 'veil of ignor-ance,' a construct used by health ethicists to judge principles for resource allocation, these respondents would evaluate the relevant health states from an *ex ante* perspective in terms of their relative desirability compared with other possible health states.

9.4.2.3 Approaches to obtaining health-state utilities

Preferences are frequently assessed by presenting respondents with holistic vignettes, describing all domains of health that comprise a particular health state. So, for example, for a scenario describing mild arthritis, the vignette would describe the patient's role function, mental health, cognitive function-ing, and other domains, whether or not they are affected by the condition, giving a full picture of the health state. The respondent would then provide preferences for the state as a whole. This contrasts with elicitation of prefer-ences that are based on descriptions – possibly more detailed – that focus on the problems specific to the illness. For example, the arthritis example would be comprised of scenarios characterizing the joint pain and mobility directly associated with the condition.

The health status scales to which preferences are assigned can be either disease-specific (or condition-specific) or generic. Disease-specific scales, such as in the examples above that use either the problem-specific or holistic vignette approach to getting utilities for arthritis, gather data for scenarios where a condition or a disease is explicit in the description. An example of such a scale is the Functional Capacity Index, used to classify health states associated with traumatic injuries (14).

Disease-specific scales contrast with *generic* measures, which characterize the domains of health (for example, ability to do self-care, mobility, sensory function, aspects of social function, and health perceptions) without relating them to any particular illness. Generic scales provide an important level of convenience and standardization in the derivation of QALYs. Community or patient preferences can be obtained for health states comprised of the various levels of each health domain. An analyst studying a particular illness can then 'map' health states associated with that illness on to the generic scale. Given this type of assessment – which is usually much easier to accomplish than elicitation of preferences – the analyst can look up the population preferences that have already been surveyed.

Well-known examples of generic scales used to compute QALYs include the Health Utilities Index (HUI) (15), the 5-Item EuroQOL Scale (16), and the Quality of Well-Being (QWB) Scale (17). The HUI, developed in Canada, is a multiattribute (multiple domain) scale that has been used in clinical studies, cost-effectiveness studies, and population health surveys. Preferences have been elicited for its health states for a general population sample of Canadians, using the standard gamble, and applying methods of multiattribute utility theory to infer utilities for the complete set of states from elicited utilities for a subset. The EQ-5D, which also combines multiple domains, contains approximately 250 health states. Preferences have been elicited using the time trade-off from general populations in the UK and the USA. Preferences for the QWB were obtained for a general population sample of Americans. The QWB scale differs from the HUI and EQ-5D in that preferences were assessed for it using a category scaling method (a psychological scaling approach) rather than a utility-based approach.

Health utility measures such as the EQ-5D are increasingly being incorporated in clinical trials. However, it is still much more common in trials to use a descriptive quality of life measure, such as the SF-36, or one of a number of disease-specific measures. Therefore, algorithms have been developed to convert descriptive QoL data to a utility-based instrument, or to 'map' the data onto one of the existing generic instruments. For example, Brazier et al. developed an algorithm to convert the SF-36 to a new utility instrument, the SF-6D (18). In addition, Brazier et al. present a review of 30 studies that map (or cross-walk) non-preference-based measures of health to generic preference-based measures (19). (Issues relating to the development and use of quality-of-life measures are discussed in much more detail in Chapter 4.)

The disadvantage to using a generic health-state classification system is that, if it is general enough and simple enough to apply to health states across diseases, conditions, and interventions, it may not be sensitive enough to the variations in health status associated with a particular disease. As a result, depending on the analysis, disease- or condition-specific measures may be preferred. In countries where economic evaluation is formally used in making decisions about the reimbursement or use of health-care treatments and technologies, decision makers tend to prefer a generic utility measure, since they are attempting to make resource-allocation decisions across all aspects of health care (4). (The use of economic evaluation in decision making is discussed further in Section 9.11 below.)

9.4.2.4 A note on disability-adjusted life-years (DALYs)

In 1993, the World Bank published a report on the global burden of disease using the disability-adjusted life-year (DALY) as the measure of health (20, 21). This measure deserves mention in any discussion of measures of health benefit. The DALY is a combined measure of health like the QALY, incorporating both length and quality of life. In the QALY, years of life lived are adjusted for the level of health, whereas DALYs are the number of years of life lost due to premature death or disability. Disabilities in the original specification of DALYs were categorized as falling into one of six levels of severity, with each level having an assigned weight. For example, about half of the cases of pelvic inflammatory disease examined in the World Bank study fell into class 4, which has a severity weight of 0.22; other cases of this disease fell into categories associated with higher and lower levels of disability and corresponding severity weights. In addition to an adjustment using disability weights, in the original DALY, years of life were adjusted based on age. The age weights reflect a higher valuation of years of life for a young or middle-aged adult than for a child or an elderly person. The first and last years of life are given a very low weight, while the highest weight is given to a year at age 25. The age weighting is intended to account for the fact that people are supported by others during infancy and advanced age. However, this approach has been questioned on grounds of equity and now most analysts calculate DALYs without the age weighting, at least for purposes of cost-effectiveness analysis (22).

Initially the DALY was not generally used in CEA, because it was not developed as a preference-weighted measure. (The disability weights used to adjust life-years were chosen by a panel of experts.) The DALY's preferred uses were in describing the impact of morbidity and mortality, in the developing world (23, 24). In countries where analysts have access to local preference weights for health states, the DALY is also used in examining the relative cost-effectiveness of health-care interventions, e.g., through the CHOICE program of the World Health Organization (25). Recently methods for assigning preference weights to disability states have been developed based on transformations of subjective community-based rankings of health states. Although ordinal rankings are not valid as utilities, there is some evidence that weights based on transformed ordinal preferences correspond reasonably well to EQ-5D weights derived from standard gambles (26, 27).

Some of the issues in calculating and presenting DALYs are discussed by Rushby and Hanson (28), who suggest a set of minimum reporting criteria. Comparisons between QALYs and DALYs and the implications for health policy decisions are discussed in the papers by Airoldi and Morton and by Robberstad (22, 29).

9.4.2.5 Calculating life expectancy in cost-effectiveness models

So far in this section, our discussion has focused on the measurement of the quality-of-life benefits of health interventions. Life-years are the base unit to which quality weights are applied in the QALY. In addition, as noted earlier, measures of life expectancy are sometimes used as the single measure of outcome. Differences in survival in CEA capture the life-saving and life-extending benefits of interventions, while in the QALY, the differences in weighted life-years capture the duration of health effects.

Most CEAs that use long-term measures of health benefit (length and quality of life) model the full life expectancy for the target population of the analysis with and without the intervention, comparing the two results to obtain differences in costs and health outcome to calculate the cost-effectiveness ratio. Calculations of life expectancy can be based on age-specific mortality rates derived from population life tables, adjusted for mortality differences attributable to specific procedures or illnesses under study. These calculations are typically done using Markov models and using methods for survival analysis described in Chapter 10.

9.5 Discounting costs and health outcomes

Leaving aside issues of inflation, alternative programs that require the same total investment over the life of the project may differ in their requirement for funds from year to year. Consider, for example, three programs that each consume $100 000 worth of resources over five years, but program A entails uniform investment each year, B requires more resources in the early years, and C is weighted more heavily in the later years. If these programs produce identical benefits, should we be indifferent among them? There is general agreement that future costs should be weighted less heavily than present ones. Although somewhat more controversial, there is also general agreement that future health consequences should be weighted less heavily than present ones. In this section we discuss the reasons for such time preferences and describe a method, *discounting*, to quantify the magnitude of this preference. Discounting enables us to compare future costs and health consequences with those in the present.

DEFINITION   *Discounting* is a process for computing how much a quantitative measure of resource cost or health outcome at some point in the future is worth today. *The present* value, or value today, of a future dollar or QALY depends on how far into the future it is obtained and on the rate at which it is discounted, the *discount rate*.

9.5.1 The mechanism of discounting

One dollar invested at an interest rate of 3% will bring $1.03 a year from now. We use discounting, the reverse of this 'interest' process, to compute the *present value (PV)* of a dollar that we will obtain a year from now. The *PV* is the amount of money that, if invested, will yield $1 one year from now, so $PV \times 1.03 = \$1.00$. Doing the division, we find that

$PV = \$0.97$. At a 3% discount rate, then, the present value of $1.00 next year is 97 cents.

In the same way, we can calculate that the value of a dollar spent or received *two years* from now has a present value of 94 cents:

$1.00 two years from now is worth $\$1.00/1.03 = \$0.97$ one year from now, and $0.97 one year from now is worth $\$.97/1.03 = \$0.94$ today.

The general formula for present value is:

$$PV = \frac{FV}{(1+r)^t} \qquad (9.3)$$

where *PV* is present value, *FV* is the future value, r is the discount rate expressed as a decimal fraction (e.g., $r = 0.03$), and t is time (such as two years in the previous example). Using this formula, the present value of a $500 check that will be received ten years from now, given an 8% discount rate, is $PV = \$500/(1 + 0.08)^{10} = \$232$.

Table 9.1 Current cost and discounted cost (amounts are assumed to be incurred at the end of each year)

	Current cost or income (2013$)	Discounted (3%) cost or income (2013$)
Year 0	− 50 000	− 50 000
Year 1	− 4500	− 4369
Year 2	5000	4713
Year 3	10 000	9151
Year 4	10 000	8885
Year 5	10 000	8626
Total		− 22 994

When costs or income are incurred in different amounts over a stream of years, they are discounted according to when they occur, and then summed as shown in Table 9.1. Note that Table 9.1 indicates the currency year in which *all* the dollars are reported (as it always should be), i.e., '2013$.' This has nothing to do with discounting; instead it tells the reader the value of the currency considering inflation.

In Table 9.1, there is a three-year period during which the income stream is $10 000 per year. There is a shortcut method of calculating present value for a constant amount of money, C, spent or received in each of the next N years:

$$PV = \frac{C}{r} \cdot [1-(1/(1 + r)^N)] \tag{9.4}$$

This formula can be derived from the standard formula for the sum of a geometric series, with the geometric proportion equal to $1/(1 +r)$.

In the example above, the present value of the three-year stream can be calculated by recognizing that it is the difference between a five-year stream and a two-year stream, each beginning at time zero. The value of the five-year stream is:

$$PV_5 = \$10\,000/0.03 \times (1-1/1.03^5) = \$45\,797 \tag{9.5}$$

The value of the two-year stream is:

$$PV_2 = \$10\,000/0.03 \times (1-1/1.03^2) = \$19\,135 \tag{9.6}$$

For the value of the three-year stream beginning in year three, we subtract the value of the two-year stream from the value of the five-year stream: $26\,662.

This method is handy for estimating present values or double-checking other methods.

Note that the assumption underlying the present-value calculations in Table 9.1 is that all dollar amounts are incurred at the end of each year, and that the present value is calculated as of the end of year 0 (which is the beginning of year 1). In discounting costs, it matters whether costs are counted at the beginning or the end of the year. If $10 000 payments are received at the beginning of the year for five years, the first payment should not be discounted. The calculation of present value would look like this:

$$PV = \$10\,000 + \$10\,000/(1.03) + \$10\,000/(1.03)^2 + \$10\,000/(1.03)^3$$
$$+ \$10\,000/(1.03)^4 = \$47\,171 \tag{9.7}$$

In contrast, if each payment is received at the end of the year, the present value calculation should reflect this difference in timing. The first payment is discounted for the first year, the second payment for the second, etc.:

$$PV = \$10\,000/(1.03) + \$10\,000/(1.03)^2 + \$10\,000/(1.03)^3$$
$$+ \$10\,000/(1.03)^4 + \$10\,000/(1.03)^5 = \$45\,797 \tag{9.8}$$

Note that the formula above discounts the first payment in the stream – it makes the assumption that costs are received at the end of each year.

If costs are spread evenly over the year, or if they occur in the middle of the year, a half-cycle correction may be used. This approach 'corrects' for the underestimate in present value that would result from assuming the payments were received at the end of each year and the overestimate that would result from assuming they were received at the beginning of each year. The calculation of present value with a half-cycle correction looks like this:

$$PV = \$10\,000/(1.03)^{0.5} + \$10\,000/(1.03)^{1.5} + \$10\,000/(1.03)^{2.5}$$
$$+ \$10\,000/(1.03)^{3.5} + \$10\,000/(1.03)^{4.5} = \$46\,479 \tag{9.9}$$

with 0.5 year of discounting for the first payment, 1.5 years for the second payment, and so forth. Present values can be calculated easily using spreadsheet software. Financial calculators can also be used.

9.5.2 The rationale for discounting

One reason for discounting future costs is that a dollar that is not spent today can be invested productively to yield a larger number of real dollars in the future. Investment occurs through building factories and equipment, research and development, and training of personnel. The simplest evidence that investors can earn returns on resources over time is that you can take a dollar to the bank and deposit it in a money market account that pays, for example, 5% interest, and get $1.05 a year from now. The bank's interest rate reflects not only the anticipated rate of inflation but also the real value of investments – the opportunity cost of money – in the national economy. A dollar's worth of resources in the national economy, if not spent this year, can be put to productive use to yield $1.05 worth of goods and services next year. If this includes 2% inflation, then the inflation-adjusted value would be $1.03, or a 3% return.

A second reason for discounting is that you may prefer to have the goods and services a dollar can buy now rather than to wait. This may be true either because you genuinely prefer immediate gratification, or because of potential risks – such as the failure of the bank holding your money – associated with delay. If neither of those motivations applies, then the fact that you could have earned interest from an investor – who can earn a return on your money – would lead you to demand interest from the bank. For any of these reasons, you demand a premium in the form of interest if you must postpone consumption.

The arguments for discounting health outcomes differ somewhat from the rationale for discounting costs. Clearly, there is no 'bank' for health benefits and no interest rate to demonstrate differences between present and future value. Arguments for discounting health benefits are generally made on the basis of normative theory, which specifies that the discount rate should be positive, and on the basis of people's observed time preferences for health, although studies investigating these have found discrepancies with theory on a number of variables (30–32).

There are, in addition, two frequently cited 'proofs' of the need to discount health benefits, the Keeler–Cretin paradox and Weinstein and Stason's consistency argument (33, 34). Keeler and Cretin use an example that shows that a logical paradox develops if one discounts costs and health benefits at different rates. The paradox is that, if a program's costs and effectiveness are discounted at different rates, it is possible to improve the program's performance (health benefit per dollar spent) simply by delaying its implementation. As a result, it is always preferable to wait rather than begin the program.

Weinstein and Stason's consistency argument holds that the basic reason for discounting future health benefits is because they are being valued relative to dollars that could be invested to yield even more dollars in the future. They show that it is equivalent (a) to calculate the future value of a stream of dollars for comparison with a future health benefit and (b) to calculate the present value of a stream of QALYs for comparison with a present cost. Since (a) is clearly correct, the equivalence of (a) and (b) proves that discounting of QALYs is required for consistency.

Several arguments have been advanced against discounting health benefits. Some merely rest on distaste for the implications of discounting. For example, with discounting, prevention programs generally have a lower net value because the benefits occur in the more distant future. Other arguments rest on the notion that health is different from many commodities. For example, unlike many commodities, the marginal utility of health does not decline as income rises. Gravelle and Smith argue that when health effects are measured in QALYs, as opposed to monetary terms, discounting effects at a lower rate is a valid way of taking account of the likely increase in the future value of health effects as individuals become richer (35). In a recent paper, Claxton et al. argue that whether one discounts health at a lower rate depends on whether the objective is to maximise health or welfare, whether the budget for health is fixed and appropriately set, whether the cost-effectiveness threshold and the consumption value for health is constant over time, and finally whether the social time preference for health is the same as that for consumption (36). Notwithstanding the objections to discounting, the discounting of both costs and health effects – and at the same rate – is standard practice in CEA.

9.5.3 The discount rate

Because the purpose of the discount rate is to account for the opportunity cost of money, it is appropriate to choose a market-based rate for discounting. There are other considerations, however. When possible, it is important for analysts to choose a rate that is consistent with other analyses in the field and consistent over time, in order to facilitate the comparability of analyses.

Over the past two decades, discount rates used in economic evaluation have ranged from as low as 1 or 2% to 10%. Perhaps the most common discount rate in CEA has been 5%; however, this rate was initially used when market-based interest rates were significantly higher than they were around the turn of the century. As of 2001, a lower rate of 3% was recommended for the USA, to reflect the trend toward lower interest rates and to be consistent with published guidelines (37). In some other jurisdictions, a discount rate is recommended by the Ministry of Finance, or the agency that requests economic evaluations (4, 38). Many analysts include the 5% rate when conducting sensitivity analyses on the discount rate, in order to facilitate comparability with older analyses. It is recommended that analysts follow the literature for current recommendations on the choice of a discount rate.

9.6 Incremental cost-effectiveness analysis

All health applications of CEA involve a comparison between at least two alternatives. For example, CEA might be used to compare two drug regimens for patients following myocardial infarction. As discussed earlier, the main use of CEA is in situations when one alternative is both more costly and more effective than the other (upper-right quadrant of the cost-effectiveness plane – Figure 9.1). The cost-effectiveness ratio describing this alternative is the ratio of the difference in net cost to the difference in net health effectiveness, compared to the other choice. Notice that the ratio is a ratio of differences – an incremental ratio.

This paradigm of alternatives is always embedded within the basic cost-effectiveness model. In the example of exercise 9.1 of physicians' choice of clinical preventive services, each clinical service on the 'menu' could either be performed or not performed. The clinician's problem is to decide which combination of services to perform, and which ones not to perform. The yes/no decisions for each option can be made independently, so as to maximize health benefit given a budget constraint.

In many health applications of CEA, however, the choices involve two or more interventions that, by definition, cannot be selected at the same time – not just a yes/no choice for each alternative. The choice among four strategies for breast cancer screening, each involving a different screening interval, is such a choice among mutually exclusive, or *competing choices*. Another is the choice between two different surgical procedures. This situation contrasts with the choice facing a public health agency of whether to implement an antismoking campaign and/or a skin cancer screening program, since the decision to perform one service does not inherently preclude a decision to perform the other one (although the budget might constrain the decision).

The basic difference between these situations is that in competing choice situations such as that among breast cancer screening methods, the alternatives are not independent. In other words, the choice of the first alternative influences the benefit to be gained (or the cost incurred) by the second. In a non-competing situation – such as the public health agency with a financial budget or the clinician with a time budget – the benefits of each program can be added. In the competing choice situation, they cannot. The benefit of Program A – annual mammogram – clearly will depend on whether the alternative is no mammogram, biannual mammogram, or mammogram every five years. The decision algorithm for using CEA differs in these two situations. We provide an example of each below.

9.6.1 The shopping spree problem

The shopping spree problem is an example of the basic (non-competing choice) cost-effectiveness model. In this problem, there are a number of available programs, for which net costs and net effectiveness have been

Table 9.2 Non-competing programs: a 'shopping spree' problem

Program	QALYs gained	Cost ($)
A	100	1 800 000
B	100	5 000 000
C	500	1 000 000
D	100	2 200 000
E	100	1 200 000
F	500	2 000 000
G	100	10 000 000
H	200	1 200 000
I	150	4 500 000
J	50	800 000
K	250	2 000 000

QALYs: quality-adjusted life-years.

evaluated, relative to the alternative of no program (Table 9.2). There is a limited budget; that is, the total net cost of the programs that are selected cannot exceed a specified amount. The decision maker's objective is to maximize the total net effectiveness (health benefit) of the programs selected.

Program alternatives in this problem are assumed to be independent. Any combination of programs is feasible – limited only by the budget constraint. Neither the net cost nor the net effectiveness of any program depends on what other programs are selected. Programs are also assumed to be divisible, with proportional costs and effectiveness. (In other words, a program that costs $1.0 million and saves 500 QALYs can be partially implemented, such as at the $500 000 level, and the benefit achieved will be proportional [250 QALYs].)

In the shopping spree problem, the decision maker first rules out any programs that cost money but have negative effectiveness. These programs, which would fall into the lower-right quadrant of Figure 9.1, are said to be *dominated* by their alternative of no program. No $/QALY threshold can make such programs cost-effective; they would not be selected under any scenario. Similarly, the decision maker would select any programs that are cost-saving and offer some benefit. Because they do not require resources, these programs can be selected regardless of the specified budget.

Table 9.3 Non-competing programs in order of cost-effectiveness

Program	Cost ($)	QALYs gained	C/E
C	1 000 000	500	2000
F	2 000 000	500	4000
H	1 200 000	200	6000
K	2 000 000	250	8000
E	1 200 000	100	12 000
J	800 000	50	16 000
A	1 800 000	100	18 000
D	2 200 000	100	22 000
I	4 500 000	150	30 000
B	5 000 000	100	50 000
G	10 000 000	100	100 000

QALYs: quality-adjusted life-years; C/E: cost-effectiveness ratio.

Furthermore, their net cost savings could be added into the budget, thus increasing the resources available for other programs on the list. Neither of these types of programs (dominated or cost-saving) appears in Table 9.2.

The other programs, those with positive cost and positive effectiveness, are ranked in ascending order of their cost-effectiveness ratio in Table 9.3. (Alternatively, the programs could be ranked in descending order of their effectiveness-to-cost ratio.) Programs are then selected from the least to the most expensive until the budget is expended. The final array of programs selected will depend on the budget constraint. In Table 9.3 with a $3.0 million budget, only Programs C and F could be selected. A total of 1000 QALYs would be gained and the $3.0 million budget limit would be reached. Also note that if the budget is $3.0 million, the last program selected, F, has a cost-effectiveness ratio of $4000 per QALY. The significance of this 'marginal cost-effectiveness ratio' associated with a budget constraint will become clear when we turn to the competing choice situation. If the budget were instead $10.0 million, the decision maker would again begin with Programs C and F, but could also add Programs H, K, E, J, and A before reaching the budget ceiling. With the $10.0 million budget, the marginal cost-effectiveness ratio (for Program A) is $18 000 per QALY. Not surprisingly, programs with higher (less desirable) cost-effectiveness ratios can be adopted as more resources are added to the budget.

Table 9.4 The distinction between average and incremental cost-effectiveness ratios

Program alternative	Effectiveness	Cost	Average cost-effectiveness ratio (C/E)	Incremental cost-effectiveness ratio ($\Delta C/\Delta E$)
M1	10	$100 000	$10 000/QALY	$10 000/QALY
M2	10.001	$110 000	$10 999/QALY	$10 000 000/QALY

QALYs: quality-adjusted life-years.

9.6.2 The competing choice problem

In the competing choice problem, there are again a number of available programs. As with the shopping spree problem, the programs are assumed to be divisible. The decision maker's objective is the same: to maximize the total net effectiveness of programs selected subject to a limited budget.

In the competing choice problem, however, a subset of the available programs are mutually exclusive: if you select Program M1 you cannot select Program M2. For example, M1 and M2 might be two dosages of the same drug; if you chose to administer M1, which requires giving 5 mg of Drug A per day, you could not at the same time implement M2, 10 mg of Drug A. By definition, one of these choices (in this case presumably M2) is more effective but more costly than the other, and the decision between the two depends on whether the extra benefit is worth the extra cost.

Because the choices are mutually exclusive, it becomes necessary to look at the incremental cost-effectiveness ratio as a basis for decisions, rather than at average cost-effectiveness ratios such as those calculated for each option in Table 9.3. This is exactly what we were doing in the shopping spree, although we may not have recognized it, but in the shopping spree, each program was being compared to a null alternative. Now we have two or more active alternatives for some of the options, in addition to the null option. The incremental cost-effectiveness ratio gives the added cost per unit of added benefit of an option, relative to the next less expensive choice. Use of the incremental cost-effectiveness ratio permits the decision maker to account for the fact that there was a less expensive option when selecting programs.

For example, consider two programs, M1 and M2 (Table 9.4). Option M1 yields ten QALYs at a cost of $100 000. Its average cost-effectiveness ratio is $10 000 per QALY. The second program, M2, costs $10 000 more. It is also more effective, but the difference in effectiveness between the two programs is tiny: 0.001 QALY. Its incremental cost-effectiveness ratio is $10 000/0.001 = $10 000 000 per QALY.

If the decision maker were to use Option M2's average cost-effectiveness ratio of $10 999 in making program selections, M2 would be selected in a line-up of programs before Program E in the previous example, with its cost-effectiveness ratio of $12 000.

But is that really a good choice? A check of the potential QALYs gained shows that it is not. If $1.2 million were spent on Program E, 100 QALYs would be gained (Table 9.5). This is in fact less than would be gained if the decision maker purchased M2 and then used the remaining funds on Program E. But this calculation overlooks M1, which we know will yield almost as many QALYs as M2. If we select M1, we would gain slightly fewer QALYs than if M2 were chosen, but the remaining funds spent on Program E would purchase more QALYs. The final total of QALYs gained with the $7.4 million would be greater if we chose M1 rather than M2.

The calculation of incremental cost-effectiveness (Table 9.4) gives the true ratio of cost-effectiveness for mutually exclusive programs, allowing us to 'see' the relative worth of programs that we arrived at in the example of M1 and M2. This calculation gives the ratio of *additional* cost per unit of *additional* benefit when programs are mutually exclusive. The incremental cost-effectiveness ratio of Program M2 reveals that, although the dollar and QALY amounts do not differ radically in the context of the programs A through M2 in our examples (Table 9.5), the decision maker is actually paying $10 million per QALY in selecting M2 over M1. Even though it yields more total QALYs than M1, M2 should not be selected over M1 until all programs which yield health benefit at a rate less expensive than $10 000 000 per QALY have been exhausted.

9.6.3 Extended dominance

The consideration of mutually exclusive programs reveals a final pitfall in comparing programs. This is that a program may look like a reasonable choice on the basis of its incremental cost-effectiveness ratio *only* if a more expensive but more efficient option has not yet been considered. Once all options are considered, this program can be shown to cost more per additional unit of benefit than another option, and thereby be ruled out by *extended dominance*. Extended dominance differs from simple dominance described earlier, because with simple dominance a program is less advantageous on two dimensions than its alternative – that is, it is more costly and yields less benefit. This is not true in extended dominance, where the program is more costly but yields more benefit. The problem is simply that it doesn't yield as much *extra* benefit as a third, more expensive, option.

Consider Programs L1, L2, L3, L4, and L5 shown in Table 9.6. These are mutually exclusive programs. To calculate their incremental cost-effectiveness,

Table 9.5 Total quality-adjusted life-years (QALYs) gained: a check on selection of competing choice M1 vs. M2

Original choice:

Program	Program cost ($)	QALYs gained	C/E ($/QALY)	Cumulative QALYs	Cumulative program cost
C	1 000 000	500	2000	500	1 000 000
F	2 000 000	500	4000	1000	3 000 000
H	1 200 000	200	6000	1200	4 200 000
K	2 000 000	250	8000	1450	6 200 000
E	1 200 000	100	12 000	**1550**	7 400 000

Choose M2:

Program	Program cost ($)	QALYs gained	C/E ($/QALY)	Cumulative QALYs	Cumulative program cost
C	1 000 000	500	2000	500	1 000 000
F	2 000 000	500	4000	1000	3 000 000
H	1 200 000	200	6000	1200	4 200 000
K	2 000 000	250	8000	1450	6 200 000
M2	**110 000**	**10.001**	10 999	1460.001	6 310 000
E (partial)	1 090 000	90.833	12 000	**1550.834**	7 400 000

Choose M1:

Program	Program cost ($)	QALYs gained	C/E ($/QALY)	Cumulative QALYs	Cumulative program cost
C	1 000 000	500	2000	500	1 000 000
F	2 000 000	500	4000	1000	3 000 000
H	1 200 000	200	6000	1200	4 200 000
K	2 000 000	250	8000	1450	6 200 000
M1	**100 000**	**10**	10 000	1460	6 300 000
E (partial)	1 100 000	91.667	12 000	**1551.667**	7 400 000

Table 9.6 Incremental cost-effectiveness with dominance and extended dominance

Program	QALYs	Cost ($)	Incremental cost-effectiveness ratio ($/QALY) ($\Delta C/\Delta E$)
L1	10	50 000	5000
L2	15	150 000	20 000
L3	20	450 000	60 000
~~L4~~	~~35~~	~~800 000~~	
L5	40	750 000	15 000

QALYs: quality-adjusted life-years.

Table 9.7 Recalculation of incremental cost-effectiveness program eliminated by extended dominance

Program	QALYs	Cost ($)	Incremental cost-effectiveness ratio ($/QALY) ($\Delta C/\Delta E$)
L1	10	50 000	5000
L2	15	150 000	20 000
L5	40	750 000	24 000

QALYs: quality-adjusted life-years.

the programs are arranged in the order of increasing cost and increasing effectiveness. A dominated program, L4, with higher cost but lower effectiveness than L5, can be eliminated immediately. This leaves Programs L1, L2, L3, and L5. The incremental cost and incremental effectiveness are calculated for each program relative to the preceding program. Then the incremental cost-effectiveness ratio for each option compared to the next most effective option is calculated.

At this point, Program L3 can be ruled out by extended dominance. It stands out in Table 9.6 because its incremental cost-effectiveness ratio, $60 000, is higher than that of Program L5. We reason as follows: 'If we are willing to spend additional resources at a rate of $60 000 per QALY for L3, then surely we would spend more resources to pay for L5, which can buy QALYs more cheaply than L3.' Removing this program and recalculating the incremental cost-effectiveness ratios (Table 9.7) confirms that L5 indeed achieves additional benefit at a lower per-unit cost than L3 did.

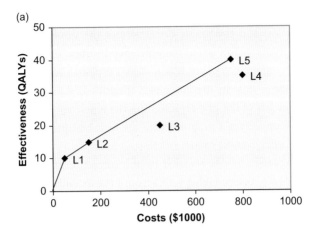

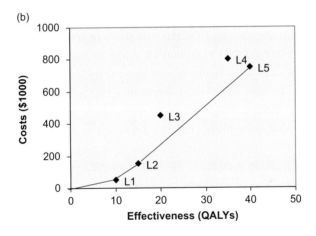

Figure 9.2   Costs vs. effectiveness for five competing programs L1–L5 plotted in cost-effectiveness space. L4 is inferior by simple dominance and L3 is ruled out by extended dominance. (a) In cost-effectiveness space, with costs on the x-axis and effectiveness on the y-axis, (extended) dominated programs fall below the line representing the efficiency frontier. This plot demonstrates the diminishing marginal returns of programs as you go up the efficiency frontier. The Panel on CEA recommends presenting results with this plot. (b) In cost-effectiveness space, with effectiveness on the x-axis and costs on the y-axis, (extended) dominated programs fall to the left and above the line representing the efficiency frontier. In this plot the slope of the line connecting a program with the next best program equals its incremental cost-effectiveness ratio. QALYs, quality-adjusted life years.

A graph illustrates both forms of dominance. Costs vs. effectiveness for the five competing programs L1 to L5 have been plotted in *cost-effectiveness space* (Figure 9.2). Some recommend presenting cost-effectiveness space with costs on the x-axis and effectiveness on the y-axis (Figure 9.2a) (37). In this plot, dominated and extended dominated programs (L4 and L3 respectively) fall below the line of potentially optimal programs (also known as the *efficiency frontier*) and the graph demonstrates the diminishing marginal returns of programs as you go up the efficiency frontier. Many analysts use the reverse plot (Figure 9.2*b*)(1) in which costs are plotted on the *y*-axis and effectiveness on the *x*-axis. In the latter plot (extended) dominated programs fall to the upper left of the line representing the efficiency frontier and the slope of the line connecting a program with the next best program equals its incremental cost-effectiveness ratio.

Another trap is revealed by the correction of the incomplete analysis in Table 9.6, before taking into account the extended dominance of the extravagant L3 option. At this stage, it might appear that L5 has an incremental cost-effectiveness ratio of $15 000/QALY. If the cutoff is $18 000/QALY, then L5 might seem to be cost-effective. But it is not! After eliminating L3, the true incremental cost-effectiveness ratio of L5 is revealed to be $24 000 per QALY. Evidently, Option L1 is the cost-effective option if we can only afford up to $18 000 per QALY. Option L5 would be most cost-effective only if our next best uses of the resources cost more than $24 000 per QALY gained.

The issue of extended dominance highlights an important analytical concern in CEA. A suboptimal program can be made to look reasonable if better options are omitted. For this reason, it is important that cost-effectiveness analysts carefully consider the choice of program options to be included in an analysis. In particular, the best available option and the most widely used option should always be considered.

9.6.4 Combining the shopping spree and competing choice problems

To review the steps in selecting among programs, let us look at the full array of programs we have considered in this section, including some that are not mutually exclusive (Programs A–K) and some that are (L1, L2, and L5). To select among these programs, the decision maker first rules out any dominated programs, and selects any programs that save money and yield positive effectiveness. (If we have been lucky enough to have cost-saving options, we can add the money saved to the budget before selecting from the remaining programs.) The next step is to rank the independent programs (those that are not mutually exclusive) in the order of their cost and effectiveness and calculate their cost-effectiveness ratios (Table 9.3). Looking at the list of programs, we can do a preliminary selection of programs, establishing which programs our budgeted amount of funds will cover. The cost-effectiveness ratio of the final (marginal) program demonstrates the opportunity cost of resources.

At this point, we arrange the competing programs in the increasing order of their cost, and calculate incremental cost-effectiveness ratios. We exclude

Table 9.8 Non-competing and competing programs in order of cost-effectiveness

Program	Cost ($)	QALYs gained	Incremental cost-effectiveness ratio ($/QALY) ($\Delta C/\Delta E$)
C	1 000 000	500	2000
F	2 000 000	500	4000
L1	**50 000**	**10**	**5000**
H	1 200 000	200	6000
K	2 000 000	250	8000
E	1 200 000	100	12 000
J	800 000	50	16 000
A	1 800 000	100	18 000
L2–L1	**100 000**	**5**	**20 000**
D	2 200 000	100	22 000
L5–L2	**600 000**	**25**	**24 000**
I	4 500 000	150	30 000
B	5 000 000	100	50 000
G	10 000 000	100	100 000

QALYs: quality-adjusted life-years.

options that are ruled out by extended dominance, and then recalculate the incremental cost-effectiveness ratios for the remaining options (Table 9.7). With this new set of ratios, it may again be necessary to rule out options that are dominated by extended dominance. Once the options are in increasing order of incremental cost-effectiveness ratios, this step is complete.

The final selection of programs from among both the independent and the mutually exclusive options will depend on the overall budget that is available. The decision maker will begin with Program C and continue selecting until the budget is exhausted. L1, L2, or L5 will be selected in the order they appear in the table; however, because these programs are mutually exclusive, only one of them may be included in the final package of programs.

In Table 9.8, we use the notation 'L2–L1' to denote the *substitution* of L2 for L1, thus adding its *incremental* QALYs relative to L1 but absorbing its *incremental* cost in the budget. The cost-effectiveness ratio for this transaction is the ratio of the incremental cost to incremental QALYs: $20\,000$/QALY.

9.6.5 Comparing cost-effectiveness studies

The hypothetical examples above demonstrating incremental CEA make use of tables presenting various program or intervention alternatives and their respective cost-effectiveness ratios. These tables became known in the UK as *league tables* – a reference to listings of soccer teams and their performance – and the name has stuck. The 'textbook' case for using CEA for resource allocation indeed implies the use of such tables for making decisions across alternative uses of resources.

The CEAs have traditionally referenced other cost-effectiveness studies as points of comparison for cost-effectiveness ratios presented. For example, a cost-effectiveness study of a new drug to decrease mortality from myocardial infarction might provide cost-effectiveness ratios obtained for a widely used antihypertensive medication as a point of reference. A widely used benchmark in the USA is the cost-effectiveness ratio for dialysis for end-stage renal disease, the first and only intervention for many years to have been singled out for coverage under the Medicare program for citizens of all ages.

As the field of CEA has grown, tools to facilitate comparisons among interventions in health and medicine are becoming more available. Some projects have devoted a great deal of effort to developing league tables, dissecting and adjusting analyses to assure their comparability. An example is a study of CEA of breast cancer screening by Brown and Fintor (39). Other projects have developed databases of studies to make cost-effectiveness information more accessible and to assess the studies' quality. The most comprehensive efforts of this type are the National Health Service Economic Evaluation Database compiled in the UK, an ongoing database which analyzes approximately 400 cost-effectiveness studies annually (Centre for Reviews and Dissemination [40] and a database housed at the Tufts Medical Center [41]).

A key issue in comparing CEAs is the standardization of methods, which became the primary motivation of published guidelines of economic evaluation methods (see Section 9.8 below). In addition, as economic evaluations have increasingly been used in health-care decision making, the establishment of a benchmark, or threshold, of what might be deemed 'cost-effective' has gained importance (see Section 9.11 below).

9.7 Handling uncertainty in cost-effectiveness analysis

In modeling and calculating the changes in discounted costs and health benefits needed for a cost-effectiveness study, there are many areas where uncertainty can enter the analysis. The most evident of these is uncertainty surrounding the various estimates that are used as inputs to the analysis – estimates of the size of a treatment effect or the cost of an hour of a practitioner's time, for example. Uncertainty of this type includes sampling variability around a central estimate of a parameter's value, uncertainty about the generalizability of estimates obtained from a particular sample, and uncertainty caused by lack of data on which to base certain estimates. A range of assumptions also underlies the structure of cost-effectiveness models – their methods of combining various data – and this is another source of uncertainty in calculations of cost-effectiveness.

All CEAs should contain sensitivity analyses that test the robustness of results given plausible ranges for important parameter values. Sensitivity analyses may examine high and low values, specific alternative values, or they may be threshold analyses that determine the value of a parameter that would change a decision.

Probabilistic sensitivity analysis (42) explores the parameter uncertainty around CEAs by assigning explicit probability distributions to the uncertain parameters. These distributions may be estimated from parametric sampling distributions of empirical data, from bootstrap analyses of data from clinical trials and databases, or from Bayesian and meta-analytic approaches that combine data with subjective prior distributions. Analysis and presentation of uncertainty in CEA will be discussed in more detail in Chapter 12.

9.8 Guidelines for the conduct of cost-effectiveness analysis

The standardization of methods has been an important concern in the cost-effectiveness field. Guidelines provide analysts and users of CEA with benchmarks for ensuring the quality of analyses. Equally important, standardization promotes the comparability of analyses, a feature central to the usefulness of CEAs, taken as a group, for assessing the relative value of programs and interventions.

Early guidelines for CEA were published by individual authors and by the Office of Technology Assessment. These guidelines tended to be somewhat general, and a lack of quality and consistency persisted in the field.

9.8.1 The US Public Health Service Guidelines

The US Public Health Service (USPHS) took an important step in addressing these issues during the 1990s. It convened the Panel on Cost-Effectiveness in Health and Medicine, a group of experts in cost-effectiveness and related fields, to develop guidelines with the input of US federal agencies that fund and use CEA in the health arena. The Panel developed a set of consensus recommendations referred to as the Reference Case to serve as a point of reference for analysts seeking comparability with other analyses in the literature (37, 43–45).

The Reference Case is comprised of recommendations concerning the nature and limits of CEA, components to be included in the numerator and denominator of the cost-effectiveness ratio, measuring terms in the numerator, estimating effectiveness of interventions, valuing health consequences, discounting, handling uncertainty, and reporting the analysis. These recommendations are included in the appendix to this chapter. Although the panel based its recommendations on theoretical grounds when possible, many recommendations reflect the practical constraints (and budget limitations) facing analysts, and others are somewhat arbitrary, generated for the purpose of establishing a consistent convention in the field.

The Reference Case analysis is recommended for analyses intended to inform broad resource-allocation decisions, and, for this reason, it takes the societal perspective. The panel recommends that a Reference Case be included in other analyses as well, to contribute to the pool of studies using a comparable methodology and to serve as a point of comparison between perspectives.

As this book goes to press, the National Institutes of Health is sponsoring an updated version of the Panel's report, possibly including changes to some of its recommendations. Readers are urged to keep abreast of the most recent recommendations as they are developed.

9.8.2 International methods guidelines

Methods guidelines for economic evaluation have now been developed in several jurisdictions. Some, like those produced by the USPHS Panel (37), have been developed with a general purpose of maintaining or improving methodological standards of economic evaluation. Other sets of guidelines in this category are those developed in Canada by the Canadian Agency for Drugs and Technologies in Health (46) and those developed for authors and editors of the *British Medical Journal* (47).

In addition, because of the growth in the use of economic evaluation in decisions about the funding and use of health-care treatments and technologies (See Section 9.11 below), some methods guidelines have been developed to assist manufacturers and sponsors of technologies in the submission of evidence to decision makers. A good example of this category of guidelines is the Academy of Managed Care Pharmacy format (48). This was produced in order to facilitate an organized and comprehensive presentation of evidence on new drugs to health plans in the USA. Other examples of methods guidelines for formal submissions of evidence are those produced by the National Institute for Health and Clinical Excellence in the United Kingdom

(NICE) (4), and the Health Care Insurance Board (CvZ) in The Netherlands (38). In some jurisdictions (e.g., Canada) the guidelines developed for more general purposes are also used as a basis for formal submissions of evidence.

As more international methods guidelines have been produced, there have been several attempts to classify and compare them. An up-to-date taxonomy is maintained by the International Society for Pharmacoeconomics and Outcomes Research (International Society for Pharmacoeconomics and Outcomes Research) (49). The similarities between the various guidelines far outweigh their differences. The biggest differences are in (i) the choice of perspective (either societal or health-care payer); (ii) the role of modeling (either generally encouraged for evidence synthesis, or only for extrapolation of costs and benefits into the future), and (iii) the measure of benefit (QALYs, monetary valuation, or presentation of disaggregated clinical outcomes).

In general those guidelines produced to assist in the formal submission of evidence tend to be a little more prescriptive, since there is a greater need for standardization of methods, given the decision maker's need to compare the relative cost-effectiveness of different treatments and technologies. To this end, some jurisdictions (e.g., the United Kingdom) have followed the 'reference case' approach, first proposed by the US Panel. This is useful because it facilitates standardization without stifling methodological development, since analysts are allowed to submit results produced by different methods, as long as they also submit those produced by the reference case methods.

9.9 Transferring economic data or analyses from one setting to another

It is quite common for a potential user of economic evaluations to encounter a published study undertaken in a different setting. Most commonly this will be a different location (e.g., country or jurisdiction), but it could also be a different practice setting (e.g., private for-profit as opposed to public not-for-profit). The question thus arises as to how the data used, or analyses conducted, could be interpreted for use in decisions in the new setting.

Individual physicians, or formulary decision makers, frequently use clinical data from other settings. After all, it is not possible to repeat major clinical trials in every conceivable location or practice modality. Often, data on relative clinical effect is considered to be generalizable, although in some clinical trials tests of heterogeneity in clinical effect across treatment centers are performed prior to the data being pooled.

In contrast, the generalizability of economic data cannot be assumed, since it is known that several factors, thought to vary between settings, could impact upon study results. These include, but are not confined to, differing demography and epidemiology of disease, differing practice patterns, differences in the availability of health-care resources, differences in relative prices, and differences in the values being placed on the various dimensions of health improvement (e.g., health utility gains) (50). The different international methods guidelines recognize the importance of these factors to differing extents. In an analysis of 26 sets of guidelines, Barbieri et al. found that all those that recognized the distinction between relative treatment effect and baseline risk considered the former to be highly transferable across settings and the latter not (51). In addition, there was agreement that prices/unit costs of resources are not transferable across settings. There was less agreement on whether data on resource utilization or health utility values could be transferred across settings.

If an economic evaluation is conducted alongside a multinational clinical trial, involving resource-use data collection in several countries, statistical analyses can be conducted, either to demonstrate that the data can be pooled, or to generate country-specific cost-effectiveness estimates. These include tests of heterogeneity (similar to those performed on the clinical data) and multivariable regression (with and without the use of hierarchical models) (52).

9.10 Distributive justice and equity issues in cost-effectiveness analysis

The CEA is not an ethically neutral methodology. It contains assumptions that, although defensible, influence the results of analyses and may raise moral questions as a result. The ethical implications of CEA may conflict with important values that decision makers hold or adopt with respect to decision making in the public interest.

Some important critiques derive from the assumption in CEA that years of life are equal – apart from distinctions reflecting quality of life. Although this approach seems 'fair,' it can be argued that society may or should value years of life differently based on a variety of factors. Thus, some may argue with a CEA that finds an intervention that saves five years of life for a healthy 80-year-old to be of equal value as an intervention saving the same number of QALYs for a healthy 50-year-old. Others may argue with the assumption that one QALY provided to a severely ill person has the same societal value as one QALY for a mildly ill person. Similarly, it is not clear that an intervention that confers small benefits on many people is equally desirable to one that confers large benefits on a few individuals, even if the total QALYs conferred by each is identical.

Another issue in the valuation of health benefits concerns the use of utility weights to determine the value of life extension in terms of QALYs. There are strong arguments against using lower values of quality of life for those with disabling conditions. If a year of life in a wheelchair is given a quality weight of 0.8, interventions that save a year of the life of the wheelchair-bound person will be worth less than interventions that save a year of life for a non-disabled person – a disturbing result. Yet, if analyses do not assign a lower quality weight to a year of life with a disability, an intervention to prevent or cure that disability will appear to have no value. Analysts have used a variety of approaches to address this dilemma, but ethical objections or logical inconsistencies seem to persist.

The CEA can inadvertently insert existing patterns of social inequality and health risk into resource allocation recommendations. For example, the analysis that examines a successful HIV prevention intervention for intravenous drug abusers will find that the intervention is less cost-effective than a successful intervention for another population subgroup, because the intravenous drug users have a higher mortality from other causes. Similarly, on the cost side, an analysis that uses women's average wage rate to determine the opportunity cost for family caregivers will have assigned a lower value to time than if an overall average rate were used, because of the gender-based discrepancy between women's and men's wages.

It is important that analysts and users of CEA be cognizant of its assumptions, including those of CEA generally and those that are specific to a given analysis. A good cost-effectiveness study will present sensitivity analyses on variables that may be problematic, as well as discussing the effect of the assumptions on the results and implications of the analysis.

9.11 Using economic evaluation in health-care decision making

The analytical approaches outlined in this book can be used in making treatment decisions at the individual patient level and/or the health-care program level. Most readers will be familiar with the issues of application at the individual patient level, but use at the program level requires more discussion. Essentially this involves decisions about which treatments or technologies should be reimbursed, or covered, by insurance plans or by the health-care system operating in the jurisdiction.

Since decisions at the program level typically involve the consideration of the relative costs, as well as the relative benefits, of health-care treatments and technologies, economic evaluation is being increasingly used. However, the extent of the uptake of economic evaluation varies greatly across jurisdictions. In more 'socialized' health-care systems, such as those existing in Canada, Australia and New Zealand, the United Kingdom, and several other European countries, economic evaluation is becoming widely used. In the USA, the formal use of economic evaluation has so far been restricted to several large prevention programs and some health plans. It is not currently formally incorporated in decisions made by the Centers for Medicare and Medicaid Services (CMS), although some researchers argue that the availability of cost-effectiveness evidence is an important factor in Medicare coverage decisions (53).

The reasons for the differences in attitude to the use of economic evaluation are many and varied (54, 55). It is certainly clear that making a central decision about which health technologies should be reimbursed makes more sense in a socialized health-care system like that existing in the UK, than it would in a system like that existing in the USA, with its multitude of health plans and substantial patient co-payments for some services.

In those jurisdictions where economic evaluation has been widely used, several issues have emerged. First, in order to make a decision based on a cost-effectiveness study, the decision maker needs to refer to a cost-effectiveness threshold. For example, in the United Kingdom, NICE currently has a threshold of 20 000 GBP per QALY gained, rising to 30 000 GBP if other arguments can be made in support of the technology concerned (56). The threshold can be interpreted as the maximum amount the jurisdiction concerned would be willing to pay to adopt the new technology.

In budget constrained health-care systems, like that existing in the UK, the threshold can also be interpreted as the shadow price of the budget constraint; namely, the likely value of the technology that would be displaced in order to accommodate the adoption of the new technology. (This is the interpretation based on the stylized 'shopping spree' problem presented earlier in this chapter.) Few health-care systems announce an explicit threshold, although implicit thresholds can be estimated by reference to past decisions by the agency or organization concerned.

Secondly, although the application of a cost-effectiveness threshold does lead to some technologies being denied reimbursement altogether, these are in the minority. For example, in a study of the decisions made by NICE on new anti-cancer drugs between 2000 and 2008, 15 per cent of drugs were rejected altogether (57). It is much more common for technologies to be restricted to subgroups of the patient population, based on characteristics such as severity of disease, or whether the patient responds to therapy. However, even this can prove controversial.

Thirdly, although decision makers in these jurisdictions do apply a cost-effectiveness criterion, it is clear that other factors are considered in the decision. For example, George et al. noted that, in an evaluation of decisions taken by the Pharmaceutical Benefits Advisory Committee (PBAC) in Australia, a general cost-effectiveness logic was being applied (58). However, a closer examination of the data showed that there were several 'outliers'; namely, technologies that appeared to be cost-effective but were rejected and vice versa. They speculate on the reasons for this and cite seriousness of the condition, size of the budgetary impact, the presence or absence of other effective therapies for the condition concerned, and equity considerations. In addition, several of the multivariable analyses of reimbursement decisions in different jurisdictions, while stressing the importance of cost-effectiveness as an explanatory variable, point out that the strength of the clinical data and the overall budgetary impact of adopting the new technology are equally important, if not more important, factors (59).

The use of economic evaluation in health-care decision making is likely to evolve in the future, especially in the USA, following the advent of comparative effectiveness research. All that can safely be concluded at this point is that decision makers in several jurisdictions find evidence on the relative cost-effectiveness of health technologies to be useful, but consider this evidence alongside several other factors that they deem to be important in their jurisdictions.

9.12 Economic evaluation in health care – a final note

Cost-effectiveness assists a decision maker or contributes to a policy discussion by summarizing large amounts of information and by clarifying the decision-making process. It provides information concerning the relative worth of an intervention per unit of cost. Although CEA can make a significant contribution, it is far from sufficient for most decisions regarding health and medical interventions.

The appropriate use of CEA depends on the recognition of what this tool provides. A cost-effectiveness ratio, as distinct from a measure like that of net monetary benefit found in cost–benefit analysis, does not give an absolute measure of value that can be used in a decision of whether or not to undertake a program. The cost-effectiveness ratio alone cannot determine whether the benefit of an intervention is worth its cost. Instead, 'cost-effective' is a relative term reflecting the 'price' of additional units of benefit. An intervention can only be cost-effective as compared to another use of resources or as compared to some recognized standard. Annual cervical cancer screening for 50-year-old women can be more cost-effective – cost less per unit of health benefit – than annual cervical cancer screening for 40-year-old women. It can also be incrementally cost-effective compared to semi-annual screening for 50-year-old women. However, the decision about which intervention is appropriate must be made on the basis of available resources and the values associated with the decision context.

Misinterpretations of cost-effectiveness information are frequently evident in the way cost-effectiveness results are communicated. One often hears statements that, 'Program X is cost-effective.' This general statement is technically without meaning, because it does not identify either the comparator or the $/QALY standard by which the cost-effectiveness ratio is judged. A program that costs $75 000 per life-year saved might or might not be cost-effective – depending on what available alternatives exist for saving lives.

It is most accurate in describing cost-effectiveness results to state the full comparison that is being made, for example, that 'Program X has an incremental cost-effectiveness of $40 000 per QALY saved as compared with Program Y.' The user of general claims about cost-effectiveness may mean to imply that Program X is a cost-effective use of resources compared to available or widely used alternatives. Although an argument of this type may sometimes serve in a political context, it is rarely appropriate in a research or decision-making forum.

Although it can be an important aid to decision making, CEA is not intended to be a decision-making algorithm. Decisions must be made within the context of the decision makers' values and considering a variety of influences and inputs, of which CEA may be one. Values and goals relevant to a decision – political, social, religious, and ethical – are often excluded from a CEA. This is particularly the case for decisions at the societal level, since, in decisions at the patient level, the patient's values can be directly incorporated into the QALY or other measure of health outcome, while outcomes in societal level analyses are aggregates. The methods of CEA do not of themselves prevent an analyst from trying to incorporate specific values into an analysis, for example, by adjusting the weights used to calculate a measure of health outcome or even weighting costs differently based on who ultimately pays them. However, the values entering into decisions are too complex – and not well enough known – to make their systematic incorporation into CEA a feasible practice. In addition, including them would make analyses less transparent, less consistent, and more difficult for users to understand and interpret.

Finally, in applying CEA, it is always important to be aware of the scope of other interventions to which a program is being compared. In a good-quality analysis, the analyst will take stock of all the relevant alternatives and include them in the analysis. For example, a surgical cardiac procedure should be compared to available medical procedures, not only to other surgeries. However, because of space limitations, most cost-effectiveness reports will be unable to take a truly broad view, with the result that certain patterns of resource allocation are left unchallenged. It is left to users of CEA to bear in mind that there may be important preventive approaches to the same problems that are in search of cures, and that interventions in the arenas of public health, medicine, education, criminal justice, and environmental safety may have widely different cost-effectiveness. Similarly, from the standpoint of good policy, it may sometimes be better to challenge a budget constraint than to ration resources within the constraint.

Appendix

Summary recommendations of the Panel on Cost-Effectiveness in Health and Medicine

These framing propositions and recommendations are compiled from the report of the Panel on Cost-Effectiveness in Health and Medicine (37). Although these guidelines were developed more than 15 years ago, they remain very influential in shaping the methods that analysts use. A database containing structured reviews of studies published using methods consistent with the Panel's recommendations has been established (41).

The Panel's recommendations are classified as follows: framing propositions (F) describe the nature and limits of CEA and serve as basic starting points in defining CEA. Reference Case recommendations (R) are intended for use in a Reference Case analysis as defined by the Panel, which seeks to improve comparability for analyses that will be done to inform resource allocation. Guidance recommendations (G) are intended to improve the conduct of analyses, but are not explicitly required for a Reference Case analysis. An 's' indicates instances when a sensitivity analysis would be of particular importance. Additional recommendations, including recommendations for future research, may be found in the Panel's report.

I. The nature and limits of CEA and of the Reference Case

1. Cost-effectiveness analysis (CEA) is a methodology for evaluating the outcomes and costs of interventions designed to improve health. F
2. The CEA evaluates a given health intervention through the use of a 'cost-effectiveness ratio.' In this ratio, all health effects of the intervention (relative to a stated alternative) are captured in the denominator, and changes in resource use (relative to the alternative) are captured in the numerator and valued in monetary terms. F
3. The CEA is an aid to decision making, not a complete procedure for making resource-allocation decisions in health and medicine, because it cannot incorporate all the values relevant to such decisions. F

4. The CEA, cost-consequence analysis, and cost–benefit analysis are complementary, rather than mutually exclusive, forms of analysis. The use of one does not preclude the use of any of the others in a given study. F

5. When a CEA is intended to contribute to decisions on the broad allocation of health resources, a Reference Case analysis should be done to enhance comparability across studies. The Reference Case includes not only the associated baseline computation but also a meaningful set of sensitivity analyses. F

6. The Reference Case is based on the societal perspective. This perspective requires that an analysis consider all health effects and all changes in resource use. R

   6.1 Evaluation of effectiveness should incorporate both benefits and harms of alternative interventions. R

   6.2 The boundaries of a study should be defined broadly enough to encompass the range of groups of people affected by the intervention and all types of cost and health consequences. R

   6.3 The time horizon adopted in a CEA should be long enough to capture all relevant future effects of a health-care intervention. R

   6.4 Decisions about costs and health effects to include in a CEA, such as the precision with which costs and effects are measured, the time horizon of the study, and the definition of the study boundaries, should strike a reasonable balance between expense and difficulty, and potential importance in the analysis. R

7. The Reference Case analysis should compare the health intervention of interest to existing practice (the 'status quo'). If existing practice appears not to be a cost-effective option itself, relative to other available options, the analyst should incorporate other relevant alternatives into the analysis, such as a best-available alternative, a viable low-cost alternative, or a 'do-nothing' alternative. R

   7.1 When varying levels of program intensity are relevant, alternative program options (e.g., as defined by variation in duration or frequency of the intervention) should be included in the analysis and compared using the incremental cost-effectiveness algorithm. R

8. The estimates of resource consumption and effects of relevance for a CEA are those for the population or group that is actually affected by the health intervention. R

II. Components belonging to the numerator and the denominator

1. The major categories of resource use that should be reflected in the numerator of a C/E ratio include costs of health-care services; costs of

patient time expended for the intervention; costs associated with caregiving (paid or unpaid); other costs associated with illness such as childcare or travel expenses; and costs associated with non-health impacts of the intervention (e.g., on the education system or the environment). R

2. Effects of a health intervention on length of life are incorporated in the denominator of the C/E ratio. A monetary value should not be imputed for lost life-years and should not be included in the numerator of the C/E ratio. R

3. For a Reference Case analysis, health-related quality of life should be captured by an instrument that, at minimum, implicitly incorporates the effects of morbidity on productivity and leisure. Effects of a health intervention on subsequent morbidity, including the full value of morbidity time to patients, are incorporated in the denominator of the C/E ratio. R

   3.1 Effects of lost productivity borne by others (e.g., employers, co-workers) including 'friction costs,' when significant, should be included in the numerator. R

4. Time spent seeking care or undergoing an intervention is a resource and a component of the intervention. It should be valued in monetary terms and incorporated in the numerator of a cost-effectiveness ratio. R

   4.1 In some instances (e.g., when recuperating from surgery), time could be categorized either as morbidity time (valued in the denominator) or as input to the intervention itself (costed out in the numerator). As a general rule, in a Reference Case analysis, this time should be considered as morbidity time. G

   4.2 In some instances, time may be a clear input to a health intervention, but the intervention will, in addition, produce a significant impact on health status. When relevant to a Reference Case analysis, the impact on health status should be captured in the denominator, leaving the time component (costed out) in the numerator. G

III. Measuring terms in the numerator of the C/E ratio

1. Changes in the use of resources caused by a health intervention should be valued at their opportunity cost. R

   1.1 Costs should reflect the marginal or incremental resources consumed. R

   1.2 Resource consumption should be assessed from a long-term perspective. R

2. To the extent that prices reflect opportunity costs, they are an appropriate basis for valuing changes in resources. R

2.1 When prices do not adequately reflect opportunity costs because of market distortions, they should be adjusted appropriately. R

2.2 When substantial bias is present in prices, and adjustment is not feasible, more suitable proxies for opportunity costs should be considered. G

3. In aggregating resource costs across time, CEAs should be conducted in constant dollars that remove general price inflation. If the prices of the goods in question change at a rate different from general price levels, this variation should be reflected in the adjustment used. R

4. 'Transfer payments' (e.g., cash transfers from tax payers to welfare recipients) associated with a health intervention redistribute resources from one individual to another. While administrative costs associated with such transfers are included in the numerator of a C/E ratio, the transfers themselves are not since, by definition, their impact on the transferor and the recipient cancel out. R

5. For individuals in the labor force, wages are generally an acceptable measure of time costs. Wages corresponding to the target population should be used to approximate time costs. In general, age- and gender-specific wage estimates will provide adequately specific estimates. R

5.1 Use of group-specific wages may influence the conclusions of the analysis in ways that are ethically problematic. In these instances, sensitivity analysis should be conducted to explicitly indicate the nature of this influence. R s.

5.2 The wage rate generally does not adequately reflect the value of time for persons engaged primarily in leisure or in activities for which they are not compensated. For individuals not engaged in compensated employment, wages, used as proxies, must be adjusted to reflect the full opportunity cost of time. R

6. In theory, the numerator of a C/E ratio should include the net costs of health care and non-health consumption during years of life added by the intervention. However, because of problems in measuring these costs, and because of unresolved issues concerning the role of non-health costs in CEA, the Reference Case may either include or exclude health care costs associated with diseases other than those affected by the intervention, in added years of life. R

6.1 Whenever the inclusion or exclusion of health care costs of unrelated diseases makes a significant difference to the analysis, a sensitivity analysis should be performed to assess the effect on the C/E ratio. R s

IV. Measuring terms in the denominator of the C/E ratio

1. For a Reference Case analysis, incorporation of morbidity and mortality consequences into a single measure should be accomplished using QALYs. R

   1.1 In general, since lives saved or extended by an intervention will not be in perfect health, a saved life year will count as less than one full QALY. R

2. To satisfy the QALY concept, the quality weights must be preference-based, interval-scaled, and measured or transformed onto the interval scale where the reference point 'death' has a score of 0.0 and the reference point 'optimal health' has a score of 1.0. C

3. A CEA should be based on a health-state classification scheme which reflects domains (attributes) that are important for the particular analysis. R

   3.1 If the CEA is intended for Reference Case use, the preference measure used should be a generic one, or be capable of being compared to a generic system. R

4. In general, community preferences for health states are the appropriate ones for use in the Reference Case analysis. R

   4.1 When adequate information is unavailable regarding community preferences, patient preferences may be used as an approximation, but the manner in which they might differ from community preferences should be discussed and, where relevant, sensitivity analyses that reflect likely differences should be included. R s

   4.2 If distinct subgroup preferences are identified that will markedly affect a C/E ratio, the study should provide this information and conduct sensitivity analyses that reflect this difference. R s

5. The health-related quality of life of those whose lives have been saved or extended by a health intervention may be influenced by characteristics such as age, gender, or race. This may affect the Reference Case analysis in ways that are ethically problematic. In these instances, sensitivity analyses should be conducted to indicate explicitly how the results are affected by these characteristics. R s

6. When designing primary data collection efforts, or deriving the necessary probability estimates from secondary data sources for estimation of effectiveness in a CEA, outcome probability values should be selected from the best-designed (and least-biased) sources that are relevant to the question and population under study. G

7. Evidence for estimation of effectiveness may be obtained from: randomized controlled trials, observational data, uncontrolled experiments, descriptive series, and expert opinion. G

7.1 Good quality meta-analysis and other synthesis methods can be used where any one study has insufficient power to detect effects, or where results conflict. G

7.2 Expert judgment should only be used to fill in values where no adequate data sources exist, or when the parameter is of secondary importance in the analysis. G

8. Where direct primary or secondary empirical evaluation of effectiveness is not possible (e.g., in important subpopulations or in differing time frames), the use of modeling to estimate effectiveness is a valid mode of scientific inquiry for CEAs. G

V. Discounting

1. Costs and health outcomes should be discounted to present value. R

2. Costs should be discounted to present value at a rate consistent with the shadow-price-of-capital (SPC) approach to evaluating public investments. This rate (often termed the *social rate of time preference*) can be approximated by the real rate of return on long-term government bonds. R

3. Costs and health outcomes should be discounted at the same rate. R

    3.1 A real, riskless discount rate of 3% should be used. R

    3.2 Because of the large number of CEAs that have adhered to a discount rate of 5%, analysts should perform sensitivity analyses using 5% as well as a reasonable range of rates (drawn from 0% to 7%). R s

    3.3 The discount rate should be subject to review, and possible revision, over time in light of significant changes in the underlying economic data. However, to retain comparability with other analyses, both 3% and 5% should continue to be used in analyses for at least the next ten years. R s

VI. Uncertainty

1. At a minimum, univariate (one-way) sensitivity analyses should be conducted in order to determine where uncertainty or lack of agreement about some key parameter's value could have substantial impact on the CEA's conclusions. R

2. Analysts should conduct multivariate (multiway) sensitivity analyses for important parameters. R

3. Where possible, where parameter uncertainty is a major concern, a reasonable confidence interval or credible interval should be estimated based on either statistical methods or simulation. G

VII. Reporting guidelines

(For a summary of reporting guidelines see [44].)

1. We encourage analysts to document cost-effectiveness studies in two parts, a *journal report* and a more comprehensive *technical report*, making the latter available on request to readers requiring more detail concerning the analysis. G

2. For the specific purpose of journal review, we recommend that editors request and authors submit a concise *technical addendum* with the journal report to assist reviewers assessing the study's methodology. This material may or may not be published along with the journal report. G

3. If a cost-effectiveness analysis is intended to allow comparisons among the interventions studied and health-care interventions broadly, the report should highlight the Reference Case results. Key sensitivity analyses should be conducted with respect to the Reference Case. R

4. The perspective(s) of the analysis should be explicitly identified in a cost-effectiveness report. R

5. The following information comprises a basic set of results in the journal report: total costs, total effectiveness, incremental costs, incremental effectiveness, and incremental cost-effectiveness ratios, both discounted (at the Reference Case rate of 3%) and undiscounted. G

6. An appropriate number of significant figures should be used to report C/E results; generally two significant figures unless the precision of the data warrants a greater number. G

7. In reporting incremental cost-effectiveness ratios, options ruled out because of dominance or extended dominance should be excluded. Among undominated options, incremental C/E ratios should be reported in increasing order of cost and effectiveness, starting with the lowest-cost option considered (generally the status quo or 'do nothing' option). R

8. C/E ratios should be compared to available C/E ratios for other interventions that compete for resources with the intervention under study. Such interventions may be drawn from health care broadly if the decision context is broad, or from restricted areas, such as particular diseases or intervention modalities. G

REFERENCES

1. Drummond MF, Sculpher MJ, Torrance GW, O'Brien BJ, Stoddart GL. *Methods for the Economic Evaluation of Health Care Programmes.* 3rd edn. Oxford: Oxford University Press; 2005.
2. Tilling C, Krol M, Tsuchiya A, Brazier J, Brouwer W. In or out? Income losses in health state valuations: a review. *Value Health.* 2010;13(2):298–305.

3. Tilling C, Krol M, Tsuchiya A, Brazier J, van Exel J, Brouwer W. Does the EQ-5D reflect lost earnings? *Pharmacoeconomics.* 2012;30(1):47–61.

4. National Institute for Health and Clinical Excellence (NICE). *Guide to the Methods of Technology Appraisal.* London: NICE; 2008.

5. Meltzer D. Accounting for future costs in medical cost-effectiveness analysis. *J Health Econ.* 1997;16(1):33–64.

6. Johannesson M, Meltzer D, O'Conor RM. Incorporating future costs in medical cost-effectiveness analysis: Implications for the cost-effectiveness of the treatment of hypertension. *Med Decis Making.* 1997;17(4):382–9.

7. Garber AM, Phelps CE. Economic foundations of cost-effectiveness analysis. *J Health Econ.* 1997;16(1):1–31.

8. Kruse M, Sorensen J, Gyrd-Hansen D. Future costs in cost-effectiveness analysis: an empirical assessment. *Eur J Health Econ.* 2012;13(1):63–70.

9. Farnham PG, Gorsky RD, Holtgrave DR, Jones WK, Guinan ME. Counseling and testing for HIV prevention: Costs, effects, and cost-effectiveness of more rapid screening tests. *Public Health Reports.* 1996;111(1):44–53.

10. Koopmanschap MA, van Exel JNA, van den Berg B, Brouwer WBF. An overview of methods and applications to value informal care in economic evaluations of healthcare. *Pharmacoeconomics.* 2008;26(4):269–80.

11. Van den Berg B, Ferrer-I-Carbonell A. Monetary valuation of informal care: The well-being valuation method. *Health Econ.* 2007;16(11):1227–44.

12. Koopmanschap MA, Rutten FFH, Vanineveld BM, Vanroijen L. The friction cost method for measuring indirect costs of disease. *J Health Econ.* 1995;14(2): 171–89.

13. Ware JE, Sherbourne CD. The Mos 36-Item Short-Form Health Survey (Sf-36).1. Conceptual framework and item selection. *Med Care.* 1992;30(6):473–83.

14. MacKenzie EJ, Damiano A, Miller T, Luchter S. The development of the Functional Capacity Index. *J Trauma.* 1996;41(5):799–807.

15. Feeny D, Furlong W, Boyle M, Torrance GW. Multiattribute Health-Status Classification Systems – Health Utilities Index. *Pharmacoeconomics.* 1995;7 (6):490–502.

16. The EuroQol Group. EuroQol – a new facility for the measurement of health-related quality of life. *Health Policy.* 1990;16(3):199–208.

17. Kaplan RM, Anderson JP. A general health-policy model – update and applications. *Health Services Research.* 1988;23(2):203–35.

18. Brazier J, Roberts J, Deverill M. The estimation of a preference-based measure of health from the SF-36. *J Health Econ.* 2002;21(2):271–92.

19. Brazier JE, Yang YL, Tsuchiya A, Rowen DL. A review of studies mapping (or cross-walking) non-preference based measures of health to generic preference-based measures. *Eur J Health Econ.* 2010;11(2):215–25.

20. Musgrove P. Investing in health: the 1993 World Development Report of the World Bank. *Bulletin of the Pan American Health Organization.* 1993;27(3):284–6.

21. World Bank. World Development Report 1993: Investing in Health. *Community Disease Report: Weekly.* 1993;3:137.

22. Robberstad B. QALYs vs. DALYs vs. LYs gained: What are the differences, and what difference do they make for health care priority setting? *Norsk Epidemiologi*. 2005;15(2):183–99.

23. Murray CJL, Lopez AD. Global mortality, disability, and the contribution of risk factors: Global Burden of Disease Study. *Lancet*. 1997;349(9063):1436–42.

24. Murray CJL, Lopez AD. Regional patterns of disability-free life expectancy and disability-adjusted life expectancy: Global Burden of Disease Study. *Lancet*. 1997;349(9062):1347–52.

25. Edejer TT-T. *Making Choices in Health: WHO Guide to Cost-effectiveness Analysis*. Geneva: World Health Organization; 2004.

26. Craig BM, Busschbach JJ, Salomon JA. Modeling ranking, time trade-off, and visual analog scale values for EQ-5D health states: a review and comparison of methods. *Med Care*. 2009;47(6):634–41.

27. Craig BM, Busschbach JJ, Salomon JA. Keep it simple: ranking health states yields values similar to cardinal measurement approaches. *J Clin Epidemiol*. 2009;62(3):296–305.

28. Rushby JF, Hanson K. Calculating and presenting disability-adjusted life-years (DALYs) in cost-effectiveness analysis. *Health Policy Plan*. 2001;16(3):326–31.

29. Airoldi M, Morton A. Adjusting life for quality or disability: stylistic difference or substantial dispute? *Health Econ*. 2009;18(11):1237–47.

30. Chapman GB, Elstein AS. Valuing the future – temporal discounting of health and money. *Med Decis Making*. 1995;15(4):373–86.

31. Lipscomb J. Time preference. In Gold MR, Siegel JE, Russell LB, Weinstein MC, eds. *Cost-effectiveness in Health and Medicine*. USA: Oxford University Press; 1996. pp. 214–46.

32. Redelmeier DA, Heller DN. Time preference in medical decision-making and cost-effectiveness analysis. *Med Decis Making*. 1993;13(3):212–17.

33. Keeler EB, Cretin S. Discounting of life-saving and other non-monetary effects. *Manage Sci*. 1983;29(3):300–6.

34. Weinstein MC, Stason WB. Foundations of cost-effectiveness analysis for health and medical practices. *N Engl J Med*. 1977;296(13):716–21.

35. Gravelle H, Smith D. Discounting for health effects in cost-benefit and cost-effectiveness analysis. *Health Econ*. 2001;10(7):587–99.

36. Claxton K, Paulden M, Gravelle H, Brouwer W, Culyer AJ. Discounting and decision making in the economic evaluation of health-care technologies. *Health Econ*. 2011;20(1):2–15.

37. Gold MR, Siegel JE, Russell LB, Weinstein MC. *Cost-Effectiveness in Health and Medicine*. USA: Oxford University Press; 1996.

38. College voor zorgverzekeringen (CvZ). *Guidelines for Pharmacoeconomic Research, updated version*. 2006 [cited 2012 18 August]; available from: http://www.cvz.nl.

39. Brown ML, Fintor L. Cost-effectiveness of breast-cancer screening – preliminary results of a systematic review of the literature. *Breast Cancer Res Treat*. 1993; 25(2):113–18.

40. Centre for Reviews and Dissemination. *NHS EED*. York: University of York; 2012 [cited 2012 18 August]; available from: http://www.crd.york.ac.uk/CRDWeb/AboutNHSEED.asp.

41. Tufts Medical Center. *Cost-effectiveness analysis registry*. 2012 [cited 2012 18 August]; Available from: https://research.tufts-nemc.org/cear4/.

42. Griffin S, Claxton K, Hawkins N, Sculpher M. Probabilistic analysis and computationally expensive models: Necessary and required? *Value Health*. 2006;9(4):244–52.

43. Russell LB, Gold MR, Siegel JE, Daniels N, Weinstein MC. The role of cost-effectiveness analysis in health and medicine. *JAMA*. 1996;276(14):1172–7.

44. Siegel JE, Weinstein MC, Russell LB, Gold MR. Recommendations for reporting cost-effectiveness analyses. *JAMA*. 1996;276(16):1339–41.

45. Weinstein MC, Siegel JE, Gold MR, Kamlet MS, Russell LB. Recommendations of the panel on cost-effectiveness in health and medicine. *JAMA*. 1996; 276(15):1253–8.

46. Canadian Agency for Drugs and Technologies in Health. *Guidelines for the Economic Evaluation of Health Technologies*. Ottawa, Canada: CADTH; 2006.

47. The BMJ Economic Evaluation Working Party. Guidelines for authors and peer reviewers of economic submissions to the BMJ. *BMJ*. 1996;313(7052):275–83.

48. FMCP Format Executive Committee. *The AMCP Format for Formulary Submissions*. Alexandria, VA: AMCP; 2009 [cited 2012 18 August]; 3.0:[available from: http://www.amcp.org/AMCPFormatforFormularySubmissions/].

49. International Society for Pharmacoeconomics and Outcomes Research (ISPOR). *Pharmacoeconomic Guidelines Around The World*. USA: ISPOR; 2012 [cited 2012 18 August]; available from: http://www.ispor.org/PEguidelines/index.asp.

50. Sculpher MJ, Pang FS, Manca A, et al. Generalisability in economic evaluation studies in healthcare: a review and case studies. *Health Technol Assess*. 2004;8(49).

51. Barbieri M, Drummond MF, Rutten F, et al. ISPOR Good Research Practices Economic Data Transferability Task Force: What do international pharmacoeconomic guidelines say about economic data transferability? *Value Health*. 2010;13(8):1028–37.

52. Drummond MF, Barbieri M, Cook J, et al. Transferability of Economic Evaluations Across Jurisdictions: ISPOR Good Research Practices Task Force Report. *Value Health*. 2009;12(4):409–18.

53. Chambers JD, Morris S, Neumann PJ, Buxton MJ. Factors predicting Medicare national coverage: an empirical analysis. *Med Care*. 2012;50(3):249–56.

54. Neumann PJ. *Using Cost-effectiveness Analysis to Improve Health Care: Opportunities and Barriers*. USA: Oxford University Press; 2004.

55. Sampat B, Drummond MF. Another special relationship? Interactions between health technology policies and health care systems in the United States and the United Kingdom. *Journal of Health Politics, Policy and Law*. 2011;36(1):119–39.

56. Rawlins MD, Culyer AJ. National Institute for Clinical Excellence and its value judgments. *BMJ*. 2004;329(7459):224–7.

57. Mason AR, Drummond MF. Public funding of new cancer drugs: Is NICE getting nastier? *Eur J Cancer Clin Oncol.* 2009;45(7):1188–92.

58. George B, Harris A, Mitchell A. Cost effectiveness analysis and the consistency of decision making – evidence from pharmaceutical reimbursement in Australia (1991 to 1996). *Pharmacoeconomics.* 2001;19(11):1103–9.

59. Drummond MF. *Twenty Years of Using Economic Evaluations for Reimbursement Decisions. What Have We Achieved?* University of York, York: Centre for Health Economics 2012. Research Paper No. 75.

Recurring events

Everything flows and all changes are cyclic.

Heraclitus, Greek philosopher

10.1 Introduction

In previous chapters we have seen several applications of decision trees to solve clinical problems under conditions of uncertainty. Decision trees work well in analyzing chance events with limited recursion and a limited time horizon. The limited number of sequential decisions or chance nodes allows one to capture all the necessary information to maximize expected utility. However, when events can occur repeatedly over an extended time period, the decision-tree framework can become unmanageable. Many decision situations involve events occurring over the lifetime of the patient, thus extending far into the future. Life spans vary, but conventional trees require us to specify a fixed time horizon. The probabilities and utilities of these events may change over time and must be accounted for. This is the case for most chronic conditions. Examples include heart disease, Alzheimer's disease, various cancers, diabetes, asthma, osteoporosis, human immunodeficiency virus (HIV), inflammatory bowel disease, multiple sclerosis and more. This chapter offers a methodology for dealing with recurring events and extended (variable) time horizons.

EXAMPLE

Consider a patient with peripheral arterial disease (PAD: obstruction of the arteries to the legs) for whom a decision has to be made for either bypass surgery or percutaneous intervention (PI). We assume that conservative treatment through an exercise regimen has not provided sufficient relief. A very simplified decision tree is presented in Figure 10.1. Following the choice of treatment, the patient may die as a result of the procedure (captured in the 'mortality' branches) or survive the procedure. If the patient survives, treatment may fail and the patient returns to the pre-procedure prognosis, or treatment may be successful and the patient is relieved of symptoms. If we consider some fixed time horizon like a year or five years, we can assign utilities to the three possible outcomes (success, failure, death) and calculate expected utilities to choose a preferred treatment. In the current structure, there is no explicit allowance for the time horizon we are

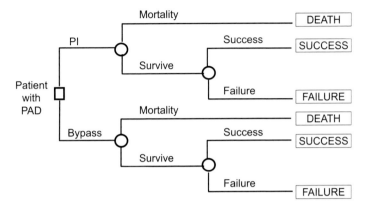

Figure 10.1   Decision tree for peripheral arterial disease (PAD). PI, percutaneous intervention.

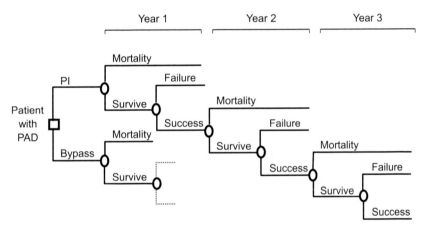

Figure 10.2   Decision tree for peripheral arterial disease (PAD) with a three-year time horizon. PI, percutaneous intervention.

considering, nor for the timing of the various events. Even if we consider a fixed time horizon of, say, five years, there surely is a different implication for prognosis if failure occurs in the first year versus the fifth year.

To incorporate the timing of events, we could break the problem into individual sequential years. Figure 10.2 depicts a partial tree with a three-year breakdown. In this tree we can see that events can occur at different time points. For example, failure can occur during the first year, or in the second year, or in the third. Similarly, the patient can die during the first year, or second or third. We can similarly proceed and expand the depth of the tree to include many more years into the future. If we were to allow for such events as a stroke or a myocardial infarction (MI or 'heart attack'), these can occur repeatedly and not only once, so we must accommodate these possibilities. Even if we have a fixed time horizon of, say, 20 years, the tree becomes very 'bushy' and unmanageable. The problems compound if we want to consider the 'lifetime' of the patient without having to specify a fixed time horizon. One clearly sees that the conventional decision tree approach has certain limitations, and we need a more complex model.

Another reason to adopt a type of decision framework having a more flexible time horizon is that some decision problems lend themselves to using life expectancy or quality-adjusted life expectancy as the outcome measure. This is especially true in cost-effectiveness analyses, in which a common outcome measure is needed to compare the benefits of different interventions to prevent or treat different conditions. The methodology offered in this chapter will enable such calculations.

There is another valuable contribution of the recursive models developed in this chapter. We often need survival curve data in modeling the choice among alternatives in a decision analysis. While it would be ideal to have such survival curve data for the alternative interventions being considered, this is usually not possible for several reasons. First, such data may not exist at all, e.g., we may have data for only a single time point such as two-year follow-up. Second, even if we have some survival curve data, there is often the need to extrapolate the results further into the future. Finally, the population from which the data were acquired may be somewhat different from the population to whom we wish to apply them. Therefore we need some general means of modeling events over time.

This chapter will focus on the simplest and most useful technique for modeling recursive events, Markov models (1–3). Markov models are a special case of wider-class, state-transition models (4). We will also introduce more advanced methods such as discrete event simulation (5, 6) and dynamic transmission models (7).

10.2 Markov models

Markov models are most useful when the decision problem involves risk over time, when the timing of events is important, and when events may happen more than once. These models differ from decision trees in that, instead of modeling uncertain events at chance nodes, the uncertain events are modeled as transitions between defined health states. In mathematical representations of Markov models, these transition probabilities are typically represented in terms of matrix algebra, but we will not need this formal representation in this book. Instead, we discuss the conceptual structure of state-transition models,

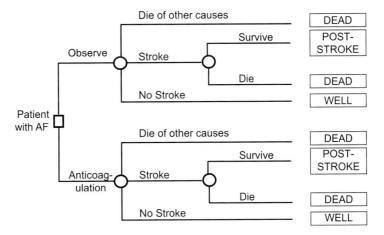

Figure 10.3   Decision tree for atrial fibrillation (AF).

including more general structures that permit us to model transition probabilities that depend on individual patient characteristics and histories. We will build on the following example.

EXAMPLE   Atrial fibrillation is a major public health problem, as it is the cause of 10–15% of all strokes. It is an irregularity of the heart rhythm that can lead to the formation of small blood clots (emboli) in the circulation. If these clots reach the brain, then a stroke occurs. Several trials have now demonstrated that anticoagulation dramatically reduces this risk of stroke. The dilemma is that it also increases the risk of bleeding, the most serious form of which is a bleed into the brain (i.e., a hemorrhagic stroke). Thus the decision problem is whether the reduced risk of embolic stroke from using anticoagulation is worth the increased risk of bleeding. Clearly this depends on the risk of emboli – the higher the risk, the greater the payoff from anticoagulation. But how high does the risk need to be to make it worthwhile? One way to approach this is to draw the simplified decision tree in Figure 10.3. The uncertainty in this problem relates to what event the patient may experience (stroke, death, no event), which then translates into one of three possible outcomes (post-stroke, dead, well). We have made some implicit simplifying assumptions that the post-stroke state is the same following a bleed (hemorrhagic stroke) or an embolus (ischemic stroke), and that dead is the same regardless of how the patient dies. We can then assign utilities to the various outcomes and roll back the tree. As in the previous example, a stroke or bleed can occur repeatedly during the lifetime of the patient, so we must model the entire uncertain life span of the patient, and allow for repeated uncertain events. Similarly, we have to allow for death to occur at any time point. The following development will relate to this example and present the Markov model.

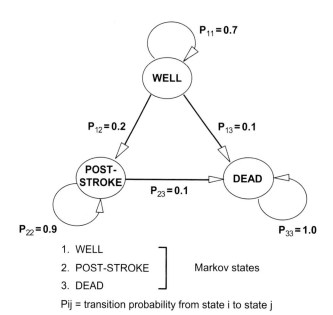

1. WELL
2. POST-STROKE   ⎤ Markov states
3. DEAD   ⎦

Pij = transition probability from state i to state j

Figure 10.4   State-transition diagram. Well, post-stroke, and dead represent the three Markov states. P_{ij}, transition probability from state i to state j.

In this problem, the patient must be in one of three mutually exclusive and collectively exhaustive *states*: well, post-stroke, or dead. The well state includes patients who are asymptomatic, but in whom the atrial fibrillation continues. Their physical functioning is normal and let's assume they have a normal quality of life in spite of the increased risk of stroke. We also assume that the risk of death from all other causes is similar to the rest of the population. The post-stroke state relates to patients who have survived a stroke. They have a reduced quality of life and an increased probability of further stroke (and hence require treatment with anticoagulation).

The time horizon of the analysis is divided into equal time intervals (e.g., year, month), referred to as *cycles*. All events of interest are modeled as *transitions* from one state to another. Figure 10.4 presents a *state-transition diagram*. The arrows represent possible transitions among the states. Notice that it is possible for a patient to remain in a given state in successive time periods. This is represented by an arrow leading from a state into itself. Also notice that some transitions are not possible (e.g., from dead to well). The model also assumes that in any given cycle, only one transition is possible. In Section 10.9, we will introduce discrete event simulation models, which require neither a fixed cycle length nor predefined states.

The length of the cycle is chosen to reflect a time interval that is clinically meaningful. If the decision problem considers the entire life span of the

Table 10.1 Probability transition matrix

		State of next cycle		
		Well	Post-stroke	Dead
State of current cycle	**Well**	0.7	0.2	0.1
	Post-stroke	0.0	0.9	0.1
	Dead	0.0	0.0	1.0

patient, and if critical events are not especially frequent, then a cycle of one year may be appropriate. For shorter time horizons, or if critical events tend to occur frequently, we may choose shorter cycles, such as one month. It is important to choose the cycle so that we can expect events to occur only once during a cycle (one transition per cycle). Another factor influencing cycle length is the availability of data. If we have only annual survival data, it is natural to use a cycle length of one year, although it is fairly straightforward to convert transition probabilities from one cycle length to another, provided that we are willing to assume that the instantaneous transition *rate* doesn't change within a cycle. (We return to the relation between rates and probabilities in Section 10.6.)

The numbers written beside each transition arrow in Figure 10.4 represent the probabilities of making that transition in one cycle. They are called the one-cycle *transition probabilities*. P_{ij} represents the probability of going from state i to state j in one cycle. For example, the probability that a well patient moves into the post-stroke state is 0.2. (We are using hypothetical numbers for this example to make the calculations more intuitive.) In any given cycle, the patient must be in one, and only one, of the states. Hence the sum of the probabilities over all arrows leading out of every state must equal 1.0.

The probabilities in Figure 10.4 can also be represented in matrix form, as in Table 10.1. The rows of the table represent the current state, and the columns represent the state of the next cycle. The probabilities in each *row* must add to 1.0. This is called the one-cycle *transition matrix*, or the *P-matrix*. In a model with many states, it is convenient to present the states and transition probabilities in matrix form.

The one-cycle transition probabilities may be constant throughout many cycles or may depend on time and thus change from cycle to cycle. If they are the same for every cycle, the Markov model is said to be a *stationary Markov model*, or a *Markov chain*. In most health applications, however, the assumption of stationarity is seldom met, if only because the probabilities of transition to 'dead' tend to increase with age and, therefore, with time. Markov chains will be useful to evaluate situations that do not evolve over a long time horizon (for example, end-stage cancer), or situations where mortality is not involved and the patient moves among various other states (for example, psoriasis, where treatment is evaluated not on patient survival but on a patient's transitions among various symptomatic stages of the disease).

Each state may be associated with a different quality of life and may involve different resource costs. Hence we can assign a different utility and cost to being in each state. Our modeling will enable the calculation of life expectancy, quality-adjusted life expectancy, expected utility, and expected resource costs.

Any process that evolves over time with associated uncertainty is referred to as a *stochastic process*, and models of such processes are called stochastic models or, equivalently, probabilistic models. If an additional restriction is applied, the process is referred to as a Markov process. This restriction states that the behavior of the process subsequent to any cycle does not depend on the history prior to that cycle. This is known as the *Markovian property* and reflects a 'lack of memory' for the process. In other words, prognosis in the above example depends only on the current state and not on how the patient reached the current state. For example, if the patient is now in the post-stroke state it doesn't matter if he or she has already spent several cycles in that state or has reached this state for the first time this cycle.

Obviously, in reality this 'memorylessness' property in Markov models does not always hold. However, we will still be able to use Markov models even for situations where the prior history or length of time spent in a state does matter. For example, the prognosis of a patient may depend on how many MIs or strokes the patient had. The trick is to create additional states to correspond to different past histories leading to the current state. This will be dealt with later in the chapter, in Section 10.4.

10.3 Evaluating Markov models

Creating a Markov model requires several steps: define the states, determine the cycle length, consider possible transitions among states, assess transition probabilities, and assess utilities (and, if you are using the model for a cost-effectiveness analysis, the costs) associated with being in each state for one cycle. Now it is time to consider the evaluation and calculation process involved with the model.

There are three basic methods to evaluate a Markov process:
1. Fundamental matrix solution (Section 10.3.1)
2. Cohort simulation (Section 10.3.2)
3. Monte Carlo simulation (Section 10.3.9)

10.3.1 Fundamental matrix solution

The fundamental matrix solution can be used only for Markov chains, when the transition probabilities are constant over time. It requires some basic knowledge of matrix algebra, which is beyond the scope of this book. This method generates values for the expected time spent in each state, yielding estimates for life expectancy in each state and overall. The mean duration in each state may be multiplied by a quality adjustment factor and summed across all the states, to yield quality-adjusted life expectancy. It also generates values for the standard deviation of the duration in each state. The matrix solution does not allow for changes in utility over time, but a modification of the fundamental matrix solution has been developed to calculate expected discounted life-years (2).

10.3.2 Cohort simulation

Cohort simulation is a very intuitive representation of a Markov process. The simulation considers a hypothetical cohort of patients who are initially distributed among the possible states and follows their transitions among the states from cycle to cycle based on the transition probabilities. In our stroke example, consider a hypothetical cohort of 10 000 patients who are all in the well state. The transition probabilities in Figure 10.4 (or Table 10.1) imply that there is a 0.7 chance the patient who is well will remain in the well state in the next cycle, a 0.2 chance the patient will go from well to post-stroke in the next cycle, and a 0.1 chance of dying. Hence, after one cycle we can expect, on average, that 7000 of the 10 000 well patients will remain in the well state, 2000 patients will be in the post-stroke state, and 1000 patients will be dead. This is represented graphically in Figure 10.5, which depicts the transitions through three cycles.

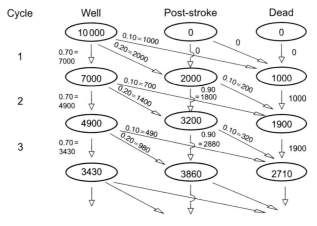

Figure 10.5   Cohort simulation.

Table 10.2 Cohort simulation

	State		
Cycle	Well	Post-stroke	Dead
0	10 000	0	0
1	7000	2000	1000
2	4900	3200	1900
3	3430	3860	2710
4	2401	4160	3439
5	1681	4224	4095
6	1176	4138	4686
7	824	3959	5217
. . .	. . .	. . .	. . .
93	0	1	9999
94	0	0	10 000

Table 10.2 presents the same information and extends the simulation for many more cycles until all (or nearly all) patients are in the dead state. The display in Table 10.2 is called the *Markov trace* for our example. The dead state is called an *absorbing state*, which means that once a patient enters that state, the probability of exiting from the state is zero. In the long run, all members of a Markov cohort end up in an absorbing state. For practical purposes, we are usually content to terminate the simulation when the fraction of the cohort remaining alive is below some small threshold (e.g., 0.1%), when a fixed age has been reached (e.g., 120), or some other criterion.

10.3.3 Calculating life expectancy

Now that we have performed the cohort simulation we are ready for some calculations of life expectancy and quality-adjusted life expectancy. Let us calculate the total number of cycles (e.g., years) that the cohort of 10 000 lived. Every cycle in which a patient is alive (either well or post-stroke) contributes one cycle 'credit' to this total. In cycle 1 there are 7000 well patients and 2000 post-stroke patients, contributing a total of 9000 cycle credits. Cycle 2 contributes 8100 (= 4900 + 3200) cycle credits, and so on. Table 10.3 presents the

Table 10.3 Calculating life expectancy

Cycle	State Well	Post-stroke	Dead	Cycle sum
0	10 000	0	0	
1	7000	2000	1000	9000
2	4900	3200	1900	8100
3	3430	3860	2710	7290
4	2401	4160	3439	6561
5	1681	4224	4095	5905
6	1176	4138	4686	5314
7	824	3959	5217	4783
. . .	. . .	. . .	. . .	. . .
93	0	1	9999	1
94	0	0	10 000	0
Total	23 333	66 667		90 000

calculations in more detail. The fifth column of Table 10.3 presents the cycle sum for that cycle.

If we now look at the total of column 5, we obtain the total number of cycles lived by this hypothetical cohort of 10 000 patients. Dividing the total number of cycles by the number of patients yields the life expectancy of an individual patient, in this case 9.0 cycles. If all we need at some point of a decision tree is life expectancy, then we have just demonstrated how this quantity can be obtained.

Moreover, the totals of columns 2 and 3 represent the total numbers of cycles (e.g., life-years) lived by cohort members in the well and post-stroke states respectively. In this example we assumed that transitions occur at the beginning of each cycle, and therefore we have not included the first entry of 10 000 in the sum. Dividing the sums by 10 000, we obtain an average duration of 2.333 cycles in the well state and 6.667 in the post-stroke state. Because patients who are alive must be either well or post-stroke, the sum of these two numbers is the total average number of cycles lived by each patient (9.0).

In this example we have used constant transition probabilities. We could have easily used time-dependent probabilities instead. In both cases – stationary or

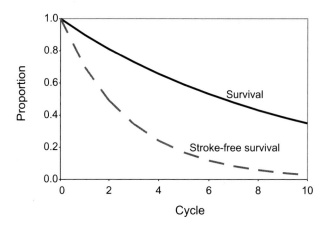

Figure 10.6   Markov survival trace.

time-dependent probabilities – the cohort simulation can easily be performed on any common spreadsheet.

10.3.4 Estimating survival curves

The cohort simulation presented in Table 10.3 can be used to plot the survival curve. This is presented in Figure 10.6 for a period of ten cycles. On the vertical axis we have the percentage of patients surviving (i.e., alive) at the end of each cycle. On the horizontal axis we plot time in cycles. For example, in Table 10.3 we see that at the beginning of cycle 3 there are 2710 patients in the dead state, implying that 7290 patients are still alive, for a survival of 72.9%. This can be seen in Figure 10.6. This curve is also referred to as a *Markov trace*. Note that it contains the same information as in the dead column of Table 10.3. Thus, by means of a Markov trace we can visually model survival and use survival data for various needs. This is especially valuable for situations when we only have one or two points on a survival curve and we need more specific data for the analysis or need to project survival into the future to estimate life expectancy. The life expectancy calculated in the previous section can be viewed as the area under the Markov trace when we follow it until it approaches the horizontal axis. We will return to the Markov trace and its relation to the 'true' survival curve later in the chapter when we discuss some 'fine-tuning' of the model.

10.3.5 Estimating partitioned survival curves

We may be interested not only in overall survival, but also in disease-free survival. We can use the information in Table 10.3 to plot a 'stroke-free'

Table 10.4 Calculating expected utility

Cycle	State			Cycle utility
	Well $U = 1.0$	Post-stroke $U = 0.6$	Dead $U = 0.0$	
0	10 000	0	0	
1	7000	2000	1000	8200
2	4900	3200	1900	6820
3	3430	3860	2710	5746
4	2401	4160	3439	4897
5	1681	4224	4095	4215
6	1176	4138	4686	3659
7	824	3959	5217	3199
...	...	...	...	...
93	0	1	9999	0
94	0	0	10 000	0
Total				63 331

survival curve for our hypothetical cohort. This curve, which lies below the overall survival curve, indicates the percentage of patients who remain well after each number of elapsed cycles. The disease-free (stroke-free in our example) survival curve is also part of the Markov trace, and is also shown in Figure 10.6.

10.3.6 Quality-adjusted life expectancy (expected utility)

As mentioned earlier, being in different states may imply a different quality of life for the patient. Let us assume that the quality of life in the well state has a utility of 1.0, dead has a utility of 0.0, and post-stroke has a utility of 0.6. The utility associated with spending one cycle in a particular state is referred to as *incremental utility*. One needs to distinguish the incremental utility, which is accrued for every cycle, from the one-time transition utility (or disutility) that is accrued when an event occurs during a cycle (see Section 10.5).

Table 10.4 presents the Markov trace for the cohort simulation in tabular form, but now with the utility calculations added. We will now assume that the cycle length is one year, so that each cycle spent in one of the 'alive' states contributes 1.0 year of life expectancy. Moreover, each cycle spent in the well state, whose utility is 1.0, contributes 1.0 quality-adjusted life-year (QALY).

Column 5 now presents the sum of utilities (or QALYs) for the entire cohort for each cycle. For example, for cycle 1, 7000 well patients have a utility of 1 QALY each, contributing a total of 7000 QALYs, and the 2000 post-stroke patients contribute 1200 QALYs ($= 2000 \cdot 0.6$), for a total of 8200 QALYs. If we now look at the total for column 5, we obtain the total expected utility for the cohort. Dividing by 10 000 we obtain an expected utility of 6.33 for an individual patient. This is equivalent to 6.33 QALYs, compared to a life expectancy of nine years when there was no consideration of quality of life.

Life expectancy can also be visualized graphically as the area under the overall survival curve. This area represents the expected number of person years lived by the members of the cohort. The area *between* the overall survival curve and the stroke-free survival curve represents the expected number of person years lived in the post-stroke state, and the area *under* the stroke-free curve represents the number of person years lived in the well state. Therefore, quality-adjusted life expectancy can be interpreted in Figure 10.6 as the weighted sum of the area *between* the overall survival and stroke-free survival curve (weighted by 0.6) and the area *under* the stroke-free survival curve (weighted by 1.0).

When we apply these types of results to cost-effectiveness analysis, we will want to weight each cycle by a factor that reflects how far it is in the future. This is called *time discounting*. If we want to discount life-years and QALYs, then every figure in column 5 should be weighted by a *discount factor* before summing them to generate discounted QALYs. As we saw in Chapter 9, a typical discount factor for the nth cycle would be $1/(1 + r)^n$, which equals $1/(1.03)^n$ if the discount rate is 3%.

We will demonstrate this procedure presently in the cost calculation.

10.3.7 Cost calculations

Let us assume that the resource costs associated with being well are $100 per year, the costs for post-stroke are $150 per year, and that being dead is costless. Table 10.5 presents the cohort simulation for the cost analysis. The first four columns represent the numbers of patients in each state for each cycle and are identical to the first four columns of Tables 10.3 and 10.4. Column 5 now represents the total costs for the respective cycle. For example, in cycle 1, 7000 patients have a cost of $100 each and 2000 patients accrue a cost of $150 each, for a total cost of $1 000 000. If we discount the costs from the nth cycle to the beginning of the simulation using a discount factor of $(1/1.03)^n$, then the present value of this sum is $970 874, as shown in

Table 10.5 Calculating expected (discounted) costs

Cycle	State			Cycle cost	Cycle PV (3%)
	Well $100	Post-stroke $150	Dead $0		
0	10 000	0	0		
1	7000	2000	1000	$1 000 000	$970 874
2	4900	3200	1900	$970 000	$914 318
3	3430	3860	2710	$922 000	$843 761
4	2401	4160	3439	$864 100	$767 742
5	1681	4224	4095	$801 700	$691 553
6	1176	4138	4686	$738 337	$618 346
7	824	3959	5217	$676 268	$549 868
...	...	...	...	...	...
93	0	1	9999	$83	$5
94	0	0	10 000	$75	$5
Total					$9 323 977

PV: present value.

column 6. Each value in column 6 is obtained by dividing the amount in column 5 by $(1.03)^n$, where n is the cycle number. The total of column 6 gives us the discounted value of all costs during the lifetime of this process. Dividing this total by 10 000 patients, we get an average discounted cost of $932 for each patient.

As we saw in Chapter 9, the total discounted quality-adjusted life years and the discounted cost data can be used to determine cost-effectiveness. In order to calculate an incremental cost-effectiveness ratio we would need to repeat the calculation for an alternative clinical strategy. Alternative clinical strategies in our example might be other treatments to prevent stroke in patients with asymptomatic AF such as newer medications (which are safer but also more expensive), catheter-guided ablation, or no treatment, which would represent the natural history of the condition. The alternative strategy would have a different set of transition probabilities, different costs and utilities associated with the health states, and different initial costs in the case of catheter-guided ablation. The incremental cost-effectiveness ratio between the two strategies would then be calculated as the ratio of the difference in expected cumulative cost, divided by the difference in quality-adjusted life expectancy.

10.3.8 Fine-tuning: the half-cycle correction

One of the basic assumptions underlying Markov models is that transitions can occur only once in each cycle. We are also assuming that the transition from state to state is instantaneous. However, we have not yet addressed the issue of when during a cycle these transitions take place. If we look at the cohort simulation of Table 10.2, we see that in cycle 1 there are 7000 patients in the well state, 2000 in the post-stroke state, and 1000 dead. Since this is cycle 1, we have evidently assumed that transitions occur at the beginning of the cycle, and membership in the cycle is counted at the end of the cycle. Alternatively, we could have assumed that transitions occur at the end of the cycle, and then the accounting would have been different. In reality, though, transitions can occur at any time during the cycle along the continuous time axis. Thus, on average, we can assume that transitions occur halfway through the cycle. If this is the case, then the 10 000 patients make the transition in the middle of the first cycle rather than at the beginning. This means that each of them contributes an additional half-cycle to the calculated life expectancy. We should add this 0.5 to the life expectancy of 9.0 cycles that we had calculated earlier, yielding a corrected life expectancy of 9.5 cycles. We should also make this adjustment in the calculation of expected utility. Since all 10 000 started out in the well state, and if transitions occur in the middle of the cycle, we have to add 0.5 units to the expected utility, yielding an expected utility of 6.83 (i.e., 6.83 quality-adjusted cycles).

The above example showed that we have underestimated life expectancy by assuming that transitions occur at the beginning of the cycle. To correct this we have added 0.5 cycles to life expectancy. This is called the *half-cycle correction*. If our accounting had transitions occurring at the end of the cycle, we should subtract 0.5 cycles.

These approximations to life expectancy can be seen graphically in Figure 10.7. The continuous curve represents the 'true' survival curve. Allowing transitions at the beginning of each cycle is equivalent to counting membership at the end of the cycle, resulting in the underestimation of survival, as shown in the top graph in Figure 10.7. Life expectancy is the area under the survival curve. The rectangles represent the area calculated by the cohort simulation. Had we assumed transitions to occur at the end of each cycle, which is equivalent to counting membership at the beginning of the (next) cycle, we would have overestimated survival, as seen in the middle graph of Figure 10.7. The half-cycle correction is equivalent to moving the graph a half-cycle to the right to simulate that transitions occur halfway through the cycle. In a practical sense we count membership at the end of the cycle and add a half-cycle for the initial

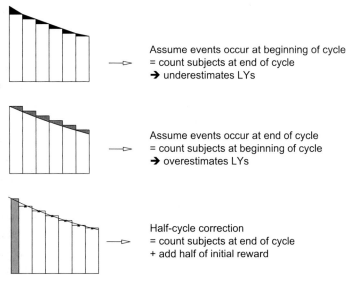

Assume events occur at beginning of cycle
= count subjects at end of cycle
→ underestimates LYs

Assume events occur at end of cycle
= count subjects at beginning of cycle
→ overestimates LYs

Half-cycle correction
= count subjects at end of cycle
+ add half of initial reward

Figure 10.7   Half-cycle correction.

membership. This yields a better approximation to the true survival curve, as seen by the lower graph in Figure 10.7.

The half-cycle correction presented above is very appropriate for situations where we follow the process to absorption (i.e., death). There are also situations where we want to calculate five-year survival, for example, or follow the process for a limited number of cycles. We must then make an additional correction for members of the cohort who are still alive at the end of the observation or simulation. To accomplish this we would subtract a half-cycle worth of utility for the surviving members of the cohort in the last cycle.

10.3.9 Monte Carlo simulation

In cohort simulation, transitions are experienced by the proportion of persons in each state corresponding to the transition probabilities. In essence, this is the 'average' experience of the patients in the cohort. In Monte Carlo simulation, instead of proportions of patients making the transitions, individual patients are simulated going from cycle to cycle one at a time, based on their transition probabilities. The transition probabilities that govern each individual transition during each cycle are realized as random events governed by computer-generated random numbers between 0 and 1. We will return to the mechanics of this random process shortly.

If a model involves an absorbing state, such as dead, then each patient is run through the process until he or she reaches that state. If the model does

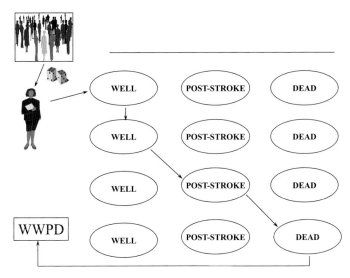

Figure 10.8   Monte Carlo simulation for a single patient. WWPD, well, well, post-stroke, dead.

not have an absorbing state, then the simulation is run a predetermined number of cycles. The process is repeated for many patients (e.g., 100 000). The appropriate number of simulated patients depends on the magnitudes of the transition probabilities in the model (smaller probabilities of uncommon events necessitate more simulations), and on the size of the difference between intervention strategies that we are expecting to find. It is not uncommon for Monte Carlo simulations of Markov models to require 1 000 000 patients.

For each patient we keep track of the number of cycles spent in each state. The average times spent in each state other than dead can be summed to yield an estimate of life expectancy. Quality adjustments can be made, and costs can be assigned to each state, so that we can calculate quality-adjusted survival and cost for each simulated patient. The averages of quality-adjusted survival and cost over the simulated patients can be interpreted as quality-adjusted life expectancy and expected cost, respectively. As in cohort simulation, discounting can be applied to both quality-adjusted life years and costs for cost-effectiveness analyses.

Returning now to the atrial fibrillation example, Figure 10.8 depicts graphically the path of one patient from the well to the dead state. The patient remains in the well state for two cycles, moves to post-stroke for one cycle and then moves to dead. This sequence of states is represented by WWPD. The dice represent the act of 'drawing probabilities' from an appropriate probability transition matrix. The technical side of performing the simulation will now be discussed.

Let us now go through a detailed example of how such a simulation is actually performed. We will use the transition probabilities of Table 10.1. To simulate each patient we need to 'simulate' the transition probabilities. This is achieved by drawing random numbers to represent the probabilities and guide transitions. Such random numbers are usually generated by a computer when the simulations are run. Our example will only involve ten patients, so it can easily be done by hand. Consider the following sequence of random numbers:

10480 15011 01536 02011 81647 22368 46573 25595 85393 30995 24130 48360

Suppose that when we start a patient is in the well state. The probabilities of 0.2, 0.7, and 0.1 in Table 10.1 are simulated by referring to the first digit in the sequence of random numbers. The digits 1–7 represent the probability of 0.7 (remaining well), the digits 8 and 9 represent the probability 0.2 (transition to post-stroke), and the digit 0 represents the probability 0.1 (death). For a patient in the post-stroke state, the probability of 0.9 is represented by digits 1–9, and the remaining 0.1 is again represented by the digit 0. (If the probabilities were in two-digit accuracy, we would have used pairs of random digits.) Drawing these numbers is like playing a lottery or a casino game, hence the name, *Monte Carlo simulation* (named after the famous casinos of Monte Carlo).

Table 10.6 presents the simulation results for ten patients. Let us look at patient number 1, generated by the first two random digits above: the first digit is 1 so it represents a transition from well to well and the second digit is 0, representing transition to death. Hence the sequence WWD. The second patient is generated by subsequent digits: 4 represents transition to well, 8 to post-stroke, 0 to dead, hence WWPD. Notice that patient number 2 is exactly the patient that is pictorially represented in Figure 10.8. Every time the sequence of digits reaches the digit 0, this indicates the death of the patient simulated.

Let us now examine Table 10.6. The second column represents the simulated sequence of states. Column 3 counts the number of cycles in the well state, column 4 is the number of cycles in post-stroke, column 5 is the total number of cycles alive (the sum of columns 3 and 4), and column 6 represents the total number of quality-adjusted cycles for each patient (where U(well) $= 1.0$ and U(post-stroke) $= 0.6$, as before). The row for 'Total' represents the sum of the ten rows and is the aggregate value for the ten patients. Taking the average (dividing the total by 10) we obtain the row for 'Mean.' Thus, the average duration is 2.9 cycles well, and 4.8 cycles in post-stroke, for a total of 7.7 cycles. The average expected utility is 5.78 quality-adjusted cycles. We could similarly add a column for costs.

Table 10.6 Monte Carlo simulation for ten patients

Patient	Sequence of states	Number of cycles in W	Number of cycles in P	Number of cycles alive (W + P)	Lifetime utility
1	WWD	2	0	2	2
2	WWPD	2	1	3	2.6
3	WWWD	3	0	3	3
4	WWWD	3	0	3	3
5	WWWWWD	5	0	5	5
6	WWD	2	0	2	2
7	WWWPPPPPPPP	3	26	29	18.6
	PPPPPPPPP				
	PPPPPPPPD				
8	WPPPPPPPD	1	7	8	5.2
9	WWPPPD	2	3	5	3.8
10	WWWWWW	6	11	17	12.6
	PPPPPPPP				
	PPPD				
	Total	29	48	77	57.8
	Mean	2.9	4.8	7.7	5.78
	Standard deviation	1.52	8.34	8.73	5.48

W, well: $U(W) = 1.0$; P, post-stroke: $U(P) = 0.6$; D, dead: $U(D) = 0.0$.

All measures (number of cycles, costs, and quality-adjusted cycles) can and should be discounted in cost-effectiveness analyses.

The Monte Carlo simulation yields another important quantity that cannot be obtained via a cohort simulation, namely a measure of variation around the mean. The standard deviation for each distribution can be calculated, because we have all individual values. In the cohort simulation, the patients do not move individually but rather as a whole cohort and therefore we cannot observe individual variation. The fundamental matrix solution mentioned earlier can also provide us with exact values for the standard deviation.

If the above simulation had been performed a very large number of times (e.g., 10 000), the numbers in the totals and means would be very close to the figures in Tables 10.3 and 10.4. The reason for the discrepancy is the small sample size. The first 20 random digits contain six zeros, three times their expected number (i.e., 2). Hence the first six patients live rather short lives, because of 'bad luck.' Over a large number of simulations, these events should balance out to their expected frequencies.

10.4 Special Markov states

10.4.1 Temporary states

In the above examples, each state had an associated utility and cost per unit of time (i.e., per cycle). There are situations where the actual event that causes a transition from state to state involves a one-time cost or temporary change in quality of life. In the atrial fibrillation example consider the transition from well to post-stroke as a result of a stroke. The stroke itself has certain morbidity and costs associated with the event: hospitalization, follow-up, recovery, etc. We cannot ignore these disutilities and costs in the utility and cost calculations.

These short-term effects can be incorporated by adding an additional state to the process, called a *temporary state*. This is depicted in Figure 10.9, where we added a state called 'stroke.' A temporary state is characterized by having transitions from it only to other states and not to itself. Thus, a patient can stay in this state for one cycle only and must move to another state for the next cycle. The presence of a temporary state enables the separate calculation of costs for that state or event and considers the separate (usually lower) utility for the period in question. The post-stroke state reflects all the years following a stroke after the patient has survived the year in which the stroke occurred. That specific year is captured in the (temporary) stroke state.

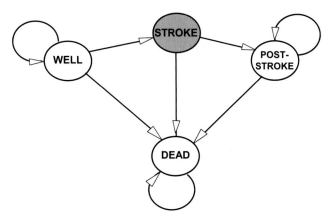

Figure 10.9   Temporary state.

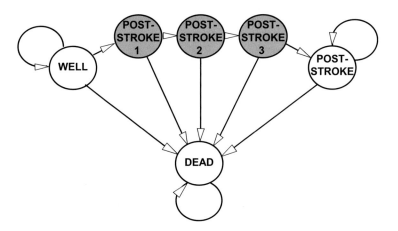

Figure 10.10   Tunnel states.

Another use of a temporary state is to be able to apply different transition probabilities following a short-term event. It is possible that the probability of dying during the 12 months following a stroke is higher than the mortality probability a year or more after the stroke. By having stroke as a separate state, we can incorporate this temporarily different transition probability into our model.

10.4.2 Tunnel states

Recall that we said that a Markov model requires that transition probabilities depend only on the current state, and possibly on time, but not on the history of prior states. This assumption has been implicit in our analysis of the atrial fibrillation example. There are situations where the history of the disease or the patient affects the transition probabilities. Fortunately, it is usually possible to modify a Markov model to incorporate this possibility.

In the atrial fibrillation example, let us assume that the annual probability of death is different in each of the first three years following a stroke. Starting from the fourth year, mortality remains constant. This can be handled by defining a series of temporary states, each leading into the next. This is depicted in Figure 10.10. The states post-stroke 1, post-stroke 2, and post-stroke 3 are temporary states and can only be visited in that particular sequence. This can be seen as analogous to passing through a tunnel; hence, these states are indeed called *tunnel states*. Thus, using tunnel states is a simple 'trick' to model the impact of history on transitions. One can enter the post-stroke 2 state *only* from the post-stroke 1 state, etc. Note that the post-stroke state, into which a patient transitions after surviving three post-stroke cycles, is not a temporary state, as a patient can remain in this state for consecutive cycles.

10.4.3 Population heterogeneity

Another example where the addition of states can help is when we are dealing with population heterogeneity. If a patient's prognosis depends on other co-morbid conditions, then decomposing one heterogeneous state into separate states for each condition will enable us to treat each subgroup of patients separately with different transition probabilities. For example, suppose that, in a patient with atrial fibrillation, survival depends on whether or not the patient had a previous MI. Thus, the well state actually contains two distinct populations: those with and those without a prior MI. For the model to reflect the differential mortality and stroke probabilities, we must partition the well state into two separate states representing the two separate patient populations. A prior MI may also influence the post-stroke patients, and this state may also require partitioning into two distinct states. Of course, the Markov model should then allow for the event MI to occur (which may require a temporary state). If we do not account for the occurrence of an MI in the model, then we can avoid the need for state partitioning by running the basic model separately on the two populations. We will return to patient heterogeneity in Chapter 12.

10.4.4 Absorbing states

The Markov models for both of our examples have a dead state. Once a patient reaches this state he or she will remain there forever. We have previously defined a state that has a transition only to itself (with probability 1.0) as an *absorbing state*, as the process is eventually totally 'absorbed' in this state. This is quite evident by the cohort simulation where all patients eventually end up in the dead state. Many chronic conditions in medicine fit such a model, and for such models the cohort simulation can be ended, for practical purposes, in a finite number of steps. These are the models usually used in published reports of decision analyses in the health and medical fields. However, there are situations where an absorbing state does not exist. If mortality is not involved we may want to follow the process for some time but may not be able to 'end' it. Models of this type are called 'non-absorbing models.'

10.4.5 Non-absorbing models

Consider the following example of a hypothetical skin disease that can either be acute or dormant. Let the cycle length be one month. The patient may bounce back and forth between the two states, as depicted in the

Table 10.7 Skin disease cohort simulation: I

	State	
Cycle	Dormant	Acute
0	10 000	0
1	8000	2000
2	7000	3000
3	6500	3500
4	6250	3750
5	6125	3875
6	6063	3938
7	6031	3969
8	6016	3984
9	6008	3992
10	6004	3996
11	6002	3998
12	6001	3999
13	6000	4000
14	6000	4000

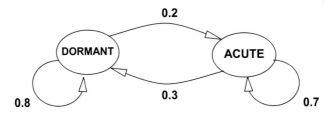

Figure 10.11 State-transition diagram for a hypothetical skin disease.

state-transition diagram of Figure 10.11. A patient whose condition is dormant has a probability of 0.8 of remaining in that state for the next cycle and a probability of 0.2 of becoming acute. Similarly, there is a probability of 0.7 of remaining in the acute state after one cycle, and a complementary probability of 0.3 for moving into the dormant state.

Let us now perform a cohort simulation of 10 000 patients. Let us assume that they all start in the dormant state. As can easily be seen in Table 10.7, after 13 cycles the number of patients in each state remains the same from

Table 10.8 Skin disease cohort simulation: II

Cycle	State	
	Dormant	Acute
0	0	10 000
1	3000	7000
2	4500	5500
3	6500	3500
4	5250	4750
5	5813	4188
6	5906	4094
7	5953	4047
8	5977	4023
9	5988	4012
10	5994	4006
11	5997	4003
12	5999	4001
13	5999	4001
14	6000	4000

cycle to cycle. From this point on, there will always be 6000 patients with a dormant condition and 4000 in an acute condition. All transitions *out* of one state are balanced by transitions *into* it. The process has reached *equilibrium*. The long-run distribution among the various states reaches a *steady state*. Let us now see what happens if all patients begin the process in the acute state. Table 10.8 presents the cohort simulation. Again, after relatively few cycles, the process reaches a steady state. Notice that we would have reached the same steady state even if we started from totally extreme initial conditions. Thus, in processes that reach steady state, the initial distribution of patients is not relevant if we observe the process long enough. In some sense, absorbing models also reach an equilibrium where all patients end up in the absorbing state and stay there. Note that not all non-absorbing models reach equilibrium. Certain conditions must be satisfied by the probability transition matrix in order to reach equilibrium. If these conditions are satisfied, we have a so-called *ergodic chain*, and the equilibrium probabilities of being in each state can be obtained by solving a series of equations that can be generated through matrix algebra. Again, this is beyond the scope of this book.

Finding the steady-state probabilities is useful in many ways. For example, if we know the percentage of time a patient will spend in each state over the lifetime, we can calculate the average utility or cost, for that patient. The information can be very useful for planning. If different medical resources are needed for patients in different states, the steady-state probabilities can tell us how to allocate proportionately various resources for the different patient groups. We can plan ahead to the steady state and make sure that supply of resources meets demand. Almost all of the applications of Markov models in health care have been in situations with absorbing states and this will continue to be the focus of this chapter.

10.5 Markov cycle trees

We started this chapter by looking at why Markov models are needed. These are situations where the time horizon in a decision problem may not be fixed and events can occur repeatedly over time. Markov models were then presented along with methods to solve them and calculate various measures that could be used in a decision analysis. It is now time to see how a basic decision tree can be combined with a Markov model to help us solve the problem without having to deal with messy and unmanageable trees, like the recursive tree in Figure 10.2.

In the presentation of calculating Markov models we treated the transition probabilities as known entities that enabled transitions from state to state. We will elaborate on obtaining some of these probabilities later in this chapter. However, for an actual clinical setting, the transition from state to state may involve different paths. In our atrial fibrillation example, a transition from well to dead may occur in several ways: the patient may die from a fatal bleed, a fatal embolus, or she may die from unrelated causes such as an accident or another disease such as cancer (known as age–sex–race [ASR]-related mortality). Similarly, the transition from well to post-stroke can be via a non-fatal bleed or non-fatal embolus (Figure 10.12). All causes of death except from a bleed or embolus have been combined into one branch: 'die of other causes.' There will be a similar tree representing the possible transitions from the post-stroke state. There is no tree for the dead state, because no transitions are possible to other states. These one-cycle subtrees can be grafted on to one special node, referred to as a *Markov node*. There is one branch emanating from this node for every possible Markov state. This node, along with the (different) probability trees emanating from it, is called a *Markov cycle tree* (Figure 10.12). A cycle tree enables the decomposition of a complex uncertain

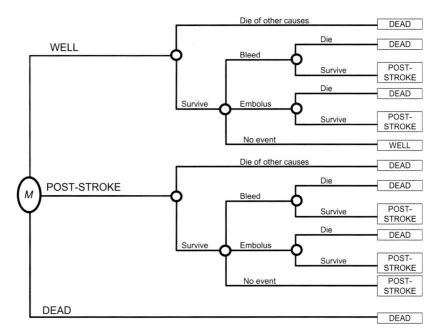

Figure 10.12   Markov cycle tree. *M*, Markov node.

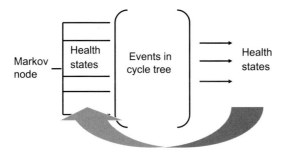

Figure 10.13   General concept of a Markov model.

situation into smaller, more manageable problems. It lends itself to available data for the various events, whereas data needed for the composite transition probabilities may be very difficult to obtain. The general concept of the Markov model is presented in Figure 10.13 with the health states emanating from the Markov node and events modeled in the cycle tree: during each cycle individuals can transition from one health state through the occurrence of events to another health state after which a new cycle begins.

Markov models with cycle trees are evaluated in a similar fashion to a Markov cohort simulation as explained above. One needs only the distribution of the initial cohort among the various states. (In our cohort simulation

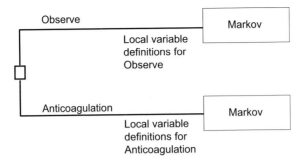

Figure 10.14   Schematic representation of the Markov decision model for atrial fibrillation. Note that the Markov model is identical in structure ('cloned') for both management options but that locally the variables have been defined so as to be applicable to the option, for example to take into account effectiveness of medication.

we assumed all patients started out in the well state.) The cohort is then partitioned among the states according to the probabilities of each subtree and traced through the subtree, yielding a new distribution of the cohort among the states. This will be the starting distribution for the next cycle. For each cycle we can calculate the cycle sum of incremental utilities and costs. These will be accumulated over all cycles until the termination of the process (when nearly the entire cohort is in the dead state).

In addition, each time an event occurs a one-time (dis)utility and cost may be incurred in that particular cycle. These transition (dis)utilities and costs (see Section 10.4.1) need to be defined in the cycle tree. An example of transition disutilities and costs is the temporary loss in quality of life and the one-time costs for the hospital admission and rehabilitation after a myocardial infarction. A term often used for these temporary disutilities and costs is a *toll*. The idea is that when a patient 'passes through' a particular event, he or she pays a toll, in terms of quality of life and/or cost.

There may be a different cycle tree for each health state branching from the initial Markov node. Furthermore, it can be useful to make a generic type of Markov model and link each strategy to this one generic Markov model, with definitions of the variables that make the model specific for that strategy. The decision problem can then be represented as the model in Figure 10.14. Such a model structure ensures that all strategies are modeled in a similar fashion. Most decision analysis software packages include the flexibility to do this.

10.6 Estimating transition probabilities

In the above examples we have used probabilities to describe transitions from state to state. The required probabilities are sometimes directly available from the literature, possibly by means of a probability tree like the one in

Figure 10.12. This is true both for constant and time-dependent transition probabilities. If probabilities do depend on time, such as when annual age–sex–race-specific (ASR-specific) mortality increases with the age of the cohort, and if we know these probabilities, then we can easily incorporate them into the cohort analysis.

Very frequently we have only limited probability data and we have to manipulate them to be able to generate estimates of the various transition probabilities. This requires the introduction of *rates*. We have seen that a probability describes the likelihood that an event will occur in a given time period and its value ranges from 0 to 1. A *rate* describes the number of occurrences of an event per given number of patients per unit of time. For example, data have shown that over three years, 60 out of 200 patients have died. The death rate is then 60 per 200 per three years, or 20 deaths per 200 patients per year, or 0.1 deaths per patient per year. Rates range from zero to infinity. A convenient mathematical property of rates, which is not true of probabilities, is that we can add and subtract rates (for the same time interval). Another convenient property of rates is that we can divide and multiply a given rate by a factor reflecting risk factors or interventions. We can also divide rates to change the units of time (e.g., divide the annual rate by 12 to convert it to a monthly rate). We cannot do these things to probabilities unless they are very small, in which case they behave much like rates. For example, suppose we wanted to reflect the fact that a particular risk group had ten times the risk of developing a disease as the general population. If the baseline probability in the general population reached more than 10% at some age, we would end up with a probability greater than 100%!

Occasionally, data in the literature will be reported as rates, and so we will need to convert rates into probabilities. If an event occurs at a constant rate r per time unit t, then the probability that an event will occur during time t is given by the equation:

$$p = 1 - e^{-rt} \tag{10.1}$$

This relates nicely to the survival curve, like the one shown in Figure 10.6 (if we label the vertical axis as probability rather than proportion). At any given time point (cycle), the height of the curve is e^{-rt}, which represents the probability of survival to time t. The complement, $1 - e^{-rt}$, is the probability of dying before time t, as described above.

On the other hand, if we have a probability and want to convert it to a rate, we use the equation:

$$r = -\frac{1}{t}\ln(1-p) \tag{10.2}$$

The reason we may wish to convert probabilities to rates is to exploit the additive properties of rates. For example, suppose we have a constant annual disease-specific mortality probability, $p_D = 0.2$, and that we also have mortality rates for the population by age (the 'A' of ASR). We then calculate the disease-specific mortality rate, r_D, using Equation 10.2. In this case $r_D = -\ln(1 - 0.2) = 0.223$. Suppose the age-specific annual mortality rate for a person of age 85 is 0.1, as before. Now we have two mortality forces acting on an 85-year-old with the disease: age-specific and disease-specific. We can add the two rates to obtain the total mortality rate of $r_D + r_A = 0.323$ and then convert this rate to a total mortality probability using Equation 10.1. This yields $p = 0.276$. This probability can now be used in the appropriate place in a Markov model or decision tree. We will revisit estimation of probabilities in Chapter 11.

A word of caution: when changing the cycle length in an analysis, transition probabilities must be adjusted. If we consider moving from an annual cycle to a monthly cycle, the probabilities *should not* be divided by 12! We have to convert the annual probability to an annual rate using Equation 10.2, divide the annual rate by 12 to obtain the monthly rate, and then convert the monthly rate to a monthly probability by using Equation 10.1. From a practical programming perspective it is useful to be able to vary cycle length without having to adjust all sorts of variables in the model. This can be facilitated by expressing all rates per person year and expressing cycle length in units of years.

10.7 Cohort vs. Monte Carlo simulation: which should I use?

One advantage of the Monte Carlo method, compared to cohort simulation, is that it also yields estimates for the entire frequency distribution of survival values for each state. These enable the estimation of variation around the expected values. However, this is not the most important advantage, nor the one that usually leads analysts to use a Monte Carlo simulation.

The most important reason to use a Monte Carlo simulation arises out of the need to retain variables that determine transition probabilities. Among such variables are aspects of patient history. In such situations, we would like to sidestep the Markov assumption that transition probabilities depend only on the current state. Such variables may include fixed characteristics, such as age, sex, and genetic risk factors. These fixed predictor variables could be accommodated by running the analysis with separate sets of transition probabilities for each relevant subpopulation, and then re-aggregating, but it might be more efficient to do a single simulation in which the population characteristics are drawn from a distribution.

More problematic are situations where the variables that influence transition probabilities are characteristics of the prior history within the decision model, such as previous occurrence of disease, response to treatment, and others. In other words, we may want the transition probabilities in a given cycle to depend on the states experienced in previous cycles. We have seen that devices such as tunnel states can be used to accommodate some such features of case histories in cohort analyses, but each such device adds to the number of states. Imagine a situation in which future transition probabilities depend on the *order* in which clinical events have been experienced, or on other complex functions of past history such as the time between events. The number of states we would have to add to shoehorn such a model into the Markovian template could fill the memories of many desktop computers. So we use Monte Carlo simulation, which enables us to define transition probabilities as functions of as many variables as we can build into the model. Such variables, when used in the simulation of an individual patient in a Monte Carlo simulation, are called *tracker variables*. The advantage of Monte Carlo simulation is that we need only retain tracker variables in memory during the simulation of one individual at a time. For each new patient, the tracker variables are 'reset,' and we begin a new simulation.

Using Monte Carlo simulation to model variability in each individual patient's disease history and to model uncertainty in the results is discussed further in Chapter 12.

10.8 Sensitivity analysis

It is inconceivable to address any modeling topic without emphasizing the importance of sensitivity analysis. This definitely holds true for Markov models. After we have obtained various measures, with or without using the models in a decision analysis, we must perform sensitivity analyses on the various parameters used. These include the determination of cycle length, the estimation of transition probabilities among states, estimation of probabilities for cycle trees, and the various costs and utilities for the different states. Even the consideration of changing the structure of the model, such as adding temporary states or tunnel states, can be included in sensitivity analysis. The nature of such analyses is not different from that which has been extensively discussed earlier in the book and will be discussed further in Chapter 12.

10.9 Discrete-event simulation

The Markov models described in this chapter complement and extend the framework of decision trees and enable an elegant way to accommodate a distant time horizon and a clinical history that evolves over discrete time cycles where the patient can be in one of several mutually exclusive states. However, in some situations, both decision trees and Markov models lack the flexibility for a more realistic representation of a clinical decision problem.

Sometimes the course of a disease may be more realistically represented by a model of continuous time, in which multiple events can occur at any point in time. In the atrial fibrillation example of Section 10.2, we can think of events such as stroke, MI, and other illnesses as occurring over time in any possible order, and not limited to one occurrence during a fixed cycle length. If we want to model such a process, we do not require the existence of states nor of mutually exclusive occurrences of events. Even if we want to consider states such as various levels of blood pressure, we face a continuum of states or a very large number of discrete states. These limitations can be overcome by other model structures that are more flexible than Markov models. We point the reader to one specific approach, discrete event simulation (DES) (5). As the name indicates, events occurring over time are simulated for a target population. Instead of specifying the probability that an event will occur within a particular time interval, as in a Markov model, one specifies the probability distribution for the time until the next event of a particular type occurs. Random numbers are used to determine the length of time until the next event of each type. Each patient is simulated individually (similar to the discrete time Monte Carlo simulations described in Section 10.3.9). Events can occur at any time point on the continuous time scale. Events can include actual clinical events such as stroke or MI, changes in clinical conditions, changes in disease status such as cancer progression, adverse effects of medication, and even administrative events such as discharge from the hospital.

The DES involves much more complex modeling as compared to decision trees and Markov models and could perhaps be considered as a more natural way to represent the course of a disease. However, it is well beyond the scope of this chapter and this book. The reader is further referred to review papers on the subject (6).

10.10 Markov decision process models

Standard Markov models can become extremely cumbersome in the context of sequential decision making since this may involve multiple embedded decision nodes in the branches of the decision tree or multiple complex strategies explicitly stating future decisions. Think of repetitive decisions such as whether or not to start on/continue/stop lipid-lowering medication, the optimal timing of initiating HIV treatment, abandon/extract decisions for failed cardiac leads, or the accept/reject decision for a patient with end-stage liver disease on a waiting list in various possible states of health offered various qualities of livers based on location and waiting time (8). In each of these problems the number of combinations of possible states and possible decisions becomes enormous, making a standard Markov model intractable. Markov decision-process models provide the analytical tools to cope with such situations. Markov decision processes are widely used in industrial and manufacturing applications, robotics, automated control, and economics but not (yet) in medical decision making. They generalize standard Markov models by embedding the sequential decision process in the model and allowing multiple decisions in multiple time periods. Two types of models can be distinguished depending on the timing of the decisions. A discrete-time Markov decision process allows for decisions only at discrete-time intervals. In a continuous-time Markov decision process the decisions can occur at any time. The analytical process involves iteratively solving a set of recursive equations which is done with dynamic programming (8).

10.11 Dynamic transmission models

Most applications of decision analysis and Markov models in health care relate to such non-communicable diseases as heart disease, stroke, cancer, and many other chronic conditions. For such conditions it is sufficient to model the outcomes for one patient at a time, since what happens to one patient does not affect the outcomes of other individuals. By contrast, in many infectious diseases the health status of one person may affect the health of others. For example, a person immunized by a vaccine is less likely to acquire, and therefore transmit, the infection to other people. Policy decisions involving such interventions as vaccinations, treatments that reduce infectivity, masks, and quarantines therefore require consideration of an entire population of individuals, not just one infected patient at a time. Examples include HIV and other sexually transmitted diseases, influenza, pneumonia, pertussis (whooping cough), hepatitis A, B, and C, tuberculosis, malaria, and more. The transmissible nature of such diseases makes them different from the non-communicable ones that have been customarily modeled in decision analyses. An intervention (e.g., vaccination) can reduce the number of cases in the community, and this will result in a reduced risk of infection for other (non-vaccinated) individuals. In order to address the effects of an intervention we need to model the transmission of disease and incorporate the changing susceptibility of the population at risk. In treating heart disease, for example, the risk reduction of individuals does not affect the risk of others. With pneumococcal disease, in contrast, reducing risk for a sub-population through vaccination strongly affects the risk of others. The class of models that address issues specific to communicable diseases fall under a class of models generally referred to as 'dynamic transmission models.' For more details and exposure to these models, the reader is referred to a review (7).

10.12 Summary

Markov models provide a framework to model recurring events and to extend models to encompass the lifetime of a patient. These models are useful when a decision problem involves risk over time, when the timing of events is important, and when events may happen more than once. In a Markov model uncertain events are modeled as transitions during defined time intervals (cycles) between defined health states (Markov states). Essential to a Markov model is the Markovian property of 'lack of memory' conditional on the health state: the events subsequent to any cycle depend only on the Markov state of that cycle and not on the history prior to that cycle. In a Markov chain the transition probabilities are constant over time. In a Markov process the transition probabilities may change over time.

Markov process models can be evaluated with a cohort simulation or a Monte Carlo simulation. A Markov cohort simulation considers a hypothetical cohort of patients who are distributed among the possible states and followed over time as they transition among the states from one cycle to the next. The model keeps track of what proportion of the cohort was in which state over time. In a Monte Carlo simulation, individual patients are simulated going through various transitions from one cycle to the next and the model keeps track of the number of cycles spent in each state per patient.

Markov models can be used to estimate (partitioned) survival curves, (quality-adjusted) life expectancy, (lifetime) costs, and any other cumulative outcome such as clinical events. Heterogeneity of the population can be modeled by increasing the number of states, using temporary states or tunnel states, or by Monte Carlo simulation, in which history is modeled with tracker variables.

Discrete-event simulation, Markov decision-process models, and dynamic transmission models are more advanced approaches that accommodate situations not fully addressed by standard Markov models. Discrete-event simulations are used to model events, such as disease progression, in continuous time. Markov decision-process models embed sequential decisions in the model and allow multiple decisions in multiple time periods. Dynamic transmission models are used to consider the health outcomes in a population at risk for a communicable disease.

REFERENCES

1. Kemeny JB, Snell JL. *Finite Markov Chains*. New York: Springer Verlag; 1976.
2. Beck JR, Pauker SG. The Markov process in medical prognosis. *Med Decis Making*. 1983;3(4):419–58.
3. Sonnenberg FA, Beck JR. Markov models in medical decision making: a practical guide. *Med Decis Making*. 1993;13(4):322–38.
4. Siebert U, Alagoz O, Bayoumi AM, et al. State-transition modeling: a report of the ISPOR-SMDM Modeling Good Research Practices Task Force-3. *Med Decis Making*. 2012;32(5):690–700.
5. Caro JJ. Pharmacoeconomic analyses using discrete event simulation. *Pharmacoeconomics*. 2005;23(4):323–32.
6. Karnon J, Stahl J, Brennan A, Caro JJ, Mar J, Moller J. Modeling using discrete event simulation: a report of the ISPOR-SMDM Modeling Good Research Practices Task Force-4. *Med Decis Making*. 2012;32(5):701–11.
7. Pitman R, Fisman D, Zaric GS, et al. Dynamic transmission modeling: a report of the ISPOR-SMDM Modeling Good Research Practices Task Force Working Group-5. *Med Decis Making*. 2012;32(5):712–21.
8. Alagoz O, Hsu H, Schaefer AJ, Roberts MS. Markov decision processes: a tool for sequential decision making under uncertainty. *Med Decis Making*. 2010;30(4):474–83.

Estimation, calibration, and validation

Essentially, all models are wrong, but some are useful.

George E. P. Box

11.1 Introduction

As discussed in Chapter 8, 'good decision analyses depend on both the veracity of the decision model and the validity of the individual data elements.' The validity of each individual data element relies on the comprehensiveness of the literature search for the best and most appropriate study or studies, criteria for selecting the source studies, the design of the study or studies, and methods for synthesizing the data from multiple sources. Nonetheless, Sir Michael David Rawlins avers that 'Decision makers have to incorporate judgements, as part of their appraisal of the evidence, in reaching their conclusions. Such judgements relate to the extent to which each of the components of the evidence base is "fit for purpose." Is it reliable?'(1) Because the integration of a multitude of these 'best available' data elements forms the basis for model results, some individuals refer to decision analyses as black boxes, so this last question applies particularly to the overall model predictions. Consequently, assessing model validity becomes paramount. However, prior to assessing model validity, model construction requires attention to parameter estimation and model calibration. This chapter focuses on parameter estimation, calibration, and validation in the context of Markov and, more generally, state-transition models (Chapter 10) in which recurrent events may occur over an extended period of time. The process of parameter estimation, calibration, and validation is iterative: it involves both adjustment of the data to fit the model and adjustment of the model to fit the data.

11.2 Parameter estimation

Survival analysis involves determining the probability that an event such as death or disease progression will occur over time. The events modeled in survival analysis are called 'failure' events, because once they occur, they cannot occur again. 'Survival' is the absence of the failure event. The failure

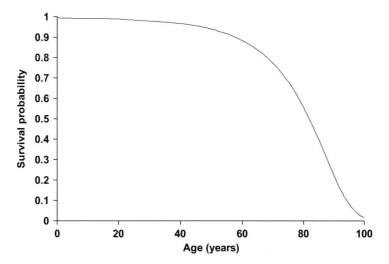

Figure 11.1   Example of a survival curve plotting the survival probability as a function of time since inception of the cohort. In this case time is since birth, expressed as age in years.

event may be death, or it may be death combined with a non-fatal outcome such as developing cancer or having a heart attack, in which case the absence of the event is referred to as event-free survival. Commonly used methods for survival analysis include life-table analysis, Kaplan–Meier product limit estimates, and Cox proportional hazards models. A survival curve plots the probability of being alive over time (Figure 11.1).

11.2.1 Estimating survival at a particular time

11.2.1.1 Life table analysis

Clinical trials typically involve patients who enroll in the study at variable times (so have variable duration of observed follow-up), and who, at study conclusion, either (a) have experienced the failure event (endpoint, e.g., death), or (b) are lost to follow-up, or (c) are still alive without having experienced the event. The term *censoring* applies to individuals who are either lost to follow-up or who complete the follow-up without experiencing the failure event (endpoint). In life table analysis, time is divided into intervals, and censoring or failure events are assumed to occur halfway through each interval. For each interval, the table tracks the number entering each interval, the number censored, the number exposed during the interval, and the number failing. Those numbers are used to calculate the proportion failing and surviving without the event during each interval (interval survival), surviving without the event through all intervals including the most recent

Interval		Entering	Censored	Failures	Exposed	Cond prop failing	Cond prop surviving	Cumulative survival	Person-years	Hazard
t_i	t_{i+1}	n'	$l+w$	d	n	q	p	$S(t)$	PY	$h(t_{mid})$
0	1	200	67	20	166.5	0.120	0.880	1.000	156.5	0.13
1	2	113	33	5	96.5	0.052	0.948	0.880	94.0	0.05
2	3	75	23	1	63.5	0.016	0.984	0.834	63.0	0.02
3	4	51	12	1	45	0.022	0.978	0.821	44.5	0.02
4	5	38	16	1	30	0.033	0.967	0.803	29.5	0.03
5		21						0.776		

Number entering interval	$n'_i = n'_{i-1} - l_{i-1} - w_{i-1} - d_{i-1}$
Number exposed	$n_i = n'_i - \frac{1}{2}(l_i + w_i)$
Conditional proportion failing	$q_i = d_i / n_i$
Conditional proportion surviving	$p_i = 1 - q_i$
Cumulative survival at start	$S(t_1) = 1$
Cumulative survival	$S(t_i) = p_{i-1} \cdot S(t_{i-1})$
Person-years during interval	$PY_i = (t_{i+1} - t_i) \cdot (n_i - \frac{1}{2}d_i)$
Hazard rate at midpoint	$h(t_{mid}) = d_i / PY_i$

Figure 11.2   Example of a life table analysis. Abbreviations: t_i beginning of the interval, t_{i+1} end of the interval, n' number of persons entering the interval, l number lost to follow-up (censored), w number withdrawn without a failure event (censored), n number exposed, q proportion failing conditional on having survived until the beginning of the interval, p proportion surviving conditional on having survived until the beginning of the interval, $S(t)$ cumulative survival at time t, PY person-years, $h(t_{mid})$ hazard (incidence) rate at midpoint of the interval.

one (cumulative survival), the number of persons alive, censored or having an event during each interval, and the hazard rate for each interval (Figure 11.2). The hazard rate is the instantaneous analog of the probability of failure during a time interval, assuming that the individual has survived event-free until the beginning of the interval. The hazard rate is also referred to as the instantaneous failure rate or, in the case where death is the failure event, the force of mortality (see Section 10.6).

11.2.1.2 Kaplan–Meier analysis

In contrast to life table analysis, Kaplan–Meier survival analysis does not require defined intervals, but the exact failure times are necessary. Using exact failure times, the Kaplan–Meier analysis produces a survival curve where each interval is the time from the last event until the next one. Each failure causes a decreasing step in the survival curve, which can occur at any point in time. The survival curve is the product of these probabilities of surviving each interval, and hence the alternative term for Kaplan–Meier analysis, product-limit analysis. If censoring occurs, the denominator for the calculation of the probabilities of survival in subsequent intervals is reduced.

11.2.1.3 Cox proportional hazard model

Cox proportional hazard models involve determining a set of survival curves that depend on multiple risk factors (2). The basic underlying hazard function, $h(t)$, which corresponds to a reference set of risk factors, may vary over time and is estimated non-parametrically, i.e., not bound by any functional distribution such as exponential. Cox models assume constant hazard rate *ratios* (*HRR*) relative to the reference combination of risk factors that are reflected in $h(t)$. For example, when using a Cox model, the hazard rate of an intervention group is assumed to be a constant multiple of the hazard rate of the control group. A Cox model is essentially a log-linear model (a linear regression after logarithmic adjustment) where the dependent variable is the natural logarithm of the 'relative hazard function' $h(t)/h_0(t)$, where $h_0(t)$ is the hazard function in the reference group and the independent variables are the sum of the regression coefficients each multiplied by their respective covariates. All covariates act multiplicatively on the hazard at any point in time, so hazard curves for groups cannot cross. Exponentiating the beta coefficients ($\exp(b_i)$) yields the hazard rate ratios for each covariate, so if the beta coefficient (b_i) equals zero, then that covariate does not affect survival (i.e., $\exp(0) = 1$) and any hazard rate ratio that exceeds one will reduce survival. In parametric proportional hazard models, the hazard function follows a specific statistical distribution such as Exponential, Weibull or Gompertz (2). Weibull and Gompertz models are often used to estimate survival and excellent textbooks explain the details (3). Accelerated failure time models are alternative types of statistical survival models in which the baseline survival function is multiplied by an 'acceleration factor' that depends on the covariates (2). Covariates then stretch or shrink the survival curve.

11.2.2 Estimating life expectancy

The area under the survival curve equals life expectancy. Consequently, life expectancy, which accounts for the differential impact of earlier versus later mortality, has become the preferred effectiveness outcome measure, especially in cost-effectiveness analyses that may also account for quality of life. A variety of methods to estimate life expectancy have evolved for use with decision models. We turn to some of those methods presently. But bear in mind that using life expectancy as the effectiveness measure assumes that the decision maker is risk neutral on life years. As discussed in Chapter 4, in order to reflect the decision maker's risk aversion on longevity, a utility function would have to be used to transform life years to utility before calculating expected values.

11.2.2.1 Declining exponential approximation of life expectancy

The Declining Exponential Approximation of Life Expectancy (DEALE) was developed in an era when computing power was limited, and so a convenient and easily calculated approximation of life expectancy was needed (4). Even in an era of rapid computing, the DEALE is useful in integrating evidence on the several forces of mortality affecting patients. The DEALE assumes a constant hazard function (i.e., the hazard function $= h(t) = \mu$). Under such an assumption, the probability of survival at time t then equals $\exp(-\mu \cdot t)$ and life expectancy equals simply $1 / \mu$.[1] Moreover, total mortality (μ_{Total}) from all causes can then be decomposed into a general population mortality rate due to age, sex, and race (μ_{ASR}) and a disease-specific excess mortality ($\mu_{Disease}$). (For example, cardiac mortality might be represented by $\mu_{Cardiac}$.) So

$$\mu_{Total} = \mu_{ASR} + \mu_{Disease} \tag{11.1}$$

These assumptions enable one to estimate the life expectancy of patients with multiple co-morbidities, by piecing together separate survival data for the different causes of death. Consider, for instance, a 42-year-old man with renal failure on hemodialysis and a Clark's level 2 superficial spreading melanoma (5). We use this example to illustrate the various methods that might be suitable, depending on the form in which the survival data are available.

What if the data are provided as probabilities of survival at a particular follow-up time?

First, assume we have data showing that two-year survival $S(2)$ of patients on hemodialysis is 77%. Using the relationship between rates and probabilities (see Section 10.6) then

$$S(2) = \exp(-\mu_{Total\_1} \cdot 2) = 0.77 \tag{11.2}$$

which implies that

$$\begin{aligned}
\mu_{Total\_1} &= -\ln(S(2))/2 \\
&= -\ln(0.77)/2 \\
&= 0.131
\end{aligned} \tag{11.3}$$

To calculate the *excess* mortality due to hemodialysis we need to subtract the general population mortality. If the mean age of the hemodialysis patients in

---

[1] The survival function $S(t)$ then equals $\exp(-\mu \cdot t)$, and the integral of the survival function from zero to infinity yields the area under the survival curve or life expectancy, which is simply $1 / \mu$.

the study is 45 years, then their life expectancy, available from the total population life table (6), is about 35.5 years, so

$$\mu_{ASR\_1} = 1/35.5 = 0.028 \qquad (11.4)$$

We can now solve for the excess mortality rate for hemodialysis by subtracting the background (ASR) mortality rate from the total mortality rate:

$$\begin{aligned}
\mu_{Hemodialysis} &= \mu_{Total\_1} - \mu_{ASR\_1} \\
&= 0.131 - 0.028 \\
&= 0.103
\end{aligned} \qquad (11.5)$$

What if the data are provided as median survival at a particular follow-up time?

Similarly, suppose we have data showing that the median survival for Clark's level 2 melanoma is 16.45 years. Then survival at 16.45 years is 50%, or 0.5. Therefore,

$$\begin{aligned}
\mu_{Total\_2} &= -\ln(S(t))/t \\
&= -\ln(S(16.45))/16.45 \\
&= -\ln(0.5)/16.45 \\
&= 0.042
\end{aligned} \qquad (11.6)$$

To adjust for general population mortality, if the mean age of the melanoma study patients is 40 years, their life expectancy is 40.1 years, so

$$\mu_{ASR\_2} = 1/40.1 = 0.025 \qquad (11.7)$$

We can now solve for the excess mortality rate for melanoma by subtracting the background mortality rate from the total mortality rate:

$$\begin{aligned}
\mu_{Melanoma} &= \mu_{Total\_2} - \mu_{ASR\_2} \\
&= 0.042 - 0.025 \\
&= 0.017
\end{aligned} \qquad (11.8)$$

Because the life expectancy for a 42-year-old white male is 36.4 years (6), combining this with the disease-specific mortality rates calculated above allows us to estimate the life expectancy of a 42-year-old white man with renal failure on hemodialysis and a Clark's level 2 superficial spreading melanoma.

First, we convert the background life expectancy into an annual mortality rate in the general population,

$$\mu_{ASR\_3} = 1/36.4 = 0.027 \qquad (11.9)$$

Next we calculate the total mortality rate as the sum of its three components

$$\begin{aligned}
\mu_{Total\_3} &= \mu_{ASR\_3} + \mu_{Hemodialysis} + \mu_{Melanoma} \\
&= 0.027 + 0.103 + 0.017 \\
&= 0.147
\end{aligned} \qquad (11.10)$$

Finally, we convert the total mortality rate to life expectancy:

$$
\begin{aligned}
\text{Life Expectancy} &= 1/\mu_{Total\_3} \\
&= 1/0.147 \\
&= 6.8 \text{ years}
\end{aligned}
\tag{11.11}
$$

What if the data are provided as relative survival?

Suppose that, instead of data on absolute survival in a study population, we have data on relative survival (*RS*), defined as the ratio of survival of the population with disease relative to an age-, sex-, and race-matched general population (the reference group). In that case, excess disease-related mortality simply equals

$$
\mu_{Disease} = -\ln(RS(t))/t
\tag{11.12}
$$

How to avoid underestimating disease-specific mortality

The above calculation of disease-specific mortality uses life expectancy in the general population to estimate general population mortality using the DEALE. In the near term, however, the DEALE underestimates survival and overestimates mortality in the general population, because the population mortality rate increases with age. Life tables that provide relative survival estimates avoid this overestimation. For example, out of 100 000 individuals in a birth cohort, 95 602 survive to age 45 years, and 95 038 remain alive after two more years. So, in the hemodialysis study above,

$$
\begin{aligned}
RS(2 \text{ yrs}) &= 0.77/(95\,038 \div 95\,602) \\
&= 0.775
\end{aligned}
\tag{11.13}
$$

Therefore,

$$
\begin{aligned}
\mu_{Hemodialysis} &= -\ln(RS(t))/t \\
&= -\ln(0.775)/2 \\
&= 0.127
\end{aligned}
\tag{11.14}
$$

Note that the disease-specific mortality of 0.127 calculated using RS is higher than the 0.103 calculated previously, because the DEALE overestimated general population mortality and thus led to a lower hemodialysis-specific mortality rate.

11.2.2.2 Estimating life expectancy in state-transition models

Actuarial data for large populations have been used by demographers to show that mortality rates increase (approximately) exponentially with increasing age. Demographers have found that age-specific mortality follows a statistical distribution called the Gompertz function, through which the mortality rate itself increases at an exponential rate. Consequently, as a cohort ages, it is possible to use a hazard rate for the general population that increases exponentially during each time interval or cycle. Alternatively, a Gompertz function relating age to an exponentially increasing hazard rate with a specified growth parameter can be used within Markov and, more generally, state-transition models.

In 11.2.2.1 we introduced a model in which cohort members are exposed to both a background risk of death as occurs within the general population and a risk from any additional disease-specific mortality. In a state-transition model, the general population mortality rates may be combined with disease-specific mortality and treatment efficacy, using either additive or multiplicative relationships (7). Treatment can reduce the disease-specific mortality rate, measured either as an absolute (additive) reduction or as a relative (multiplicative) reduction. It is essential to clarify exactly which method the authors are using and its applicability to the source data before applying it in a model.

For example, if treatment efficacy is reported as a relative risk (RR) or a relative risk reduction (RRR) of all-cause mortality, then this would apply to the probability of death ($pDie$) in a model with cycle length dt:

$$pDie = (1 - \exp(-\mu_{ASR}[Current\ Age] + \mu_{Disease}) \cdot dt) \cdot RR \tag{11.15}$$

or

$$pDie = (1 - \exp(-\mu_{ASR}[Current\ Age] + \mu_{Disease}) \cdot dt) \cdot (1 - RRR) \tag{11.16}$$

If treatment efficacy is reported, instead, as an absolute mortality rate reduction (ARR), then this would be subtracted from total mortality as follows:

$$pDie = (1 - \exp(-\mu_{ASR}[Current\ Age] + \mu_{Disease} - ARR) \cdot dt) \tag{11.17}$$

Treatment efficacy reported as a hazard rate ratio (HRR) can conveniently be incorporated in a multiplicative model by multiplying it by the general population mortality rate and the disease-specific hazard rate ratio ($HRR_{disease}$) that typically emerges from Cox proportional hazard models:

$$pDie = (1 - \exp(-\mu_{ASR}[Current\ Age] \cdot HRR_{disease} \cdot HRR) \cdot dt) \tag{11.18}$$

Treatment efficacy reported as a relative hazard rate reduction can easily be converted to a hazard rate ratio (HRR) using:

$$HRR = 1 - \text{relative hazard rate reduction} \tag{11.19}$$

11.2.3 Estimating cumulative events

The above equations apply for mortality, but identical methods can be used to estimate probabilities of non-fatal event rates, such as myocardial infarctions

or strokes, and the effect of therapies such as aspirin on reducing cardiovascular risk. For example, the number of myocardial infarctions (MIs) can be
calculated by defining a variable that tracks the cumulative number of MIs
and by adding one unit to this variable each time an MI occurs. When
running the model this variable would equal the cumulative number of MIs
experienced in the population under consideration and can be compared
across strategies. These tracker variables can be created for any model event.
Similarly, in a cancer model, defining a tracker variable for incident cancers
results in the cumulative incidence of cancer for each strategy; or in a
diagnostic test model, tracker variables could be applied for true-positive
and for false-positive test results (or for true-negative or false-negative test
results). Thus, these tracker variables can be used to capture surrogate outcomes, morbidity events, and disease incidence, as well as mortality. Tracking
events and outcomes will be discussed in more detail in the next chapter.

11.2.4 Extrapolating measures of effect

Randomized clinical trials are typically of limited short-term duration, yet the
recommended time horizon for economic analyses is lifetime. Hence, extrapolation beyond the end of the randomized clinical trial typically involves
the application of observational data to estimate the long-term outcomes. In
the absence of observational data, subsequent prognosis beyond the end of the
trial involves three possible assumptions, represented in Figure 11.3 (8).

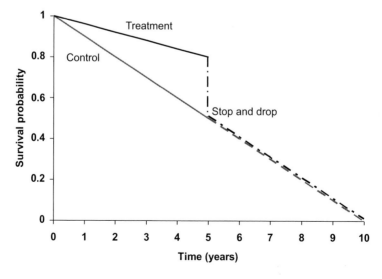

Figure 11.3 (a)   'Stop and drop' assumption: survival with treatment drops to equal that of the
control group immediately at the end of the trial, so no persistent long-term
benefit accrues.

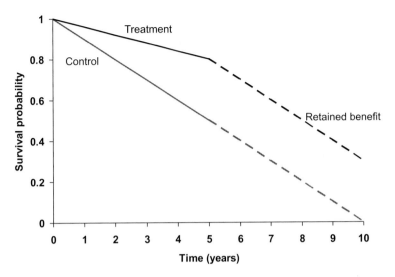

Figure 11.3 (b)   'Retained benefit' assumption: subsequent mortality rates equal that of the control group and thus survival is parallel to that of the control group, but the accumulated survival gain to that point in time is retained (i.e., 'no drop').

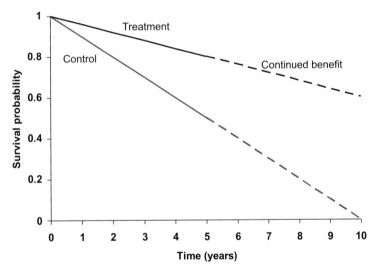

Figure 11.3 (c)   'Continued benefit' assumption: subsequent mortality rates are extrapolated from the observed treatment survival outcomes, so the incremental survival benefit continues to accrue long term. Sometimes analysts carry forward the mortality rates in the last year of observation, or an average of the last several years.

An example of 'stop and drop' can be found in an analysis of biologic agents for rheumatoid arthritis (9). An example of the 'retained benefit' assumption can be found in an analysis of thrombolytic therapy for acute myocardial infarction (10). Lastly, an example of 'continued benefit' can be found in an analysis of anticoagulation for atrial fibrillation, in which the benefit of continued use of warfarin is assumed to extend beyond the time frame of observed reduction in thromboembolic events occurring in random-ized trials (11).

Many variants of these three basic methods exist. A method intermediate between 'stop and drop' and 'retained benefit' would assume that the accu-mulated survival gain is retained for some period of time after the end of follow-up, and is then lost, either instantaneously (i.e., 'drop') or gradually over time. A method intermediate between 'retained benefit' and 'continuing benefit' would assume that the difference in mortality *rates* persists for some time interval after the end of follow-up, and then drops to no difference, either instantaneously or gradually over time.

11.3 Calibration

Calibration examines which set of alternative estimates of model parameters results in model outputs that are most consistent with available observed outcome data (e.g., epidemiologic incidence or prevalence data). Calibration is also known as fitting, although some investigators consider fitting a more limited form of calibration (12). Calibration becomes necessary either when multiple sources of data exist from which to choose from or when no data are available (12–18). The latter situation often arises in models of cancer pro-gression, because the underlying rates of pre-cancerous and tumor growth and spread are not directly observable. For example, in the USA, widespread cervical cancer screening precludes monitoring the rates of progression of pre-cancerous cervical lesions to cancer. Moreover, such a study would be considered unethical. Therefore, models of cervical cancer require indirect methods of inferring what the unobservable rates of progression must be in order to have resulted in the observed rates of cancer incidence (i.e., detec-tion) and mortality (13). In this example, population incidence and mortality are the observed epidemiologic outcome data, and the rates of progression from pre-cancerous lesions (CIN1, CIN2, CIN3) to cancer are the calibrated parameters in the model. Calibration can also be used to simultaneously adjust all epidemiologic parameters in the model (12).

Input parameters that are typically estimated through a calibration method include setting-specific parameters and input parameters with large uncer-tainty. If a risk function is included in the model, one would first calibrate the intercept, which would be a setting-specific parameter, and only if that does not provide adequate results would one calibrate the beta coefficients.

Calibration targets refer to the particular events being evaluated, and calibration for any given model may involve one or more targets. Depending on the particular type of question being examined by a model, potential data sources for observed events (the calibration targets) include incidence or prevalence of disease or mortality from trial data, observational studies, registries, vital statistics, discharge data, or hospital information systems, and may consider multiple ages or follow-up durations (19). In calibrating to outcome data, it is important to set the model's parameters to the values that would have been applicable over the time frame reflected by the outcome data. For example, in calibrating a model of cervical cancer to current disease-specific incidence and mortality in older women, the model should be set to reflect the historical screening practices that were in effect in those age cohorts, and not current screening practices (14). Ideally, the data sources for the calibration targets should be separate from the data sources used to estimate the parameters (probabilities, relative hazards, etc.) of a model (also referred to as out-of-sample prediction)(20). Calibration can also be used to establish sets of alternative parameter values, providing an additional type of sensitivity analysis.

In the absence of standard practices for model calibration, subjective decisions must be made about calibration targets, objective functions, and calibration methods (12,15,17). Consequently, a calibration checklist has been developed to facilitate methodological transparency for modelers and peer reviewers (19), and based on the checklist, seven steps necessary for performing calibration have been described (12).

11.3.1 Assessing agreement (goodness-of-fit)

Multiple methods exist for assessing the degree of agreement between the observed events (calibration targets) and the expected events (predicted by the model). Typically termed goodness-of-fit determination, these methods can be qualitative or quantitative. A qualitative *goodness-of-fit* measure between the observed and the expected could be a visual measure (12). For instance, in a model for cardiovascular disease, examination of the Rotterdam Ischemic heart disease & Stroke Computer (RISC) model showed graphically that the expected outcomes agreed closely with the observed outcomes by plotting the observed event rates against the average simulated event rates (21,22). Another straightforward method is to define acceptable windows, that is, bounds on the outputs (such as 95% CI intervals) within which results are considered acceptable. This provides a simple yes–no answer as to whether the input parameters are adequate but does not capture the magnitude of goodness-of-fit.

Quantitative methods generally assess the difference between model predictions and the empirically observed target data. The measure of goodness-of-fit can be absolute distance, relative distance, or likelihood. A simple, commonly used, absolute distance method is to minimize the sum of squared deviations. A simple relative distance method is to minimize the percentage deviation of the predicted (expected) from the target (observed) value: $\sum_i \dfrac{E_i - O_i}{O_i}$

Another relative distance method is to minimize the sum of the squared target (observed) minus predicted (expected) outcomes divided by predicted (expected) outcomes (Pearson's chi-squared test): $\sum_i \dfrac{(O_i - E_i)^2}{E_i}$

An example of relative distance is provided in the development of a breast cancer model involving a complicated simulation model that sought to calibrate their model to the incidence of four stages of breast cancer and 26 time points over 15 years for a total of 104 points (23). The modelers determined the number of simulations that fell outside of a certain range of the observed estimate by assessing the relative distance, with zero being best and 104 being the worst score. The *acceptance criteria* (convergence criteria or acceptance threshold) refer to the basis by which the modeler deems the parameter set to provide a reasonable fit (12). In the breast cancer analysis, the modelers applied non-statistically based criteria with pre-defined thresholds wherein scores of ten or less were minimally acceptable and those of five or less were exceptionally good outputs (23).

Another measure of goodness-of-fit is *likelihood*, which refers to the probability of obtaining a particular measurement of a calibration target variable, given the true value of the underlying variable. For example, if a government publishes an estimate of colon cancer incidence based on a sample of adults (such as from the United States National Health and Examination Survey), then the observed number of cases is a random variable drawn from a binomial distribution with a mean equal to the true population incidence, and a standard deviation that decreases with increasing sample size. For a given set of model parameters, the model's predicted cancer incidence will fall somewhere in the observed binomial distribution. When there are many target variables, such as disease incidence in different age-gender subgroups, mortality by age and gender, etc., the overall likelihood for a particular parameter set would be the product of the likelihoods for all the target variables. The parameter set selected would be the one that results in the highest likelihood of being consistent with the data on the target variables. This method, termed *maximum likelihood estimation*, provides statistical efficiency, but can be complicated to compute, commonly requiring simulation methods (24).

All of the above quantitative methods weight all endpoints equally even when considering more than one endpoint, but *multiobjective optimization* permits differential weighting of the calibration targets in the same goodness-of-fit analysis. For example, in a cervical cancer model, the incidence and mortality from cervical cancer received weights that were six- and three-fold greater, respectively, than the pre-cancerous incidence data (16).

Although all models strive to be accurate, the requisite modeling accuracy depends on purpose. For example, in a model of hepatitis C treatment, the observed 20-year incidence of liver cirrhosis was 28% based on a meta-analysis of five observational studies. The model predicted a nearly identical 20-year incidence of 27.5%, notably close but less than the observed incidence, making model projections likely to be conservative about the benefit of any intervention (25). Consequently, no adjustment of the probability for developing cirrhosis was made for the analysis.

11.3.2 Parameter search strategies (adjusting model parameters)

When the predicted outcomes do not match the observed data well, either parameter values or the model structure will need to be adjusted so that the simulated events approximate more closely the observed events. In univariable adjustment, one trial-and-error approach to improving fit is to vary the value of a single parameter over a range and to determine the single value of that parameter that leads to matching of the predicted with the observed outcome. For example, the probability of Barrett's esophagus leading to esophageal cancer varies broadly. In a model based on a progression from Barrett's esophagus to low-grade and then high-grade dysplasia followed by esophageal cancer, a single parameter affecting these progression rates was modified until the desired baseline lifetime risk of esophageal cancer was achieved (26).

In multivariable adjustment, multiple parameters are varied simultaneously until model predictions match observed outcomes. The *search algorithm* specifies the method used to select parameter sets for all of the possible parameter values (19). Search options (discussed further below) include manual, trial-and-error, random, grid, and directed or iterative searches, simulated annealing or genetic algorithm (12,17,19). Modelers determine the extent of the values of the parameter search and a *stopping rule* or termination criteria at which further parameter searching ceases, that is, some defined criterion of goodness-of-fit is reached or convergence occurs or completion occurs after a specific number of iterations or searches (12).

A manual search is similar to deterministic sensitivity analysis and becomes more and more like trial and error as the number of parameters that need to be calibrated increases. These methods are subject to the analyst's biases and are not as comprehensive as systematic approaches. Similar to probabilistic sensitivity analysis (discussed in Chapter 12), a random search explores combinations of randomly sampled values from distributions for all parameters. Random searches are automated but computationally inefficient. A grid search is similar to a random search but more efficient. The parameter distribution is divided into equal probability intervals and a set of random parameter values is chosen exactly once from each cell in the multidimensional parameter space. Within the best-performing cell in the grid, the process can be repeated for improved accuracy. Latin hypercube sampling is similar but even more efficient. Each parameter has a probability density function divided into intervals having the same probability area under the curve. From every interval, a random value is selected for each parameter. Efficiency occurs because a parameter value from each interval is used only once (12).

Directed or iterative search algorithms for multivariable parameter searches in model calibration have become quite sophisticated. These methods involve optimization algorithms based on numerical analysis. They are computationally more efficient and potentially more accurate than manual or random searches. The generalized reduced gradient method is based on the reduced gradient model. The latter defines a function based on a vector consisting of all parameters (12) so that moving from a particular point in the parameter space to an alternative vector along the gradient results in either the steepest ascent or descent, consequently finding the minimum point faster (12). The generalized reduced gradient method extends this approach to non-linear problem solving by using a Jacobian matrix of partial derivatives (12).

A commonly employed method is the Nelder–Mead algorithm (also known as downhill simplex) (12). Using this method, if n parameters have to be calibrated, $n+1$ initial randomly chosen parameter sets are used as inputs in the model. The model outcomes are compared to the target outcomes and ranked in order of goodness-of-fit. The worst performing parameter set is subsequently replaced with a new parameter set calculated from the previous sets so that subsequent analyses are reflected away from the worst-performing set in the direction of the best-performing sets. This is repeated until the stopping rule is attained.

Engineering search methods include simulated annealing and genetic algorithms (17). Simulated annealing provides an efficient parameter searching approach for large-scale optimization problems. Analogous to the thermodynamics of metal crystallization, simulated annealing uses temperature as an artificial parameter to assess the probability of accepting a particular set of random parameters. Think of the goodness-of-fit space in terms of peaks as poorly fitting parameter sets and valleys as better-fitting ones. At high temperatures, simulated annealing explores the parameter space broadly because the probability of accepting a new set of parameters (the peaks) is higher. Therefore, 'bigger jumps' from one parameter set to another avoids falling into or becoming mired in a local minima goodness-of-fit region (12,17). Based on the evolutionary principle of 'survival of the fittest,' the genetic algorithm generates an initial collection of candidate parameter sets and evaluates the goodness of fit for each set. The difference in goodness-of-fit between each set and the set with the largest goodness-of-fit score determines 'reproduction.' The parameter set with the largest (poorest) goodness-of-fit score is eliminated by assigning it a zero probability of reproduction. The next generation of parameter sets results from a one-point crossover method which combines two parameter sets and which also randomly changes individual parameters, e.g., within 10% of the parent values to simulate genetic mutation (17).

Increasingly, model calibration is performed using Bayesian methods. Unknown parameters are assigned prior distributions, and observed data on target variables are used to convert those prior distributions into posterior distributions using the likelihoods of the target data (12,18,27, 28). Lastly, some have proposed using multiple parameter approaches, such as a random search or grid approach to narrow the parameter space followed by more efficient methods (12).

When multiple targets are involved, searching can be done simultaneously or sequentially. For example, to calibrate a natural history model of cervical cancer through three cancer stages and two pre-cancer stages involving four different strains of human papilloma virus, all model parameters were sampled from uniform distributions over their entire range, generating 555 000 unique parameter data sets (13). Using three calibration targets and likelihood methods, the 50 'good fitting' parameter data sets were identified, and these were subsequently used in sensitivity analysis (29).

11.4 Validation

The credibility of a model's results depends on establishing the validity of the model, which subsequently affects inferences made for patients, physicians, and policymakers (20,30). Because models often integrate disparate data sources, and because of the increasing complexity of decision models due in part to the advances in computational capabilities, model predictions should be tested to ensure the accuracy and transparency of the model. Ideally, several types of validation methods are performed (22).

11.4.1 Construct validation (face validation)

Construct validity involves a conceptual understanding of the scientific basis for the approach taken at each stage in model development, including the target population, the interventions or strategies, and the health outcomes (31). Simple decision models facilitate transparency and description, yet models should also be sufficiently detailed and complex to address the problem being modeled and to appear realistic to clinical experts. For example, is the disease process for each alternative strategy represented appropriately for the proper patients? Do the disease pathways make clinical sense? Health policy models may be particularly complex because they will be used and reused to address multiple broad policy and clinical questions as they emerge (32). Face validity also involves determining whether the model provides a sufficiently convincing explanation for the results. Based on the data, assumptions, and the model structure, would the results be expected to follow logically and do the results make clinical sense (20)? Are intermediate or other outcome measures provided that would help explain the observed results? Lastly, if the model provides unexpected results, is there a 'bug' in the model (see Section 11.4.2) or can the model suggest additional research that may clarify the etiology of the discrepancy?

11.4.2 Internal validation or verification

Internal validity or verification, also referred to as internal consistency or technical validity, refers to ensuring that any mathematical calculations used in the model are accurate and consistent with the intended specifications. Any equations or parameters used in the model should be compared to the original source data. Standard methods for testing for internal validity include the following: (1) structured walk-through, wherein the model is explained to another person so that both may detect errors during that discussion; (2) manual verification, wherein the model is evaluated for a brief duration of follow-up and its outputs are compared with hand-calculated estimates or with estimates from a second modeling platform; (3) modular or simplified verification, wherein only a particular part of the model or only one particular outcome is examined; (4) sensitivity analysis by varying one parameter and ensuring that the direction of the effect is consistent with intuition (e.g., as operative mortality increases, surgery should be less favored) or that all strategies that should be affected do indeed change appropriately (33); (5) extreme analysis, wherein model behavior with input values well beyond their normal range is examined; and (6) trace analysis (or animation if appropriate), which involves detailed tracking of all individual events and their timing, a data-intensive but powerful method for detecting difficult-to-discover errors (30). Finally, good modeling practices include extensive documentation, a modular structure of the model, and a well-organized approach to programming equations and defining variables. Avoiding excessive unnecessary detail and complexity that increases the likelihood of errors will also help.

11.4.3 Cross-validation

Cross-validation, also referred to as external consistency or external convergence testing, involves comparing model results with other usually previously published models addressing the same question. For example, when examining the outcomes of different frequencies of colorectal cancer screening, two independent Cancer Intervention and Surveillance Modeling Network (CISNET) microsimulation models yielded similar results, providing not only cross-validation but also structural sensitivity analysis based on their differences (34). Similarly, when seven CISNET models used the same data on breast cancer screening, and treatment benefit, they found that 28 to 65% of the reduction in breast cancer mortality that occurred from 1975 to 2000 could be attributed to screening (35). On the other hand, in evaluating a new drug for rheumatoid arthritis, four models yielded discrepant results (36). When adjustments were made for key input variables, two of the models yielded convergent results. For the other two models, however, disparate model structures and key assumptions affected the results, which emphasized the sensitivity of this particular decision to underlying assumptions. A similar analysis has been done to compare four coronary heart disease models (37).

11.4.4 External validation

As in calibration, external validation involves comparing model results to actual observed events such as in a clinical trial, epidemiologic incidence or mortality data, or other data source which ideally should not have been used in model construction (20). The steps involved in external validation mirror those for calibration: (1) identifying data sources for the relevant outcome or outcomes, (2) performing the model simulation for that outcome or those outcomes, and (3) comparing predicted and observed results. The identification of external data sources may involve systematic literature searching. The sources identified should be justified. Whether the external data source is independent or partially independent should be specified. When comparing results, a description of the data source characteristics (e.g., age, gender, and other clinical attributes) and the extent that the simulation can and does incorporate those characteristics when attempting external validation should be provided. Finally, the simulation results are compared with the observed results, and any discrepancy between those results should be addressed.

11.4.5 Predictive validation

Predictive validation is the strongest form of validation in that it assesses a model's ability to predict future events. This may occur when models are developed to emulate planned clinical trials prior to their results becoming available. This may also occur when a model extrapolates outcomes from a randomized trial with limited follow-up duration, but extended follow-up subsequently occurs in that randomized trial. For instance, in the Multi-centre Aneurysm Screening Study (MASS), offering abdominal aortic aneurysm (AAA) screening was shown to reduce AAA-related mortality, and subsequent cost-effectiveness analysis found borderline acceptable cost-effectiveness (38). To determine internal validity or consistency, the modelers initially extrapolated model results over the same four-year time frame as the MASS trial. However, based on the subsequently available five- to seven-year data not used in developing the original model, the modelers assessed the predictive validity of their four-year model. They found that the four-year model overestimated the predicted number of AAA deaths in years five to seven for both groups, although the absolute difference was similar. They went on to identify the likely source of the divergence (unexpectedly time-invariant parameters, i.e., unaffected by time elapsed or age). Incorporating these changes into the model accounted for much of the discrepancy. Of course by incorporating these data, the modified model no longer provided an independent comparison with the MASS trial data, so the modelers went on to perform external validation with another recently completed trial. As in the case of the extension of the MASS trial, not surprisingly, further parameter modification was necessary to better approximate the results of the other trial.

11.5 Summary

When considering recurrent events as described in Chapter 10, estimation of time-dependent probabilities from hazard rates becomes necessary. A variety of methods including statistical survival models and meta-analysis of survival data are available for estimating and combining these survival estimates. For a model to be credible and to enhance transparency, increasing attention has focused on model calibration and validation. Calibration provides estimates of probabilities and other model parameters that cannot be observed directly from data, and ensures that the combined model structure and parameter values yield model predictions that approximate observed data. Validation facilitates acceptance of model results as being credible. When clinicians deem a model to have face validity, the constructs that underlie the model are acceptable. Internal validation or verification is an essential process for determining that the model constructs perform as intended, free of 'bugs.' Cross-validation compares model results with results from other models that examine the same question, not only to determine consistency but also to explore alternative structural, clinical or parameter assumptions that may account for any observed discrepancy. External validation with independent data sources provides credible evidence that a model is reliable. Lastly, predictive validation yields the strongest evidence that a model is trustworthy. Thus, the merit of a decision analysis depends not only on the structuring of the problem, the data sources, the quality and accuracy of the probabilities and values used, and the choice of model type, but also on model estimation, calibration, and validation.

REFERENCES

1. Rawlins M. *De testimonio*: on the evidence for decisions about the use of therapeutic interventions. *Lancet*. 2008;372(9656):2152–61.

2. Bradburn MJ, Clark TG, Love SB, Altman DG. Survival analysis part II: multivariate data analysis – an introduction to concepts and methods. *Br J Cancer*. 2003;89(3):431–6.

3. Kleinbaum DG, Klein M. *Survival Analysis: A Self-learning Text*. 2nd edn: Springer; 2005.

4. Beck JR, Kassirer JP, Pauker SG. A convenient approximation of life expectancy (the "DEALE"). I. Validation of the method. *Am J Med*. 1982;73(6):883–8.

5. Cuchural GJ, Jr., Levey AS, Pauker SG. Kidney failure or cancer. Should immunosuppression be continued in a transplant patient with malignant melanoma? *Med Decis Making*. 1984;4(1):82–107.

6. Arias E. *United States Life Tables, 2008. National Vital Statistics Reports*. Hyattsville, MD: National Center for Health Statistics; 2012.

7. Kuntz KM, Weinstein MC. Life expectancy biases in clinical decision modeling. *Med Decis Making*. 1995;15(2):158–69.

8. Weinstein MC. Recent developments in decision-analytic modelling for economic evaluation. *Pharmacoeconomics*. 2006;24(11):1043–53.

9. Barton P, Jobanputra P, Wilson J, Bryan S, Burls A. The use of modelling to evaluate new drugs for patients with a chronic condition: the case of antibodies against tumour necrosis factor in rheumatoid arthritis. *Health Technol Assess*. 2004;8(11):iii, 1–91.

10. Mark DB, Hlatky MA, Califf RM, et al. Cost effectiveness of thrombolytic therapy with tissue plasminogen activator as compared with streptokinase for acute myocardial infarction. *N Engl J Med*. 1995;332(21):1418–24.

11. Eckman MH, Rosand J, Greenberg SM, Gage BF. Cost-effectiveness of using pharmacogenetic information in warfarin dosing for patients with nonvalvular atrial fibrillation. *Ann Intern Med*. 2009;150(2):73–83.

12. Vanni T, Karnon J, Madan J, et al. Calibrating models in economic evaluation: a seven-step approach. *Pharmacoeconomics*. 2011;29(1):35–49.

13. Kim JJ, Kuntz KM, Stout NK, et al. Multiparameter calibration of a natural history model of cervical cancer. *Am J Epidemiol*. 2007;166(2):137–50.

14. Taylor DC, Pawar V, Kruzikas D, et al. Calibrating longitudinal models to cross-sectional data: the effect of temporal changes in health practices. *Value Health*. 2011;14(5):700–4.

15. Taylor DC, Pawar V, Kruzikas DT, et al. Incorporating calibrated model parameters into sensitivity analyses: deterministic and probabilistic approaches. *Pharmacoeconomics.* 2012;30(2):119–26.

16. Taylor DC, Pawar V, Kruzikas D, et al. Methods of model calibration: observations from a mathematical model of cervical cancer. *Pharmacoeconomics.* 2010;28 (11):995–1000.

17. Kong CY, McMahon PM, Gazelle GS. Calibration of disease simulation model using an engineering approach. *Value Health.* 2009;12(4):521–9.

18. Rutter CM, Miglioretti DL, Savarino JE. Bayesian calibration of microsimulation models. *J Am Stat Assoc.* 2009;104(488):1338–50.

19. Stout NK, Knudsen AB, Kong CY, McMahon PM, Gazelle GS. Calibration methods used in cancer simulation models and suggested reporting guidelines. *Pharmacoeconomics.* 2009;27(7):533–45.

20. Garnett GP, Cousens S, Hallett TB, Steketee R, Walker N. Mathematical models in the evaluation of health programmes. *Lancet.* 2011;378(9790):515–25.

21. Nijhuis RL, Stijnen T, Peeters A, et al. Apparent and internal validity of a Monte Carlo-Markov model for cardiovascular disease in a cohort follow-up study. *Med Decis Making.* 2006;26(2):134–44.

22. van Kempen BJ, Ferket BS, Hofman A, et al. Validation of a model to investigate the effects of modifying cardiovascular disease (CVD) risk factors on the burden of CVD: the Rotterdam ischemic heart disease and stroke computer simulation (RISC) model. *BMC Med.* 2012;10:158.

23. Fryback DG, Stout NK, Rosenberg MA, et al. The Wisconsin Breast Cancer Epidemiology Simulation Model. *J Natl Cancer Inst Monogr.* 2006;(36):37–47.

24. Chia YL, Salzman P, Plevritis SK, Glynn PW. Simulation-based parameter estimation for complex models: a breast cancer natural history modelling illustration. *Stat Methods Med Res.* 2004;13(6):507–24.

25. Wong JB, Koff RS. Watchful waiting with periodic liver biopsy versus immediate empirical therapy for histologically mild chronic hepatitis C. A cost-effectiveness analysis. *Ann Intern Med.* 2000;133(9):665–75.

26. Provenzale D, Schmitt C, Wong JB. Barrett's esophagus: a new look at surveillance based on emerging estimates of cancer risk. *Am J Gastroenterol.* 1999;94(8):2043–53.

27. Whyte S, Walsh C, Chilcott J. Bayesian calibration of a natural history model with application to a population model for colorectal cancer. *Med Decis Making.* 2011;31(4):625–41.

28. Kennedy MC, O'Hagan A. Bayesian calibration of computer models. *J R Stat Soc: Series B (Statistical Methodology).* 2001;63(3):425–64.

29. Kim JJ, Ortendahl J, Goldie SJ. Cost-effectiveness of human papillomavirus vaccination and cervical cancer screening in women older than 30 years in the United States. *Ann Intern Med.* 2009;151(8):538–45.

30. Eddy DM, Hollingworth W, Caro JJ, et al. Model transparency and validation: a report of the ISPOR-SMDM Modeling Good Research Practices Task Force-7. *Med Decis Making.* 2012;32(5):733–43.

31. Roberts M, Russell LB, Paltiel AD, et al. Conceptualizing a model: a report of the ISPOR-SMDM Modeling Good Research Practices Task Force-2. *Med Decis Making*. 2012;32(5):678–89.

32. Hunink MG, Goldman L, Tosteson AN, et al. The recent decline in mortality from coronary heart disease, 1980–1990. The effect of secular trends in risk factors and treatment. *JAMA*. 1997;277(7):535–42.

33. Wong JB. Pharmacogenomics of hepatitis C and decision analysis: a glimpse into the future. *Hepatology*. 2002;36(1):252–4.

34. Zauber AG, Lansdorp-Vogelaar I, Knudsen AB, et al. Evaluating test strategies for colorectal cancer screening: a decision analysis for the U.S. Preventive Services Task Force. *Ann Intern Med*. 2008;149(9):659–69.

35. Berry DA, Cronin KA, Plevritis SK, et al. Effect of screening and adjuvant therapy on mortality from breast cancer. *N Engl J Med*. 2005;353(17):1784–92.

36. Drummond MF, Barbieri M, Wong JB. Analytic choices in economic models of treatments for rheumatoid arthritis: What makes a difference? *Med Decis Making*. 2005;25(5):520–33.

37. Turner D, Raftery J, Cooper K, et al. The CHD challenge: comparing four cost-effectiveness models. *Value Health*. 2011;14(1):53–60.

38. Kim LG, Thompson SG. Uncertainty and validation of health economic decision models. *Health Econ*. 2010;19(1):43–55.

Heterogeneity and uncertainty

Medicine is a science of uncertainty and an art of probability.

Sir William Osler

12.1 Introduction

Decision trees and Markov cohort models, as described and illustrated in the previous chapters, are essentially macrosimulation models. Such models simulate cohorts or groups of subjects. A number of limitations exist to the use of these models. Markov cohort models, for example, have 'no memory', implying that subjects in a particular state are a homogeneous group. Techniques to overcome these limitations, such as expanding the number of states, using tunnel states, or using alternative modeling techniques, were discussed in Chapter 10. These techniques can get very complex when dealing with extensive heterogeneity within a population. Microsimulation using Monte Carlo analysis provides another powerful technique to account for heterogeneity across subjects. Microsimulation with Monte Carlo analysis was introduced in Chapter 10 as an alternative method for evaluating a Markov model. In this chapter it will be discussed at greater length in the context of simulating heterogeneity.

In the previous chapters we represented uncertainty with probabilities. Implicitly the assumption was that, even though we were unsure of whether an event would take place, we could nevertheless predict or estimate the probability (or relative frequency) that it would occur. In essence we were using deterministic models. In reality, however, we are also uncertain of the degree of uncertainty. In other words, rather than dealing with a fixed probability we are actually dealing with a distribution of possible values of probabilities. Not only are we uncertain about the probabilities we use in our models, but we are also uncertain about the effectiveness outcomes and cost estimates included in the analysis. Thus, every parameter value we enter into our models is better represented as a probabilistic variable rather than a deterministic variable. If there is a single uncertain parameter, e.g., the relative risk reduction of an intervention, then the 95% confidence interval (CI) of this parameter is commonly used to indicate the uncertainty of the effect. Uncertainty in two or more components requires more complex methods, such as Monte Carlo probabilistic sensitivity analysis, which we will also discuss in this chapter.

Patient-level heterogeneity and parameter uncertainty have very different implications for decision making, so it is not surprising that the methods used to deal with them in decision models are also very different. This chapter explores those differences, as well as the methods used to reflect them in decision analysis. One common feature is that exploration of the influence of heterogeneity and uncertainties in the model can be performed with sensitivity analysis (1). Two fundamentally different reasons exist for doing sensitivity analysis in these two situations. Heterogeneity across subgroups requires that the analyst perform a calculation for each identifiable subgroup to evaluate whether the decision might change depending on the characteristics of the subject/subgroup. Unidentifiable heterogeneity and uncertainty require some estimate of the uncertainty of the overall outcome measure of the model, i.e., the expected values of the competing strategies. These two types of analysis can be considered simultaneously, using computational methods that super-impose parameter uncertainty on top of underlying patient-level heterogeneity. Such computational methods are examples of what are known more generally as 'hierarchical' methods in statistical analysis (2).

The immediate goal of analyzing uncertainty is to obtain an interval (or region) of the outcome measure of the model that, with some probability, contains the true value. The ultimate goal is to decide whether the results are adequate for decision making, or whether obtaining more information through further research is justified (3,4). This is analogous to questioning whether another diagnostic test is necessary in the clinical setting of diagnosing a disease. Two approaches are possible: that of the frequentist versus that of the Bayesian. The frequentist approach focuses on the probability of the observed data given an hypothesis about the outcome (p(data | hypothesis)). This approach provides a confidence interval (CI) around the outcome as a function of the data. The Bayesian approach focuses on the posterior probabilities of different hypotheses about the outcome given the observed data (p(hypothesis | data)). This approach provides a credible interval (i.e., a probability distribution of outcome values) as a function of the data, combined with everything known prior to the data collection (5). In the analogy with diagnostic testing, the frequentist approach focuses on sensitivity and specificity of the evidence, whereas the Bayesian approach focuses on predictive probabilities.

Many confusing terms and concepts have been used in the analysis of heterogeneity and uncertainty. The purpose of this chapter is to clarify the various types of heterogeneity and uncertainty and to explain the techniques to analyze them (6). The focus will be on Monte Carlo simulation methods. Our approach is in essence Bayesian in that it uses evidence to revise prior information.

12.2 Types of heterogeneity and uncertainty

12.2.1 Heterogeneity across subgroups

Identifiable heterogeneity across subjects, or subgroups of subjects, is based on known dependencies on observable patient characteristics, e.g., varying age, gender, risk factors, prior events, subgroup-specific treatment effects and costs, and personal utilities. Subgroups can be identified based on the subjects' characteristics, and these subgroups are, or are assumed to be, relatively homogeneous. In such cases, the analyst needs to explore the implications of this heterogeneity (Table 12.1). The optimal intervention and the incremental cost-effectiveness ratio may differ according to identifiable patient characteristics, and these differences would be obscured by focusing on the expected values averaged across all subgroups. Heterogeneity across subgroups is the type of heterogeneity that is typically of concern to clinicians and to the developers of clinical guidelines. For example, when analyzing the optimal imaging workup for suspected coronary artery disease one will want to tailor the decision depending on age, gender, and type and severity of chest pain (1).

12.2.2 Heterogeneity in a population

The public health policy maker will typically face decisions that affect a subpopulation or the population as a whole. In these situations, heterogeneity across subjects may exist, such as varying risk factors and prior events. The ensuing disease history and prognosis may vary as a result of these varying characteristics. If we want to make policy decisions for the whole group, we would need to model the heterogeneity in the population at large (Table 12.1). Note that the policy decision does not need to be a uniform management decision for every subject (e.g., prescribe lipid-lowering medication) but can be personalized (e.g., prescribe lipid-lowering medication for subjects with a ten-year cardiovascular risk of 10% or higher). In fact, it has been shown that optimizing the decision for each individual yields more cost-effective outcomes than if we advocate a one-size-fits-all approach for everybody (7).

Examples of models that take heterogeneity in a population into account in modeling policy decisions include the Coronary Heart Disease Policy model (8,9) and the Microsimulation of Screening for Cancer (MISCAN) model (10).

Table 12.1 Types of heterogeneity and uncertainty in decision models and the corresponding simulation techniques to analyze them

Type	Explanation	Simulation technique	Output
Heterogeneity across subgroups	Known heterogeneity across subgroups, e.g., varying age, gender, risk factors, prior events; each subgroup is homogeneous	Sensitivity analyses to predict results for subgroups with identifiable characteristics	Sensitivity graphs for subgroups with identifiable characteristics
Heterogeneity in a population	Heterogeneity across subjects in a population, e.g., varying age, gender, risk factors, prior events; decision needs to be made for the population as a whole	Markov cohort analysis with varying initial states, or microsimulation of a cohort of P heterogeneous individuals having different parameter values	Mean outcome for the study population aggregated across the P heterogeneous individuals in the cohort
Stochastic uncertainty	First-order uncertainty: uncertainty due to randomness about the outcome for one study population (or one individual if $P = 1$)	Microsimulation of multiple ($n = 1 \ldots N$) cloned copies of the study population of size P (or N cloned copies of one individual if $P = 1$)	Mean and standard error of mean outcomes across N study populations each of size P
Parameter uncertainty: fixed effects/ random effects	Second-order uncertainty: measurement error of the parameter values due to (1) limited sample size of studies but fixed underlying true value (fixed-effects model) or (2) due to limited sample size of studies and heterogeneity of the underlying true value across study populations (random-effects model)	Probabilistic sensitivity analysis: Monte Carlo simulation with $s = 1 \ldots S$ iterations, with each iteration s using one set of random values from the joint distribution of the parameters. Estimation of the distribution of parameter values uses fixed effects or random-effects meta-analysis, as considered appropriate	Distribution of S means, each mean derived from a simulated study population of size P, or from the expected value of a decision tree or Markov cohort model
Model structure uncertainty	Uncertainty with respect to the modeling assumptions	Sensitivity analysis by using different modeling assumptions.	Yields alternative results

12.2.3 Stochastic uncertainty

Stochastic uncertainty, or first-order uncertainty, is the uncertainty related to the possible events that may occur over the course of time; it is the uncertainty about the actual realized outcome for an individual patient or for a sample of patients (Table 12.1). This uncertainty is entirely due to chance, within the limits of our understanding of what governs these outcomes. In decision models every chance node contributes to this uncertainty (1). For example, consider a specific chance node at which a patient has an estimated probability of 5% that she will die from an invasive procedure. Stochastic uncertainty reflects the uncertainty related to the actual outcome—the patient may or may not die. This uncertainty should be distinguished from uncertainty about whether 5% is the correct probability to apply to this patient (i.e., patient heterogeneity) and from uncertainty around the 5% because of the limited sample of patients in which the parameter was estimated (i.e., parameter uncertainty).

In the setting of prescriptive decision making using models, stochastic uncertainty represents the uncertainty related to the expected outcome in the future. The smaller the sample of subjects for which the decision needs to be made, the larger the uncertainty about the actual realized outcomes. From an individual patient's perspective, stochastic uncertainty reveals the probability of a very bad individual outcome. From a hospital administrator's perspective, stochastic uncertainty may be relevant if he/she is concerned about the possibility of a very bad outcome among the small patient group for which the decision is being made. From the public policy maker's perspective, however, stochastic uncertainty is irrelevant in making decisions for a large population, so the analysis of stochastic uncertainty only contributes noise to the expected outcomes. For this reason, it is uncommon to report results in a format that reflect stochastic uncertainty, except in special situations where the uncertainty about the actual outcomes in a small population is of interest to a decision maker.

12.2.4 Parameter (variable value) uncertainty

Rather than dealing with fixed probabilities, we usually need to deal with imperfect knowledge of the probabilities. This uncertainty may be reflected by a probability distribution of possible values for the probabilities. Similarly, the utility and cost inputs are generally better represented as probabilistic parameters rather than as deterministic parameters – not because of person-to-person variation but because we are uncertain about the values of these costs and utilities in the population of interest. This uncertainty is sometimes referred to as second-order uncertainty (11).

Sometimes the uncertainty in the parameter (variable value) is thought to arise solely from measurement due to limited sample size of the studies while some fixed underlying true value is assumed to exist. These situations are also referred to as Type B uncertainty in the risk analysis literature (12) or fixed effects in the meta-analytical literature (13). When the measurement error of the parameter is due to both limited sample size of studies and due to differences across study populations, the risk analysis literature speaks of Type A uncertainty, and the meta-analytical literature speaks of random-effects models.

12.2.5 Model structure uncertainty

The structure of a model depends on assumptions made about the natural course of a disease, how interventions influence this course, the available evidence, and choices made during the modeling process. Furthermore, analysts can opt for more or less model complexity depending on the research question, time pressures, and the required validity and precision. Different research teams develop different models to represent the same decision problem, which can lead to a large variation in outcomes (14–16).

An example of model structure uncertainty is whether a multiplicative versus additive mortality function is the most appropriate (17). Another example is the choice of risk factors to include in a disease model, such as CD4 cell count for HIV, or serum lipids and systolic blood pressure for cardiovascular disease. Not knowing the exact form of the underlying mathematical model, and not knowing which risk factors are causal, may lead to uncertainty about whether the model accurately reflects the probabilities of outcomes. This is uncertainty associated with the assumptions that are made regarding how the model should work (Table 12.1).

12.3 Analyzing heterogeneity

12.3.1 Sensitivity analysis: one-way, two-way, *n*-way

Sensitivity analysis may be used to analyze heterogeneity, by determining the results for subgroups of individuals with identifiable characteristics. Univariable (one-way) sensitivity analysis, for example for age, is usually performed first to explore the robustness of the results for varying patient characteristics one at a time. Multivariable (two-way, *n*-way) sensitivity analyses are essential to further explore the robustness of the results for varying multiple patient characteristics simultaneously.

12.3.2 Markov cohort analysis with varying initial states

Modeling heterogeneity across individuals in a population may be performed by constructing a (virtual) cohort of subjects representative of the population under consideration. Thus, instead of starting out with, for example, 10 000 cloned copies of one subject or patient, we now divide the 10 000 subjects into subgroups depending on their characteristics such as risk factors and past events. Each subgroup is modeled by letting them start out in the appropriate corresponding health state in the Markov model. As the model progresses over time, the subgroups will go through the corresponding ensuing disease history. Markov cohort analyses with varying initial states can take into account that management decisions may differ depending on risk factors and past history by explicitly modeling the decision conditional on the initial health state.

For example, strategies for the prevention of cardiovascular disease can be modeled with a Markov cohort model in which initial states are defined by risk factors such as age, gender, blood pressure, smoking status, lipid levels, body weight, and family history. The incidence of cardiovascular disease in the model depends on the risk factors and is modeled specifically for each subgroup, either in a table or with an equation such as a prediction model.

A Markov cohort analysis with varying initial states within the population provides a good method to study population heterogeneity. These techniques can, however, get very complex when dealing with extensive heterogeneity within a population. Microsimulation, either in a state-transition model or a discrete-event model, provides an alternative powerful technique to account for heterogeneity across subjects.

12.3.3 Microsimulation state-transition models

A very flexible approach to modeling heterogeneity within a population is Monte Carlo microsimulation. Microsimulation state-transition models are first-order Monte Carlo simulations built into a model with a Markov-like structure, but which addresses the lack of memory in a Markov cohort model. The basic underlying principle of microsimulation is to simulate the life course of each individual separately. A microsimulation model flags subjects in order to track their characteristics and individual disease histories as they evolve over time. In a practical sense this can be done with what are often called 'tracker variables'. Tracker variables can be used to model the initial distribution of age, gender, risk factors, and prior events and are subsequently adjusted as the subjects' age, their risk factor status changes, and events occur during the ensuing disease history. The model tracks individual subjects until

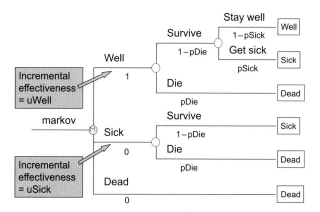

Figure 12.1   Markov model with three states: well, sick, and dead. u, utility; p, probability.

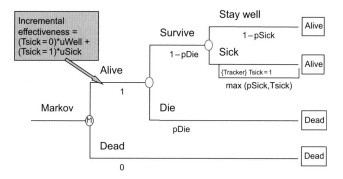

Figure 12.2   A microsimulation state-transition model that is equivalent to the Markov model in Figure 12.1. Microsimulation is performed with the tracker variable Tsick to model the sick state.

some stopping criterion – in most models the patient's death. The tracker variables are used to determine each subject's next set of probabilities of events, the utility for the health state he or she is in, and the corresponding costs associated with that health state. Continuous tracker variables permit an infinite, or continuously varying, set of health states, unlike a Markov cohort model, which requires a finite number of health states.

For example, Figure 12.1 shows a straightforward three-state Markov cohort model with the health states well, sick, and dead. The sick state has been modeled explicitly because it is associated with a lower utility than the well state. Furthermore, once a patient has become sick the model assumes he or she either stays in the sick state or dies. This same simple Markov model can be modeled using only two health states, namely alive and dead, and using a tracker variable for the sick state (Figure 12.2). To accomplish this we can, for example, add a tracker variable to the branch 'sick' that keeps track of

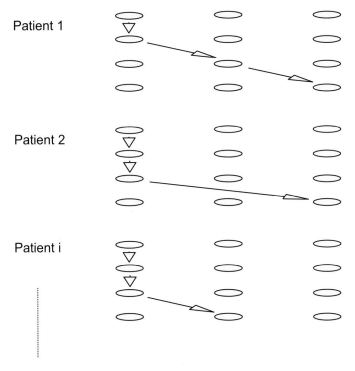

Patient 1

Patient 2

Patient i

Figure 12.3   The concept of first-order Monte Carlo microsimulation: individual disease histories are simulated one by one.

whether an individual is sick or not. If a patient becomes sick, the tracker variable changes from a value of zero to a value of one. During the next cycle the subject is known to be sick – he/she is still in the alive state but is now flagged as being sick using the tracker variable, Tsick, which is now one rather than zero. The tracker variable is used in all ensuing cycles to adjust the incremental reward by incorporating the appropriate utility, namely that for being sick rather than the utility for well. During ensuing cycles the tracker variable stays one in this particular example, the incremental reward stays the same, namely that associated with being sick, and patients are forced down the 'sick' branch.

In a Monte Carlo microsimulation, subjects representative of the population for which the decision needs to be made are followed individually through the model (Figure 12.3). Once you have decided to use tracker variables to flag patients, the calculations need to be done by simulating each individual subject, because a conventional cohort analysis cannot, by definition, keep track of the individual disease histories. Depending on what outputs are required, the model may need to keep a record of how many patients were in particular health states over time, the number of specified events per patient, and the accumulated units of utility and costs per patient.

Although this particular example may seem trivial, when modeling heterogeneity the use of tracker variables can be very powerful. Microsimulation techniques can be used to model any type of heterogeneity or disease history, either initially or over the course of time. This includes modeling, for example, the distribution of risk factors for cardiovascular disease (both initially and as they change), past events such as myocardial infarctions (MI) and strokes, tumor growth such as the growth of liver metastases, the progression of atherosclerotic disease such as in carotid artery stenosis, and the epidemiology and progression of infectious diseases such as human immunodeficiency virus.

In theory one could model everything with tracker variables and only have, for example, the states alive and dead, but such a model would be difficult to represent visually in a clear and transparent way. In practice, a compromise between health states and tracker variables is advisable. Some logical distinction can sometimes be helpful. Typically we would model post-event outcomes as health states, whereas the underlying risk factors, biomarkers, disease progression, and therapeutic procedures are modeled using tracker variables. For example, in a cardiovascular disease model the health states could be well, post-MI, post-stroke, post-MI-and-stroke, and dead, and the tracker variables could be age, gender, blood pressure, smoking status, lipid levels, family history, CT coronary calcium score, prior percutaneous coronary intervention (PCI), and prior coronary artery bypass grafting (CABG).

12.3.4 Microsimulation using discrete-event simulation

Microsimulation can also be performed using discrete-event simulation. Discrete-event simulation is a technique developed in industrial engineering to model chains of discrete stochastic events and to model competition for the available physical resources (18). Sets of equations can be used to model directly the demographic characteristics and risk factors of the subjects. The life history of each subject is simulated and the development of disease, symptoms, and disease progression can be modeled with equations that track the time to the next event. Instead of dividing time into intervals during which events may or may not occur, as in a Markov model, in discrete-event simulation the time to the next event is estimated based on the probability distribution of the time interval until that event. The variables are then updated to the point in time at which that next event occurs. Such simulations are performed for a large number of subjects, creating a file of simulated life histories that can be considered analogous to a population registry. In discrete-event simulation entities (e.g., patients) may interact and compete for resources. Queues and delay times in a queue can also be modeled, for example, being on a waiting list for an organ transplantation.

The equations are programmed in a computer simulation which directly simulates the individual life histories by aging the individual, modeling disease progression, and updating the disease status with the events that have occurred. Similar to Monte Carlo microsimulation, events are simulated by random draws from distributions describing the probability of an event. As subjects move through the model their expected survival time may change, for example, as a result of detection in a hypothetical screening program that is being analyzed. Events and the use of resources are tracked using equations that include time as a variable. The outputs of the model can be anything that is of interest, such as survival curves, life expectancy, resource utilization, costs, waiting times, and queue length.

Microsimulation using discrete-event simulation has been used extensively to model health programs for screening of cancer. It is also very useful for modeling the potential effects of policy changes or management decisions, such as the effect of buying an additional computed tomography scanner, opening another catheterization laboratory, introducing dedicated stroke units, or changing policy about liver transplantations. Discrete-event simulation can even be used to model a pathophysiological system.

12.4 Analyzing stochastic uncertainty

Performing a Monte Carlo microsimulation of each individual subject in a population has the advantage that it provides us with an estimate of the variation in outcomes across subjects that is expected to occur due to pure chance, or stochastic uncertainty (first-order uncertainty). Monte Carlo analysis was discussed previously as a method of analyzing Markov models in Chapter 10. Because we simulate individual subjects, we get a distribution of the possible outcomes across subjects and with that some measure of the degree of uncertainty of the outcome.

A Monte Carlo simulation of stochastic uncertainty should be distinguished from a microsimulation of heterogeneity in a population discussed above. The type of decision to be made dictates the type of analysis required.

If we are concerned about the decision for one type of individual, we could think of this as a population of size $P = 1$. Performing N simulations of this patient, i.e., analyzing the results for N cloned copies of this patient, will yield measures of stochastic uncertainty associated with the potential outcomes for this subject and other identical subjects. The resulting distribution might be of interest to the individual patient, but it should not be confused with uncertainty about what the expected outcome is likely to be.

We have argued earlier that an individual decision should be based on expected utility, and we have shown how utilities can be constructed to reflect risk aversion.

We could also simulate N cloned copies of a study population of size P with its heterogeneity– a two-level simulation – which yields N possible aggregate outcomes. The mean and variance across the N aggregate outcomes give us some indication of the uncertainty associated with the population outcome. This type of analysis is, however, rarely performed and stochastic uncertainty is generally considered noise in population simulations.

Conceptually, Monte Carlo simulation of stochastic uncertainty is analogous to bootstrapping a dataset. The bootstrap technique is a non-parametric method used to draw inferences from a dataset (19). A bootstrap sample is a random sample, drawn with replacement, from the dataset and equivalent in size. Patients may be represented a number of times in each bootstrap sample. Conceptually a bootstrap sample replicates the drawing of the original sample from the underlying population. The statistic of interest is calculated in every bootstrap sample and the distribution of the statistic across the entire set of bootstrap samples (e.g., $N = 1000$) provides a non-parametric estimate of the stochastic uncertainty of the statistic. For example, if you want to simulate the results of a clinical trial or clinical cohort and you have data from a representative sample that would be eligible for the trial, then you could use N bootstrap copies of that sample to represent the uncertainty about which types of patients will actually enter the simulated trial.

12.5 Analyzing parameter uncertainty

12.5.1 Sensitivity analysis: one-way, two-way, n-way

Sensitivity analysis is generally performed on plausible ranges of the parameters (variable values) using, for example, the 95% CI or some other justifiable range. Univariable (one-way) sensitivity analysis is always a good method to start exploring the robustness of the results of the analysis. A tornado diagram (Figure 12.4) can be used to present the results of many one-way sensitivity analyses in a single graph. In a tornado diagram a horizontal bar represents the range of expected outcomes (across all strategies) given the range of each parameter. A wide bar indicates that the parameter has a large effect on the expected value. The tornado shape arises by ordering the bars starting with the most influential parameter – which yields the widest bar – at the top. The bars are centered around the baseline value. A mark is used to indicate if and where the optimal strategy changes.

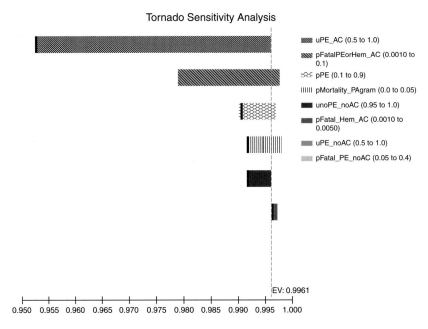

Figure 12.4   Example of a tornado diagram which presents the results of many one-way sensitivity analyses. (Based on the pulmonary embolism example from Chapter 3.)

Multivariable (two-way, *n*-way) sensitivity analyses are essential to explore the robustness of the results in more depth. Generally many parameters contain uncertainty, and an *n*-way sensitivity analysis can get unmanageable. Best-case and worst-case scenarios, in which extreme parameter values are chosen first biasing towards and subsequently biasing against the program under consideration, are useful methods to explore the extremes of *n*-way sensitivity analysis but may lead to conflicting decisions. Although several algorithms have been developed to perform n-way sensitivity analysis in a structured way (20), these are only seldom used. Conventional univariable and multivariable sensitivity analysis is limited by the subjectivity of the choice of parameters to analyze, the chosen range of values considered plausible and meaningful, the decision as to what constitutes a meaningful difference in results, and difficulties in presenting and interpreting the multiple analyses.

12.5.2 Monte Carlo probabilistic sensitivity analysis

A robust numerical technique to analyze the uncertainty of the parameter values in a model is probabilistic sensitivity analysis using Monte Carlo simulation. Monte Carlo simulation to analyze uncertainty may be used for

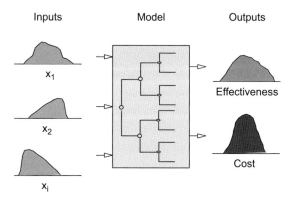

Figure 12.5   The concept of second-order Monte Carlo probabilistic sensitivity analysis.

any model, whether it be a decision tree, a Markov cohort model, a micro-simulation state-transition model, a regression equation, a model of genetic inheritance, or an astrophysical model of the universe. The basic underlying idea is illustrated in Figure 12.5. Uncertainty of all input parameters is modeled with probability distributions of their values. For each run of the model a value of each input parameter is picked at random from its distribution. So for the first simulation run of the model we pick at random a value from the distribution of the parameter x_1, a value from the distribution of the parameter x_2, a value from the distribution of the parameter x_3, etc. We run the model with these values and get one set of outputs from the model, for example, one effectiveness outcome value and one cost outcome value. A large number of iterations, S (for example, $S = 1000$) of this procedure are performed, with each iteration using one set of values from the distributions of the parameters and each iteration yielding one set of outcome values. Performing a large number of iterations yields a distribution of effectiveness and cost values. These distributions provide us with a measure of the uncertainty in the results of the model associated with the probabilistic nature of the input parameters.

If data are available from a representative study, one can bootstrap the primary data to obtain a non-parametric estimate of the distribution of the parameter values (21, 22). For public policy-making purposes the distribution of the input parameters is generally best modeled with the combined experience from various representative centers to indicate the uncertainty of the parameter values across settings (11, 23, 24). Meta-analytical techniques can help derive the appropriate probability distributions (25, 26). In general, two meta-analytical approaches can be used. One approach, a fixed-effects model, assumes that the uncertainty of the parameter values is due to only the limited sample size of the studies and that some fixed underlying true value exists. In contrast, a random-effects model assumes that the uncertainty is due to both the limited sample size of the studies and the heterogeneity of the underlying true value across study populations. In general, a random-effects model will yield wider distributions of the input parameters and thus larger uncertainty in the overall outcomes, which is a more conservative estimate.

When specifying the probability distributions of multiple parameters, it is important to specify the parameters in a way that permits the assumption that they are probabilistically independent. For example, consider an analysis evaluating statin therapy in reducing the probability of cardiovascular disease (CVD) events relative to no statin therapy. The probability of a CVD event with statin therapy and the probability of a CVD event without statin therapy may both be uncertain, but part of the uncertainty may relate to the baseline probability of CVD events and part of the uncertainty may relate to the effectiveness of statin therapy. For purposes of probabilistic sensitivity analysis, it would be best to define the two uncertain parameters as: (1) the baseline probability without treatment, and (2) some measure of the risk reduction with treatment, such as relative risk, odds ratio, or hazard rate ratio. By specifying probability distributions around the two parameters defined in this way, it would be reasonable to treat them as independent, which permits their values to be sampled independently from their respective distributions. In situations where it is impossible or impractical to define all parameters as having independent distributions, then one must specify multivariate joint distributions for sets of related (interdependent) parameters. If you have patient-level data, one can determine multivariable multivariate distributions and draw from these.

In probabilistic sensitivity analysis the relevant uncertainty to capture in the distributions is second-order uncertainty related to the sampling of the parameter, that is, the distribution of the mean. Note that this is different from the first-order uncertainty related to heterogeneity (discussed in paragraph 12.3), which is simply the distribution of the parameter value in a population. If the distribution were to be normal in both cases, second-order uncertainty would be represented by the mean and standard error of the population mean, whereas first-order uncertainty would be represented by the mean and the standard deviation of the individual values of the parameter in the population.

The normal distribution is, however, not a convenient distribution to use for most parameters, since it is not bounded whereas most parameters are bounded. A very practical example is a probability parameter, which needs to be bounded by zero and one. Beta distributions are most commonly used to

Table 12.2 Commonly used distributions to model parameter uncertainty (second-order uncertainty) in probabilistic sensitivity analysis

Distribution	Parameters modeled	Form	Comment
Uniform	Any	Range low–high	All values are equally likely. Uninformative distribution
Triangular	Any	Minimum, maximum, likeliest	
Beta	Probability Quality of life weights (utility)	Beta(r,n), where r = number of events, n = number of patients For observed mean μ and standard error s: $r = \mu n$ n = $(\mu(1\text{-}\mu)/s^2) -1$	Bounded between 0 and 1
Dirichlet	Probability in the context of multiple events		Extension of the beta distribution, for multiple events
Lognormal	Rate Relative risk Hazard rate ratio Odds ratio Costs	ln(parameter) has a normal distribution with mean and standard error	Values > 0, positively skewed
Gamma	Resource use Costs	Gamma(α, β) For observed mean μ and standard error s: $\alpha = \mu^2/s^2$ $\beta = \mu/s^2$	Values > 0, positively skewed
Histogram	Any	Non-parametric	Based on trial data: observed relative frequency per value or per interval
Bootstrap	Any	Non-parametric	Based on trial data: simulated relative frequency per value

reflect uncertainty around probabilities, in part because of the ability to revise them in a Bayesian calculation, using evidence about the proportion of times an event occurs in a study population. In general, parameter distributions may be modeled parametrically using some estimate from the available data combined with the judgment of the analyst (27,28). Distributions that are commonly used for different types of parameters are tabulated in Table 12.2.

It is widely recommended that the distributions used in sensitivity analyses be based on empirical evidence, reflecting the sampling uncertainty or between-study variation in studies (6). For that reason, artificial distributions such as the uniform (or triangular) should be avoided, unless the only available evidence about uncertainty comes from expert judgment about upper and lower bounds. Alternatively, one can construct a non-parametric distribution based on available data from an observational cohort or clinical trial using either a simple histogram or using bootstrapping.

12.5.3 Analytical probabilistic sensitivity analysis: the delta method

Uncertainty analysis for multiple parameters may be performed analytically. This entails deriving equations for the uncertainty in the results using differential calculus. To calculate the uncertainty requires the variance–covariance matrix of the parameter estimates. This is only doable if the model is straightforward with a limited number of parameters and a reliable data source to estimate the variance–covariance matrix exists. Analytical methods often become cumbersome and unmanageable with complex models. They are, however, very useful when modeling multiattribute (composite) outcomes based directly on the results of clinical trials. Analytical estimates of the overall variance in the composite outcome can be estimated with the delta method (see Appendix for general equation). For example, in paragraph 12.8.2 we define the net health benefit: $NHB = QALY\text{-}cost/WTP$, with WTP the societal threshold willingness-to-pay. For a fixed WTP, the variance of the net health benefit is a function of the variance of the QALYs and variance of the costs:

$$\text{var}(NHB) = \text{var}(QALY) + (1/WTP)^2\text{var}(cost) - (2/WTP)\cdot\text{cov}(QALY, cost)$$
$$(12.1)$$

If all the parameters in the model are independent, the delta method simplifies to a fairly straightforward equation without the co-variance terms (see Appendix), which would imply that the variance in the results can be estimated by determining the change in the outcome estimate for a small change in each parameter value, taking the square of this estimate, multiplying that with the variance of the parameter value, and summing the products for all parameters.

The delta method and assuming independence of the input parameters may provide an initial estimate of the variance in the results. Unfortunately, the method becomes complex quickly as the number of parameters increases and the variance–co-variance matrix structure of the parameters needs to be estimated.

12.6 Analyzing varying model structures

To analyze the uncertainty associated with the use of varying modeling assumptions, the simplest approach is to redo the analysis using alternative assumptions. Performing the analysis first with, for example, a multiplicative mortality function and subsequently with an additive function will shed light on how this assumption affects the results. If the alternative assumption has no major impact on the results, a sentence or two in the report will suffice. If the alternative assumptions affect the decision, there is a choice to be made: either find more evidence to justify the use of one assumption instead of the other or, if this is impossible, present the results of both analyses and let the decision maker decide which of the analyses is the more appropriate based on his/her own judgment. Alternatively we could provide a weighted combination of the results, the weights being proportional to the belief we have in the assumption, but the results of such a weighted analysis are difficult to interpret. Some analysts recommend assigning subjective probabilities to the various possible model structures, and including model structure as a parameter in a probabilistic sensitivity analysis.

On a more global level one could compare analyses performed by different analysts to determine the influence of varying model structures. An attempt to consolidate the different results depending on the underlying assumptions of the model can provide valuable insights into the decision problem and modeling process (16). Such a comparison, especially when performed across different settings and different countries, can demonstrate different perspectives on the decision problem, varying consequences of decisions, differences in costs and effectiveness, and different approaches to coping with uncertainty.

12.7 Combined analysis

Combining heterogeneity, stochastic uncertainty, and parameter uncertainty in one analysis implies performing multiple hierarchical simulations (2). How these are combined depends on the goal of the analysis, which is determined by what the simulation should reflect and what the outputs need to represent (Table 12.3). For example, analyzing parameter uncertainty in a policy decision for a heterogeneous patient population would typically use

Table 12.3 Hierarchical combined analysis: the most common types of analyses of models combining parameter uncertainty, patient heterogeneity, and microsimulation of individuals

Simulation reflects	Output represents	Outer loop	Middle loop	Inner loop	Calculate mean across	Present
Parameter uncertainty, policy decision for a heterogeneous population	Distribution of expected individual outcome	Parameter values	None	Microsimulation of heterogeneous individuals	Micro-simulated individuals (inner loop)	Distribution across parameter values (outer loop)
Parameter uncertainty, individualized decision	Distribution of expected individual outcome for one individual	Parameter values	None	Microsimulation of cloned individuals	Micro-simulated individuals (inner loop)	Distribution across parameter values (outer loop)
Patient heterogeneity, in the face of parameter uncertainty	Distribution of expected individual outcome for heterogeneous individuals	Patient charac-teristics, per iteration a different individual	Para-meter values	Microsimulation of cloned individuals	Parameter values (middle loop)	Distribution across patient characteristics (outer loop)
Patient heterogeneity, parameter uncertainty, and stochastic uncertainty	Distribution of individual outcome	Patient charac-teristics, per iteration a different individual	Para-meter values	Microsimulation of cloned individuals	Do not aggregate	Distribution across micro-simulated individuals (inner loop)

For an exhaustive review see (2).

the first type of analysis in Table 12.3 with parameter uncertainty being modeled in the outer loop and individual patient heterogeneity modeled through microsimulation in the inner loop. In this analysis the mean would be calculated across all microsimulated individuals (inner loop) for each set of parameter values (outer loop) and the distribution across the sets of parameter values (outer loop) would represent the uncertainty in the outcomes. Thus, the algorithm for the first type of hierarchical analysis in Table 12.3 would look as follows:

ALGORITHM FOR CALCULATION OF PARAMETER UNCERTAINTY IN A POLICY DECISION FOR A HETEROGENEOUS POPULATION

A1. Outer loop (parameter uncertainty):

A2. For $i = 1,2,3...I$ simulations (2nd-order parameter samples)

     B1. Randomly draw values from distributions of all parameters

     B2. Inner loop (heterogeneity):

     B3. For $j = 1,2,3...J$ simulations (1st-order microsimulation)

         C1. Randomly pick an individual from the heterogeneous population

         C2. Run the model and note the outcome for individual j

     B4. Calculate the mean of the J outcomes obtained at B3

A3. Present distribution of values across the I simulations obtained at A2.

The inner loop of simulations is always the microsimulation of individuals, which may be a heterogeneous group of individuals or cloned copies of one individual, depending on the goal of the analysis. The parameter values and individual patient characteristics should be simulated in either the inner, middle or outer loop, depending on the goal of the analysis. Aggregation is performed by calculating the mean across the microsimulated individuals if the simulation should reflect an expectation of individual outcome in the face of parameter uncertainty. Aggregation is performed across the distribution of parameter values if the simulation should reflect patient heterogeneity. No aggregation is performed if the distribution of individual outcomes is of interest.

12.8 Uncertainty in cost-effectiveness analysis

Cost-effectiveness analysis, as described in Chapter 9, is increasingly being used to evaluate medical technology and allocate scarce health-care resources. In the previous chapters dealing with cost-effectiveness we considered the input parameters to the model deterministic and thus the outputs were also assumed deterministic. Here we will consider how to deal with the uncertainty in both the costs and effectiveness when the input parameters are considered probabilistic or the analysis is being performed as a microsimulation to reflect heterogeneity across subjects in the population or stochastic uncertainty or a combination of these. In such models the outputs, in terms of incremental costs and effectiveness gained, are themselves probabilistic rather than deterministic (21,29).

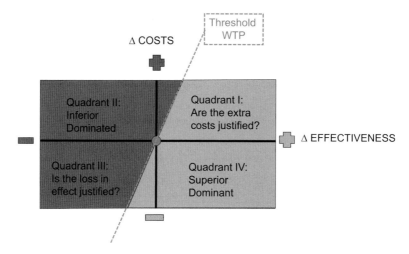

Figure 12.6   The costs-vs.-effectiveness graph with the implications per quadrant.

Comparing two health-care strategies is generally done using the incremental cost-effectiveness ratio (ICER). The *ICER* is estimated using:

$$ICER = \frac{\overline{C}_1 - \overline{C}_0}{\overline{E}_1 - \overline{E}_0} = \frac{\Delta \overline{C}}{\Delta \overline{E}} \tag{12.2}$$

where $\overline{C}_1$ and $\overline{C}_0$ are the mean values of the costs using Strategy 1 (the strategy under consideration) and Strategy 0 (the next-best strategy) respectively, $\overline{E}_1$ and $\overline{E}_0$ are the mean values of the effectiveness yielded by Strategies 1 and 0 respectively, and $\Delta \overline{C}$ and $\Delta \overline{E}$ are the mean incremental costs and mean incremental effectiveness gained.

Many analyses evaluating uncertainty in cost-effectiveness studies have focused on presenting the means, CIs, upper and lower bounds, or distribution of the ICER. There are, however, several problems with the interpretation of ICERs and all papers that report distributions or standard deviations or standard errors or CIs of cost-effectiveness ratios should be interpreted with caution (30–33).

By presenting ICERs, information is lost with regard to the distribution across the four quadrants of combinations of $\Delta \overline{E}$ and $\Delta \overline{C}$ and the position within the quadrants (Figure 12.6) (29,34). (Here we have chosen to plot the Δeffectiveness on the x-axis and the Δcosts on the y-axis. Some authors choose to reverse the axes.) Negative ICERs are meaningless: it is impossible to distinguish whether a negative ICER results from a gain in effectiveness at lower costs (superior strategy by dominance, $\Delta \overline{E} > 0$ and $\Delta \overline{C} < 0$, quadrant IV) or a loss in effectiveness at higher costs (inferior strategy by dominance, $\Delta \overline{E} < 0$ and $\Delta \overline{C} > 0$, quadrant II). These two situations have very different implications; i.e., the former strategy should be accepted, the latter rejected and in both situations the ICER is irrelevant to the decision. Likewise, given a

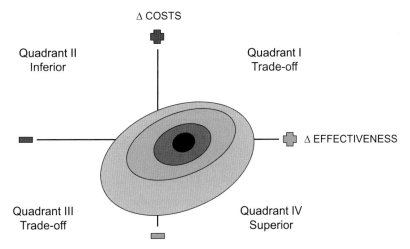

Figure 12.7   The joint distribution of incremental costs vs. incremental effectiveness from an analysis with uncertainty and/or heterogeneity.

positive ICER, it is impossible to distinguish whether this results from a gain in effectiveness at higher costs ($\Delta \overline{E} > 0$ and $\Delta \overline{C} > 0$, quadrant I) or by a loss in effectiveness at lower costs ($\Delta \overline{E} < 0$ and $\Delta \overline{C} < 0$, quadrant III). The ICERs in the quadrant I and III need to be interpreted differently. A policy maker faced with an increasing budget will question whether the increment in costs can be justified given the gain in effectiveness (quadrant I) whereas a policy maker faced with a decreasing budget will question whether the cost-savings are large enough to justify a small loss in effectiveness (quadrant III). In quadrant I we consider strategies with an ICER lower than the threshold willingness-to-pay cost-effective, whereas in quadrant III we consider strategies with an ICER higher than the threshold willingness-to-pay cost-effective. Even within the first quadrant (gain in effectiveness at higher costs), there may be different implications for health-care management depending on the purchasable units of health and the associated costs. For example, the fixed cost of a strategy may exceed the available budget, although the ratio of cost and effectiveness may be favorable.

12.8.1 The joint distribution of costs and effectiveness

Uncertainty in costs and effectiveness using the joint distribution of costs and effectiveness (Figure 12.7) displays the uncertainty in the relationship between costs and effectiveness and, therefore, in the ICER itself. The function clearly distinguishes between the four quadrants of combinations of $\Delta \overline{E}$ and $\Delta \overline{C}$, and it is an informative method to display the relationship between costs and effectiveness. The joint distribution is well defined for every value of costs and effectiveness, which implies that even for a difference in effectiveness of close to zero, or equal to zero, the method may be applied (35). The joint distribution of costs and effectiveness can be represented graphically in various ways using a scatterplot of $\Delta \overline{C}$ versus $\Delta \overline{E}$, a three-dimensional histogram (the x- and y-axes representing the $\Delta \overline{E}$, $\Delta \overline{C}$ plane and the z-axis representing the relative frequency with which a particular combination of $\Delta \overline{E}$, $\Delta \overline{C}$ occurs which yields a sort of mountain landscape), or as iso-probability contour lines in a two-dimensional contour plot (the bird's-eye view), as illustrated in Figure 12.7.

In the context of parameter uncertainty, each data point in the scatterplot of the joint distribution represents the results for a randomly chosen combination of parameter values from all possible combinations. In the context of stochastic uncertainty, each data point represents the expected outcome in a cloned (or bootstrapped) copy of the population under consideration. In the context of heterogeneity, each data point represents the expected outcome for a randomly chosen patient from the heterogeneous population under consideration.

12.8.2 Linear combinations of effectiveness and costs

An alternative to working with the joint distribution of $\Delta \overline{E}$ and $\Delta \overline{C}$ is to optimize a weighted linear combination of effectiveness and costs. In an analysis from the societal perspective, the relevant weight is society's threshold willingness to pay for the gain of one unit of effectiveness (WTP), or its inverse. One can, for example, maximize net health benefits (34) with:

$$\text{Net health benefits} = \text{effectiveness} - \text{cost} / WTP \qquad (12.3)$$

Net health benefits of an intervention are typically expressed in QALYs and can be interpreted analogously to effectiveness. The costs associated with the intervention are subtracted from the effectiveness, after expressing them in an equivalent number of QALYs by taking into consideration society's willingness-to-pay threshold. A program's net health benefit calculates the net health gain expected from the program (effectiveness) minus the health gain forgone in other programs by diverting resources (money) to the program under consideration (cost / WTP). If the net health benefit of one intervention exceeds that of another, i.e., if the *incremental* net health benefit exceeds zero, we can conclude that the intervention is cost-effective compared to its comparator given the threshold willingness-to-pay.

Similar to the net health benefit, the net monetary benefit is defined as:

$$\text{Net monetary benefit} = \text{effectiveness} \cdot WTP - \text{cost} \qquad (12.4)$$

Net monetary benefits of an intervention are measured in monetary units, with effectiveness expressed in terms of monetary units by taking into consideration society's willingness-to-pay threshold. If the net monetary benefit of one intervention exceeds that of another (the incremental net monetary benefit exceeds zero), we can conclude that the intervention is cost-effective compared to its comparator given the threshold willingness-to-pay.

Simulating heterogeneity and uncertainty will yield a probability distribution of effectiveness and cost outcomes and thus a probability distribution of the weighted combinations (i.e., net monetary benefit and net health benefit). The distributions of the weighted combinations of effectiveness and costs are straightforward to calculate and interpret when analyzing the effects of heterogeneity and uncertainty in a model. This approach is very powerful when analyzing heterogeneity and uncertainty among multiple strategies, as is often the case with the evaluation of diagnostic tests or screening strategies. Furthermore, the concept can be used very efficiently for the calculation of criteria that a new test or treatment would need to attain to be cost-effective compared to an existing technology (36–39). Furthermore, the concept can be extended to include a weighted combination of the effectiveness and costs when more than one subject is affected by the decision, as would be the case when we consider an intervention for a pregnant woman and her fetus.

12.8.3 The acceptability curve

Net health benefit and net monetary benefit have the disadvantage that society's willingness-to-pay threshold is included in the estimate. However, this disadvantage can be dealt with by performing and presenting the analysis for various values of *WTP*. A widely used method of displaying this information is called an acceptability curve (29). Having estimated the joint distribution of $\Delta\overline{E}$ and $\Delta\overline{C}$ we can construct an acceptability curve. The acceptability curve plots the relative frequency or probability that the strategy is cost-effective compared to the alternative for varying threshold values of the ICER (*WTP*). This implies summing the relative frequencies of three components (Figure 12.8) of the joint distribution (29,40):

$$\Delta\overline{E} \geq 0 \text{ and } \Delta\overline{C} < 0 \text{ (component 1 in quadrant IV)} \tag{12.5}$$

$$\Delta\overline{E} > 0 \text{ and } \Delta\overline{C} \geq 0 \text{ and the ICER} \leq \text{WTP (component 2 in quadrant I)} \tag{12.6}$$

$$\Delta\overline{E} < 0 \text{ and } \Delta\overline{C} \leq 0 \text{ and the ICER} \geq \text{WTP (component 3 in quadrant III)} \tag{12.7}$$

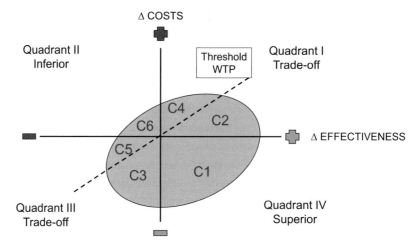

Figure 12.8   The six components of the joint distribution of costs and effectiveness.

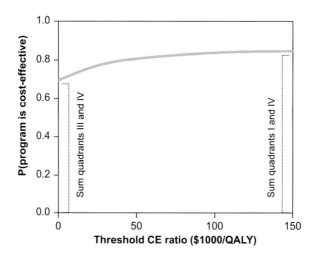

Figure 12.9   Acceptability curves. The probability that a strategy is optimal is plotted for a range of willingness-to-pay values. CE, cost-effectiveness; QALY, quality-adjusted life year.

Summing the relative frequencies of these three components of the joint distribution is equivalent to calculating the fraction of the distributions of the incremental net health benefits or net monetary benefits with values larger than zero.

The starting value of the acceptability curve (Figure 12.9) equals the sum of components 1 and 3 for a threshold ICER of zero, which is the sum of the joint distribution in quadrants III and IV, i.e., the region in which the program is cost-saving compared to its comparator. As the threshold ICER increases (Figures 12.7 and 12.8), component 2 increases and the acceptability curve rises. Simultaneously, however, component 3 of the distribution decreases and causes the acceptability curve to drop. Depending on the position and shape of the joint distribution, these two effects may cancel out or cause the curve to either increase or decrease. For large values of *WTP* the curve levels off to the relative frequency of the joint distribution in quadrants I and IV, i.e., the region in which the program increases effectiveness, irrespective of cost.

An acceptability curve as shown in Figure 12.9 applies to the situation in which there are only two alternative strategies – the strategy of interest and a comparator such as the current standard of care. In situations in which more than two strategies are being compared, the concept of an acceptability curve generalizes to a family of curves, with each curve representing the probability that the corresponding strategy is cost-effective as a function of *WTP*. Sometimes, curves are shown for all the competing strategies, in which case the ordinates of the acceptability curves sum to 1.0. Sometimes, as in Figure 12.9, curves are shown for all but one of the competing strategies, in which case the probabilities sum to less than or equal to 1.0, and the residual probability applies to the omitted strategy (e.g., the status quo).

12.9 Value of information analysis

Although acceptability curves present the probability that a new strategy will be cost-effective or not, they provide no information on the magnitude of gained versus forgone health benefit caused by the decision made (41). For example, an intervention may reach a 95% probability of being cost-effective, which is reassuring, but if the harm caused by taking the wrong decision in the remaining 5% is huge, we would still not want to adopt the intervention. Value of information analysis fills this gap by calculating the forgone net benefit of the remaining uncertainty, which is equivalent to the value of doing future research, in either monetary or health terms. Value of information analysis is particularly useful when considering optimal allocation of research funds.

More research to decrease uncertainty is justified if, and only if, the expected benefit to future patients exceeds the cost of performing the research. Thus, it is important to obtain some idea of how much future research can help us in making optimal choices. Information obtained in future quantitative research can reduce parameter uncertainty. A decrease in parameter uncertainty may avoid implementation of suboptimal interventions, and consequently is expected to benefit patients and/or reduce costs. Value of information analysis estimates the expected benefit of obtaining more information through future research. In essence it combines the probability that we make a suboptimal decision with the forgone health (or monetary) benefit of that decision (1, 42,43). The value of information is not the actual value of future research, because we cannot predict what the research will show. Instead, the value of information is the 'expected' value of future research, with the value of each possible research result weighted by its prior probability of occurring. It is expressed in the same units as the model outcome. Value of information analysis was introduced by Grundy and others in the late fifties and developed by Raiffa and Schlaifer. Since the late eighties it has received increasing attention in the risk analysis literature and more recently in health care (4).

Ideally decisions about research are made iteratively. A probabilistic model is developed based on the best available evidence. Value of information analysis is performed to determine whether future research is justified and to guide the design of a new study. The new study is performed, and the information obtained is incorporated into the model. This process is repeated over and over again until the cost of the future research is larger than the benefit that we can expect from obtaining more information.

12.9.1 Expected value of perfect information (EVPI)

The expected value of perfect information (EVPI) is the expected benefit per patient of performing a future study with an infinite sample size that would eliminate all parameter uncertainty (1, 42,43). The EVPI is calculated as the average opportunity loss across all samples in the probabilistic sensitivity analysis. The opportunity loss per sample is defined as the difference between the maximum expected benefit in that sample (had we known the parameters perfectly and made the optimal choice) and the sample's expected benefit given the strategy chosen (the choice being made based on the average expected benefit).

Suppose we face a decision in which there are several alternative strategies (i), and in which some parameters are uncertain. We perform a Monte Carlo probabilistic sensitivity analysis in which N parameter sets are drawn from their joint distribution. For each of these possible parameter sets (n), each strategy (i) has a net health benefit ($NHB_{i,n}$). If we knew that the parameters had the values drawn in the nth iteration, we would choose the strategy that gives the maximum net health benefit conditional upon that parameter set. We can denote that maximum net health benefit by $\max_i(NHB_{i,n})$. Since each of the N simulated parameter sets has a probability of approximately $1/N$ of being the true parameter set, we can calculate the expected value of the net health benefit *with perfect* *information* as the average of the values of $\max_i(NHB_{i,n})$. Without perfect information, we must choose an optimal strategy without any more information, but subject to the prior distribution of parameter values; if parameter set n is true, then the net health benefit of that optimal strategy can be represented as NHB_n^*. Note that this net health benefit is usually less than the net health benefit that could have been obtained if we knew the parameter values and chose the best strategy accordingly – $\max_i(NHB_{i,n})$. The difference between these two quantities, conditional on a set of values of the parameters, is called the *opportunity loss*.

We can now express EVPI as the average of the opportunity loss (the first line in the equations below). By separating the equation into two components, as in the second line below, we can express EVPI as the gain in expected benefit from perfect information:

$$
\begin{aligned}
EVPI &= \frac{1}{N}\sum_n \left(\max_i(NHB_{i,n}) - NHB_n^*\right)\\
&= \frac{1}{N}\sum_n \max_i(NHB_{i,n}) - \max_i \frac{1}{N}\sum_n NHB_{i,n}
\end{aligned}
\tag{12.8}
$$

In these equations, $NHB_{i,n}$ is the net health benefit of strategy i on iteration n, N is the number of iterations performed in the probabilistic sensitivity analysis, $\max_i$ is the maximum across the strategies i, and NHB_n^* is the net health benefit obtained on iteration n from the strategy that on average (i.e., using current information) is optimal. The averages are calculated across all samples from the probabilistic sensitivity analysis, which implies they are the expectations across the distributions of the parameters θ. Note that NHB_n^* averaged across the N iterations equals the maximum average NHB, using current information.

ALGORITHM FOR THE EVPI CALCULATION

A1. For $i = 1,2,3\ldots I$ simulations

    B1. Randomly draw values from all distributions of the parameters θ

    B2. Calculate net benefit for each strategy

    B3. Identify the optimal strategy and its benefit

A2. Calculate average of values obtained at B3

A3. EVPI = average from step A2 − expected net benefit with current information

---

12.9.2 Population EVPI

Thus far we have calculated EVPI per patient facing the decision of interest. The *population EVPI* is the expected benefit to all future patients. It is estimated by multiplying the EVPI per patient by the size of the future populations that are expected to benefit from the research, discounting expected benefit in future years. In equation form:

$$Population\ EVPI = EVPI \sum_t \frac{I_t}{(1+r)^t} \tag{12.9}$$

where I is the annual incidence, t is time in years, and r is the discount rate. Because it assumes perfect information, which no realistic research study can provide, the population EVPI is an upper bound on the value of the research. If the research is expected to be more expensive than the population EVPI, it is a poor investment: the uncertainty is not important enough to be resolved, given the cost of resolving it.

Population EVPI estimates are influenced by subjective choices for the annual population to benefit and the number of years that the future research results would apply. It is frequently unclear whether we should consider the local setting only, a region, a state, the whole country, the continent, or all patients worldwide. Furthermore, the period that patients will benefit from the new study is uncertain because of future improvements, novel technology, and new insights. These ambiguities are, however, inherent to the general problem of allocating resources wisely and not specific to estimating the value of information itself.

12.9.3 Expected value of partial perfect information (EVPPI)

If the population EVPI is sufficiently large, the next step is to identify the parameters with the highest informational value. The expected value of partial perfect information (EVPPI) calculates the EVPI of individual parameters or subsets of parameters. The EVPPI is particularly useful in guiding the design of a future study in that it focuses the data collection.

The calculation of EVPPI usually requires a two-level simulation. In the outer loop values are drawn for the parameters of interest, θ_I. In the inner loop values are drawn for the other parameters, θ_C (the complement of the parameters of interest). If the model is linear for each of the complementary parameters, and if there are no correlations between the parameters of interest and the complementary parameters, then the means of the (marginal) distributions of the complementary parameters can be used instead of taking the expectation over the distribution, which simplifies the simulations. Linearity of a model implies that the expected value of the model with uncertain parameters equals the model outcome when it is evaluated using the expected values of the parameters.

ALGORITHM FOR THE EVPPI CALCULATION

A1. For i = 1,2,3... I simulations

     B1. Draw a value for θ_I

     B2. For j = 1,2,3... J simulations

         C1. Draw a value for θ_C

         C2. Calculate net benefit for each strategy

         C3. Identify optimal strategy and its benefit

     B3. Average over the J values obtained at C3

A2. Average over the I values obtained at B3

A3. EVPPI = average from step A2 – expected net benefit with current information

---

12.9.4 Expected value of sample information (EVSI)

Whereas EVPI and EVPPI calculate the expected benefit of removing all uncertainty from the parameters, obtaining such perfect information is in practice impossible. We can only hope to *reduce* uncertainty. This is because of the finite sample size of every study, and limits to the generalizability of the study population to the general population. The EVPI gives a ceiling on the amount of information that can be obtained from a future study, and as such is a first hurdle that needs to be passed in justifying the need for more research. If we want a more precise estimate, we would need to calculate the expected value of sample information (EVSI) that will actually be obtained from a new study with finite sample size n. The EVSI is best presented in a graph as a function of sample size. The graph will asymptotically reach EVPI.

ALGORITHM FOR THE EVSI CALCULATION

A1. For i = 1,2,3... I simulations

     B1. Draw a sample $\theta_I(i)$ from the prior of θ_I

     B2. Draw a sample $D(i)$ from $D|\theta_I(i)$ from study with size n

     B3. For j = 1,2,3... J simulations

         C1. Draw a value for θ_C

         C2. Calculate net benefit for each strategy

         C3. Identify optimal strategy and its benefit

     B4. Average over the J values obtained at C3

A2. Average over the I values obtained at B4

A3. EVSI = average from step A2 – expected net benefit with current information

---

To estimate EVSI we consider new studies with all possible sample sizes n that will provide new data D on the parameters of interest θ_I (42). The EVSI is the difference between the expected value of a decision made with knowledge of the new data D and the expected value of the decision made with current information. Since we do not know D, we determine the expectation over the distribution of D, which in turn is based on prior knowledge of the parameters of interest θ_I. The expectation over D is an expectation of the new data D conditional on the parameters of interest θ_I, and averaged over the prior distribution of θ_I. For more extensive coverage of this calculation we refer to reference 42.

12.9.5 Expected net benefit of sampling (ENBS)

Having calculated the EVSI, we can then compare the result to the resources required to obtain the information and decide whether or not we would expect a gain in benefit (1,42,43). To perform a new study, resources will be required. The costs of a new study will consist of a fixed part plus a variable part that depends on how many individuals are included in the study. The expected net benefit of sampling (ENBS) is calculated as the population EVSI minus the cost of obtaining new information and is a function of n, the size of the new study. Typically, the ENBS goes up as sample size increases to a maximum and then decreases with further enlargement of the sample size. The sample size at the maximum ENBS is the optimal sample size, taking into account the benefit to be gained from the study and the cost of the study, and provides an elegant alternative to traditionally used sample size calculations.

12.10 Summary

When using mathematical models to estimate the expected value of alternative options we need to explore our assumptions and evaluate and present the effect of heterogeneity and uncertainty.

When heterogeneity relates to identifiable subgroups, the optimal decision may be determined for each subgroup separately through sensitivity analysis. When analyzing a decision for a population as a whole we may be concerned about the heterogeneity across subjects in the population. This type of heterogeneity can be analyzed with a Markov cohort analysis with varying initial states, with (first-order Monte Carlo) microsimulation of the individual disease histories, or with discrete-event simulation.

Uncertainty in our models includes stochastic, parameter, and model structure uncertainty. Stochastic uncertainty is the uncertainty related to the actual events and realized outcome for one study population (or one individual) and can be estimated through microsimulation of multiple cloned (or bootstrapped) copies of that study population. Stochastic uncertainty, however, is irrelevant from the perspective of the public policy maker. Parameter (variable value) uncertainty is due to the measurement error of the parameter values in the model caused by the limited sample size and heterogeneity of the studies from which the values were derived. Parameter uncertainty can be evaluated with probabilistic sensitivity analysis by performing a second-order Monte Carlo simulation, each iteration using one set of random values from the distributions of the parameters and the simulation producing distributions of the outcomes. Model structure uncertainty is related to the modeling assumptions with regard to the mathematical model used and can be evaluated by performing sensitivity analysis using different assumptions.

Heterogeneity and uncertainty in cost-effectiveness analyses can best be presented with the joint distribution of costs and effectiveness or using a weighted measure such as net health benefit or net monetary benefit.

Appendix

The delta method

Mathematically, the overall variance of function $f(X)$ with vector $\mathbf{X} = X_1$, $X_2 \ldots X_i \ldots X_n$ equals:

$$\mathrm{var}(\bar{f}) = \left(\frac{\overline{\partial f}}{\partial X}\right)^{T} \mathrm{var}\,\hat{X}\left(\frac{\overline{\partial f}}{\partial X}\right) \tag{12.10}$$

If all the parameters $\mathbf{X} = X_1, X_2 \ldots X_i \ldots X_n$ in the model $f(X)$ are independent, the delta method simplifies to a fairly straightforward equation:

$$\mathrm{var}(\bar{f}) = \sum_{i} \left(\frac{\overline{\partial f}}{\partial X_i}\right)^{2} \mathrm{var}\,\hat{X}_i \tag{12.11}$$

Value of information analysis

Mathematically, value of information can be expressed as follows (42).

Let:

E_θ = expectation over the parameter distributions θ (12.12)

$B(a,\theta)$ = net benefit obtained with strategy a and distributions θ (12.13)

max_a = maximum across the strategies a   (12.14)

Then:

$E_\theta B(a,\theta)$ = expected benefit over the parameter distributions θ
$\mathrm{max}_a E_\theta\, B(a,\theta)$ = expected benefit of optimum decision with current
information   (12.15)

max_a B(a,θ)= expected benefit of optimum decision with perfect
information   (12.16)

$E_\theta max_a B(a,\theta)$ = idem as eq. (12.16) averaged over θ   (12.17)

$EVPI = E_\theta max_a B(a, \theta) - max_a E_\theta B(a, \theta)$ (12.18)

Furthermore, let:

θ_I = subset of parameters θ that are of interest; θ_C complement of θ_I (12.19)

Then:

$max_a E_{\theta C|\theta I}B(a,\theta)$ = expected benefit of the optimum decision with
current information on θ_C given perfect information on θ_I (12.20)

$E_{\theta I}max_a E_{\theta C|\theta I}B(a,\theta)$ = idem as eq. (12.20) averaged over θ_I

$EVPPI = E_{\theta I}max_a E_{\theta C|\theta I}B(a,\theta) - max_a E_\theta B(a,\theta)$ (12.21)

Finally, let:

D = hypothetical new data on θ_I collected in a sample of n patients   (12.22)

Then:

$max_a E_{\theta C,(\theta I|D)} B(a,\theta_I,\theta_C)$ = expected benefit of the optimum decision
with current information on θ_C and with information on θ_I given
the data D   (12.22)

$E_D max_a E_{\theta C,(\theta I|D)} B(a,\theta_I,\theta_C)$ = idem as eq. (12.22) averaged over D   (12.23)

$EVSI = E_D max_a E_{\theta C,(\theta I|D)} B(a, \theta_I, \theta_C) - max_a E_\theta B(a, \theta)$ (12.24)

REFERENCES

1. Groot Koerkamp B, Weinstein MC, Stijnen T, Heijenbrok-Kal MH, Hunink MG.
   Uncertainty and patient heterogeneity in medical decision models. *Med Decis
   Making.* 2010;30(2):194–205.
2. Groot Koerkamp B, Stijnen T, Weinstein MC, Hunink MG. The combined analysis
   of uncertainty and patient heterogeneity in medical decision models. *Med Decis
   Making.* 2011;31(4):650–61.
3. Claxton K. The irrelevance of inference: a decision-making approach to the
   stochastic evaluation of health care technologies. *J Health Econ.* 1999;18(3):341–64.
4. Claxton K, Sculpher M, Drummond M. A rational framework for decision making
   by the National Institute For Health and Clinical Excellence (NICE). *Lancet.*
   2002;360(9334):711–15.
5. Manning WG, Fryback DG, Weinstein MC. Reflecting uncertainty in cost-
   effectiveness analysis. In: Gold MR, Siegel JE, Russell LB, Weinstein MC, eds.
   Cost-Effectiveness in Health and Medicine. New York; 1996. pp. 247–75.

6. Briggs AH, Weinstein MC, Fenwick EA, et al. Model parameter estimation and uncertainty analysis: a report of the ISPOR-SMDM Modeling Good Research Practices Task Force Working Group-6. *Med Decis Making*. 2012;32(5):722–32.

7. Basu A, Meltzer D. Value of information on preference heterogeneity and individualized care. *Med Decis Making*. 2007;27(2):112–27.

8. Hunink MGM, Goldman L, Tosteson AN, et al. The recent decline in mortality from coronary heart disease, 1980–1990. The effect of secular trends in risk factors and treatment. *JAMA*. 1997;277(7):535–42.

9. Lazar LD, Pletcher MJ, Coxson PG, Bibbins-Domingo K, Goldman L. Cost-effectiveness of statin therapy for primary prevention in a low-cost statin era. *Circulation*. 2011;124(2):146–53.

10. van Ravesteyn NT, Heijnsdijk EA, Draisma G, de Koning HJ. Prediction of higher mortality reduction for the UK Breast Screening Frequency Trial: a model-based approach on screening intervals. *Brit J Cancer*. 2011;105(7):1082–8.

11. Doubilet P, Begg CB, Weinstein MC, Braun P, McNeil BJ. Probabilistic sensitivity analysis using Monte Carlo simulation. A practical approach. *Med Decis Making*. 1985;5(2):157–77.

12. Hoffman FO, Hammonds JS. Propagation of uncertainty in risk assessments: the need to distinguish between uncertainty due to lack of knowledge and uncertainty due to variability. *Risk Anal*. 1994;14(5):707–12.

13. DerSimonian R, Laird N. Meta-analysis in clinical trials. *Controlled Clinical Trials*. 1986;7:177–88.

14. Brown ML, Fintor L. Cost-effectiveness of breast cancer screening: preliminary results of a systematic review of the literature. *Breast Cancer Res Treat*. 1993;25 (2):113–18.

15. Campbell H, Briggs A, Buxton M, Kim L, Thompson S. The credibility of health economic models for health policy decision-making: the case of population screening for abdominal aortic aneurysm. *J Health Serv Res Policy*. 2007;12(1): 11–17.

16. Mandelblatt JS, Cronin KA, Berry DA, et al. Modeling the impact of population screening on breast cancer mortality in the United States. *Breast*. 2011;20 Suppl 3: S75–81.

17. Kuntz KM, Weinstein MC. Life expectancy biases in clinical decision modeling. *Med Decis Making*. 1995;15:158–69.

18. Law AM, Kelton WD. *Simulation Modeling and Analysis*. 3rd edn. Boston: McGraw-Hill Higher Education; 2000.

19. Efron B, Tibshirani RJ. *An Introduction to the Bootstrap*. New York: Chapman & Hall; 1993.

20. Duintjer Tebbens RJ, Thompson KM, Hunink MG, et al. Uncertainty and sensitivity analyses of a dynamic economic evaluation model for vaccination programs. *Med Decis Making*. 2008;28(2):182–200.

21. Briggs AH, Wonderling DE, Mooney CZ. Pulling cost-effectiveness analysis up by its bootstraps: a non-parametric approach to confidence interval estimation. *Health Econ*. 1997;6(4):327–40.

22. Mennemeyer ST, Cyr LP. A bootstrap approach to medical decision analysis. *J Health Econ.* 1997;16(6):741–7.

23. Critchfield GC, Willard KE, Connelly DP. Probabilistic sensitivity analysis methods for general decision models. *Comput Biomed Res.* 1986;19(3):254–65.

24. Parmigiani G, Samsa GP, Ancukiewicz M, et al. Assessing uncertainty in cost-effectiveness analyses: application to a complex decision model. *Med Decis Making.* 1997;17(4):390–401.

25. Cooper H, Hedges LV, Valentine JC. *The Handbook of Research Synthesis and Meta-Analysis.* New York: Russel Sage Foundation; 2009.

26. Higgins JPT, Green S. *Cochrane Handbook for Systematic Reviews of Interventions: Cochrane Collaboration* 2011.

27. Briggs AH, Goeree R, Blackhouse G, O'Brien BJ. Probabilistic analysis of cost-effectiveness models: choosing between treatment strategies for gastroesophageal reflux disease. *Med Decis Making.* 2002;22(4):290–308.

28. Briggs AH, Ades AE, Price MJ. Probabilistic sensitivity analysis for decision trees with multiple branches: use of the Dirichlet distribution in a Bayesian framework. *Med Decis Making.* 2003;23(4):341–50.

29. van Hout BA, Al MJ, Gordon GS, Rutten FF. Costs, effects and C/E-ratios alongside a clinical trial. *Health Econ.* 1994;3(5):309–19.

30. Wakker P, Klaassen MP. Confidence intervals for cost/effectiveness ratios. *Health Econ.* 1995;4(5):373–81.

31. Chaudhary MA, Stearns SC. Estimating confidence intervals for cost-effectiveness ratios: an example from a randomized trial. *Stat Med.* 1996;15(13):1447–58.

32. Polsky D, Glick HA, Willke R, Schulman K. Confidence intervals for cost-effectiveness ratios: a comparison of four methods. *Health Econ.* 1997;6(3): 243–52.

33. Heitjan DF, Moskowitz AJ, Whang W. Bayesian estimation of cost-effectiveness ratios from clinical trials. *Health Econ.* 1999;8(3):191–201.

34. Stinnett AA, Mullahy J. Net health benefits: a new framework for the analysis of uncertainty in cost-effectiveness analysis. *Med Decis Making.* 1998;18(2 Suppl): S68–80.

35. Fieller EC. The distribution of the index in a normal bivariate population. *Biometrika.* 1932;24:428–40.

36. Muradin GS, Hunink MG. Cost and patency rate targets for the development of endovascular devises to treat femoropopliteal arterial disease. *Radiology.* 2001;221 (1):137–45.

37. Visser K, Kock MC, Kuntz KM, et al. Cost-effectiveness targets for multi-detector row CT angiography in the work-up of patients with intermittent claudication. *Radiology.* 2003;227(3):647–56.

38. Hunink MGM, Kuntz KM, Fleischmann KE, Brady TJ. Noninvasive imaging for the diagnosis of coronary artery disease: focusing the development of new diagnostic technology. *Annals of Internal Medicine.* 1999;131(9):673–80.

39. Phelps CE, Mushlin AI. Focusing technology assessment using medical decision theory. *Med Decis Making.* 1988;8:279–89.

40. Hunink MGM, Bult JR, de Vries J, Weinstein MC. Uncertainty in decision models analyzing cost-effectiveness: the joint distribution of incremental costs and effectiveness evaluated with a nonparametric bootstrap method. *Med Decis Making*. 1998;18(3):337–46.

41. Groot Koerkamp B, Hunink MG, Stijnen T, et al. Limitations of acceptability curves for presenting uncertainty in cost-effectiveness analysis. *Med Decis Making*. 2007;27(2):101–11.

42. Ades AE, Lu G, Claxton K. Expected value of sample information calculations in medical decision modeling. *Med Decis Making*. 2004;24(2):207–27.

43. Groot Koerkamp B, Nikken JJ, Oei EH, et al. Value of information analysis used to determine the necessity of additional research: MR imaging in acute knee trauma as an example. *Radiology*. 2008;246(2):420–5.

Psychology of judgment and choice

We are pawns in a game whose forces we largely fail to understand.

Dan Ariely

13.1 Introduction

This book has discussed a host of methods and approaches to analyzing decisions, to predicting alternate and optimal outcomes, and to applying quantitative and analytic approaches to understand and explain choices. Most of the chapters up until now have emphasized technical methods and are likely to have challenged and expanded your analytic skills. For this final chapter we will change gears to discuss the side of the brain that is commonly thought of as less analytical and more creative, the 'right brain' contribution to decision making. In this concluding chapter we will discuss the psychology underlying judgment and choice.

Think back for a moment to the example in Chapter 4 about genetic susceptibility for breast cancer. Here was the situation we were considering:

EXAMPLE 1

Genetic susceptibility for breast cancer

A 25-year-old woman has a strong family history of breast cancer, including a sister who developed the disease at age 35. Her sister has undergone genetic testing for cancer predisposition and has been found to carry a mutation in the BRCA1 breast cancer gene. The woman is concerned about her own risk of breast cancer and chooses to be tested. She is found to have the same mutation, and is told that her lifetime risk of developing breast cancer is approximately 65%. If she does nothing at all with this information, her chance of surviving to age 70 is 53% (compared with all women's survival probability of 84%). She has a number of options open to her: (1) careful surveillance, including regular mammography and magnetic resonance imaging (MRI), which would increase her chance of surviving to age 70 to 59%; (2) prophylactic mastectomy – surgical removal of both breasts – which would increase her chance of surviving to age 70 to 66%; (3) prophylactic mastectomy now plus prophylactic oophorectomy – surgical removal of the ovaries – when she turns 40, which would increase her chance of surviving to age 70 to 79%. Both surgical options increase her chance of survival beyond that of surveillance, but carry some personal costs – mastectomy can affect sexual function and body image, oophorectomy causes early-onset menopause and prevents child bearing. Does the benefit of risk reduction with surgery outweigh the personal costs of these interventions?

We considered the survival probabilities associated with the different options available to this woman, and how her values influenced her choice. We also acknowledged that the actual decision occurs in a 'black box,' where the woman combines and integrates all the available information with her own priorities to arrive at a decision. In addition to the values we discussed in Chapter 4, this 'box' includes her emotional fear of cancer, the lens through which she interprets the actual probabilities (that may be clouded because she has seen her sister endure the disease), and her personal expectations about getting cancer as a younger woman and as a woman with a family history of disease. All of these elements affect her decision from the 'right brain' perspective: the intuitive, non-analytic side. They combine with rational, structured thought in the 'black box' of decision making to arrive at a choice. In this chapter, we will consider the intuitive processes that are part of the decision-making box, the emotions, perceptions, feelings, and desires that are present in that box and are highly influential in decision making. While not part of our analytic toolbox, these psychological factors are integral to decision making and choice.

Two pioneers in the field of judgment and decision making, Daniel Kahneman and Amos Tversky, have shown through decades of work that human beings are fallible in their decision making at the most basic level: we misperceive probabilities of outcomes, a cornerstone of good decision making.[1] Not only do people misperceive probabilities, but they do so in surprisingly predictable ways. Kahneman and Tversky used simple experiments to demonstrate and describe the ways that people routinely make mistakes in estimating the chance of outcomes, and they developed a theory to describe decision making when choices involve an element of uncertainty in the outcomes. 'Prospect theory' is based on the knowledge of how people *actually* make choices, as opposed to how decision analysts believe they *should* make decisions (described in more detail in Section 13.6)(1, 2). Extending Kahneman and Tversky's theory, further research has described and broadened our understanding of the psychology of decision making and choice (3, 4). It is well accepted now that people diverge from Expected Utility

---

[1] Amos Tversky is deceased. Daniel Kahneman won the Nobel prize in economics in 2002 for their joint work in behavioral economics.

theory (discussed in Chapter 4) in their decision making; that people are oftentimes guided by emotions and in fact prioritize emotions in their decision making.

13.2 Rationality in decisions

Until now we have mostly discussed decision making as a rational endeavor, guided by theoretical constructs that follow prescribed rules. In fact, we know that individuals' decisions are oftentimes guided by emotions, biases, and even habit. Many people report being more fearful of flying than driving in a car, for example, even though the risk of dying in a car crash far outweighs the risk of dying in an airplane crash. Similarly, many people avoid flying on the 13th of the month if it falls on a Friday, and many high-rise apartment buildings have floors 12 and 14 but no floor 13. Emotion is integral to people's perception of risk and is therefore integral to decision making that involves any element of risk, including most medical decisions. Policy decisions are simply individuals making decisions for groups of people rather than for themselves, and may be influenced by the same 'irrationalities' found in individual decision making (as well as sometimes by the additional irrational forces of politics and public opinion). The foundation of the field of decision analysis is to inject rationality into decision making through careful and systematic analysis of options and weighing of benefits and costs (in terms of resources). It is important never to forget, however, that human beings are the analysts in decision analysis, performing these evaluations or providing the data inputs. So human psychology is an integral part of decision analysis despite our best efforts to inject objectivity into that work.

13.3 Importance of perspective

As we have discussed in previous chapters, it is important to consider the perspective from which a decision is being made when conducting an analysis. This holds for understanding the psychology underlying decisions as well. For clinical decision making, there are two perspectives involved: the physician and the patient (plus oftentimes the family, alongside the patient). Patients, physicians, and family members are all human beings and are affected by the same psychological forces though from different points of view. Policy decisions are similarly made by humans, informed by analyses performed by humans. At each point where people interject themselves into the decision process, human psychology has an opportunity to influence or sway the process. A systematically conducted decision analysis can eliminate some of the subjective forces of human psychology by careful choice and integration of data into an evaluation, that results in an economically defined 'rational' outcome (5). The question arises, however, of whether human psychology should intentionally be incorporated into policy analyses precisely because it is de facto included in individual decision making. Essentially, if there is an observed and consistent difference between normative and empirical decisions, which is preferred: what people actually choose or what they *should* choose per theories of rational choice? This question is the subject of debate in the field today. What is important for this discussion, however, is the understanding of how human psychology affects decision and choice, and with this knowledge, whether and when decision psychology should be considered in decision analysis.

13.4 Understanding risk

The chance that any outcome will occur is a fundamental piece of any decision, whether a clinical decision or a policy decision. Risk is simply another word for the chance that something will occur (an event, or a 'hazard' if it is potentially injurious), or the probability of occurrence.

EXAMPLE 2	**Characteristics of risks**

If you were offered a chance to go skydiving, would you go?

If you were visiting a new city in the summer and taking a walk around the main park or greenway, would you take off your shoes? Do you think each activity has any risks involved? How would you think about the risks?

Would your decision about skydiving be influenced by having the option of wearing a second, back-up parachute? What if you were being accompanied by an experienced skydiving instructor?

Would you walk barefoot in the park if you knew that no pesticides were applied to the grass? If it had 'organic only' signs posted?

Research has shown that the qualities or characteristics of a particular event influence people's perception of the risk of that event occurring (6). Characteristics of events include things like how much one can control an event, whether an event is undertaken voluntarily or involuntarily, how observable effects of the event are, and the scope of effects. More controllable and voluntary events, and those with observable and smaller scope effects, are all perceived as less likely to occur and less fearsome than events with opposite characteristics, even if their actual probability of occurrence is identical.

In the skydiving example (Example 2), most people view the activity as voluntarily undertaken, and many elements of the event as controllable.

Moreover, the risk of injury and death are limited to the person undertaking the activity, and the possible outcomes are well known and easily seen. As in the example, you could increase your safety by wearing two parachutes, or jumping accompanied by an experienced instructor; no one else is endangered during the activity (aside from the small chance of landing on another), and there is little doubt about the possibility of an injury or fatality. In contrast, exposure to pesticides by walking on treated lawns can be uncontrollable and involuntary; it can affect many people, not just one; and the effects are often unknown and not immediately observable. As in the example, pesticides may be applied in public areas without any posted warnings, you and many other people can unknowingly be exposed, and the effects may be delayed and/or confused with other causes.

The risks of these two 'hazards' are perceived differently because of their characteristics, separate from their actual probability of occurrence: harm due to pesticides is generally more on people's minds as a concern than injury from skydiving. One can protect oneself from the risk of skydiving but not necessarily from pesticides. As mentioned earlier, many people are more fearful of flying than of driving, because driving is under one's own control, in one's own vehicle, with generally known abilities and risks, while flying is controlled by a pilot, affected by abilities, weather, and equipment that is less known and less controllable compared to driving. Similarly, surgical interventions, such as in our breast cancer example, have a tangible and oftentimes visible result that can be of comfort to people because it is observable. In contrast, radiation or chemotherapy is more mysterious to people, the therapeutic effect is not visible or tangible, and even if the survival benefit is similar people *feel* differently about the risks and benefits associated with it compared to surgery.

As further example, consider cigarette smoking and exposure to second-hand smoke. The risks associated with these two events are perceived differently because of the voluntariness of the exposure: second-hand smoke exposure can be imposed upon an individual without consent, while smoking is considered a voluntary behavior, dependent on personal choice.

These examples illustrate that risk perception is a function of psychological forces as well as information. As we know, the probability of an outcome (i.e., the risk of its occurrence) is integral to decision making, and therefore risk perception is a component factor in decision making. Knowledge of the psychology of risk perception makes optimal decision making more possible, because misperceptions can be overcome through information, or alternately can be integrated as valid preferences into decisions.

13.5 Heuristics in information processing

Risk perception is affected by both the characteristics of events as well as the cognitive processes that occur when people consider probabilities of events. These processes occur in the 'black box' of decision making. Information processing is influenced by psychological forces that can introduce biases into information even before it is integrated into a decision. This section discusses some of the psychological forces that come into play in the information processing component of the decision process.

Heuristic principles are mechanisms people use to reduce complex tasks to simpler components. 'Heuristics' are mental short-cuts used to process information quickly, like 'rules of thumb.' People often resort to heuristics to speed cognitive processing, especially when faced with time pressure or with uncertainty. They are a common part of daily life: looking at a partially blocked billboard reading 'SMOKING KILLS. Q__T NOW' we can all fill in the missing letters with little thought or effort. When calculating restaurant tips people use multipliers of sales tax or drop digits off totals. Slightly more complicated short-cuts are used when processing information about probabilities of events, which are important in medical decision making. Many heuristics have been described that are relevant to decision making but we limit the discussion here to the most common ones in health-care decisions (for other examples, see *Predictably Irrational* by Dan Ariely (7)).

13.5.1 Availability heuristic

Think again of our first example of the 25-year-old woman considering genetic testing to see whether she is carrying a mutation in the BRCA1 gene as does her sister. When she is making the testing decision she is contemplating what she thinks is her risk of breast cancer, while knowing that her sister carries the mutation. Of course her risk is actually increased by her sister's status, but her *perception* of her risk is also influenced by her familiarity with her sister's status. The 'availability' heuristic explains that how *familiar* something is tends to influence peoples' perception of how likely it is to occur: people think more familiar things are more likely to occur and less familiar things are less likely to occur. Being familiar with something means that examples or knowledge of it are readily accessible or 'available' in your mind. When examples of things are easily retrieved in your mind, it makes those things seem more probable. So the accessibility, familiarity, and availability of breast cancer genetic mutations in this woman's mind may make her perceive her chances to also carry the mutation to be higher than someone who is less familiar with breast cancer genetic mutations, or does not know anyone with one, or has not thought much about them, above and beyond her actual increased chance due to her genetic make-up. Research has been shown that people who have a family member with cancer overestimate their own risk of cancer above and beyond actual hereditary risk: being familiar with someone who has cancer and being more aware of one's own risk of disease heightens the perception of risk (8).

Common examples of the availability heuristic at work include media attention to a particular event that amplifies people's perception of the chance that it will occur. The media attention leads the event to 'spring to mind,' making it more available to people. The 'availability' of the Japanese Fukushima Daiichi nuclear plant crisis in 2011 in people's minds triggered heightened worldwide attention and public concern about nuclear power safety in its aftermath. Similarly, following the Deepwater Horizon oil spill in the Gulf of Mexico in 2010 and the Sandy Hook Newtown shooting tragedy in 2012, increased attention was paid to oil drilling and to gun control in part because of the public's heightened concerns about safety, which dissipated over time as the example faded from the public view and anxiety abated. The degree to which examples of a hazard are retrievable can influence people's perception of the probability of an event.

Kahneman and Tversky illustrate the way in which people retrieve the most available information with a classic psychology experiment that asks people to estimate the chance that a randomly selected English word begins with the letter 'r' (r____) as opposed to having an 'r' in the third position (__r__) (of words with at least three letters). Because words starting with 'r' are more easily accessed, meaning easier to bring to mind, compared with words with 'r' (or any letter) in the third position, people report that the 'r' starting words are more likely to occur, even though in fact the opposite is true (as it is for 'k' as well)(9). Applied to health decisions, it would be easy to see why using familiarity with an event to gauge its probability of occurring is a mental short-cut that undoubtedly saves time, but can introduce bias into estimates of risk. For example, the estimate of pre-test probability of a rare disease may be overestimated if another patient was recently diagnosed with that disease. Similarly, the estimated probability of a procedural complication will be overestimated if recently a complication occurred.

13.5.2 Representativeness heuristic

How *similar* an uncertain event is to a larger class of events is another factor that influences people's perception of how likely an event is to occur. In other words, how much one event *resembles* or is *representative* of another group of events leads us to connect the probability of the two in our minds. This connection is often quick and simple, and can override other information or knowledge that more accurately informs the probability of the uncertain event's occurrence. This 'representativeness' heuristic underlies stereotypes: we mentally connect one person with a larger group of people whom this person resembles, and apply knowledge about the larger group to the individual. This knowledge of the larger group may or may not be accurate for the individual person, and other information may be overlooked in this process. Similarly, the word 'cancer' brings an image to mind that clumps all cancer sites together, making it difficult to distinguish between very aggressive and very slow-progressing types.

Kahneman and Tversky describe classic research in which subjects were presented with a description of an individual and asked to guess his occupation from a list of possibilities (9). Subjects were given the following description, and asked whether the individual was more likely to be a farmer, salesman, airline pilot, librarian, or physician:

> *'Steve is very shy and withdrawn, invariably helpful, but with little interest in people, or in the world of reality. A meek and tidy soul, he has a need for order and structure, and a passion for detail.'*

Subjects most often chose librarian as Steve's profession because he most resembles our perception of what a librarian is like; he is most similar to the larger class of librarians, therefore the probability that he is a member of that class is perceived to be the highest. What subjects overlooked is the underlying probability that anyone has any one of these occupations: in the USA, the prevalence of farmers is far greater than the prevalence of librarians, so based on probability alone it is more likely that Steve belonged to the most prevalent occupational group than any other, farmers. Note that this is the same as confusing sensitivity–specificity with predictive values which we discussed in Chapter 5. In this example Steve's personality is the analogy of the diagnostic test result (T) and his occupation is the analogy of the disease (D). Subjects are asked to consider the probability of his occupation conditional on his personality ($p(D|T)$) which they confuse with the probability of his personality conditional on his occupation ($p(T|D)$). Racial profiling is an example of the representativeness heuristic in use.

The representativeness heuristic also describes how people associate the probability of events with their similarity to a more general *process*. This is most commonly seen in people's misunderstanding of chance and the laws of statistics. The 'gambler's fallacy' is a classic example of how people misunderstand chance. After a long series of one type of outcome, such as ten 'heads' in coin flips, most people erroneously believe that the next flip is more likely to be 'tails' than 'heads' based on the rationale that it would be more representative of a chance sequence than yet another 'heads.' People want randomness to prevail, so it seems more likely and thus *fair* that tails should show up even though we all know that each flip has an equal and independent 50% chance of 'heads' and 'tails.' The representativeness heuristic explains how people in this situation assess probabilities based on similarity with a process rather than an objective assessment of chance.

13.5.3 Anchoring and adjustment heuristic

When people don't have information about something, or are unsure about it, they often make initial estimates based on some initial piece of information that they intend to later replace or update with better information. We find, however, that people get 'stuck' or *anchored* on these initial values and don't sufficiently *adjust* at a later point in time. Our 25-year-old woman in example one had some idea of her risk of breast cancer before undergoing genetic testing. Afterwards, she was given objective information about her risk of developing disease that she used to update her pre-testing belief, and then proceeded to make decisions based on this revised assessment of her own risk. Studies of women receiving genetic testing results have confirmed that we generally fail to adequately adjust our pre-testing risk beliefs to accord with our post-testing objective risk information: women who underestimated their risk of disease prior to testing become more accurate with the addition of new information but still remained too low in their assessment of risk. Similarly, women who overestimated their risk prior to testing tended to lower their risk in accord with their objective testing results but still remained too high (10–12).

Initial or provided values or thoughts are extremely influential when people's opinions are unformed or there is uncertainty, as is often the case in clinical decision making. Anchoring tends to bias assessments of probability *toward* the anchor, even if attempts are made to adjust based on more information or thought. A striking example in health care is that physicians tend to stick to their initial diagnosis giving undue weight to confirmatory evidence and despite emerging evidence to the contrary. This has been shown to be a common source of diagnostic error (13). This happens to patients as well: HIV-positive men presented with a hypothetical scenario involving sexual activity with a failed condom estimated the risk of HIV transmission much higher if first asked if it was greater or less than 90% than if they were first asked if it was greater or less than 1%. The high initial anchor of 90% pulled transmission estimates to 64%, while the low anchor at 1% pushed them down to 43%, for the exact same hypothetical scenario (14). Anchoring and adjustment results in biased estimates of risk or chance when adjustment from the initial anchor is inadequate, and affects us all.

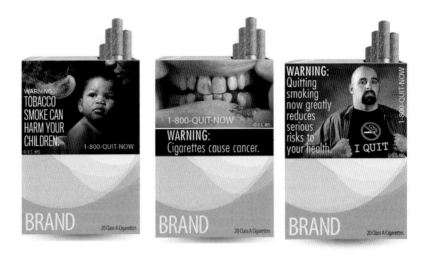

Figure 13.1   U.S. Food and Drug Administration proposed cigarette warning labels.

13.5.4 Affect heuristic

The last heuristic that we will describe is foundational to all the rest: the affect heuristic explains how people are influenced by the positive or negative emotions (i.e., affect) associated with mental representations of events. This heuristic is very easy to understand and relate to for most people. When strong emotions are involved, we tend to focus on the characteristics of an event, *not* the probabilities of occurrence. Fear associated with cancer motivates treatment decisions which oftentimes overrides evidence of limited benefit, as for patients at the end of life when chemotherapy tends to be overused (15), and for men with prostate cancer who shy away from watchful waiting (16,17). The affect heuristic is widely called upon in social marketing and has led to the field known as behavioral economics. Marketing attempts to link emotions with products to transfer that emotional response to the product they are trying to sell or encourage consumption of, such as in the advertising field equating lust for scantily clad women with lust for sports cars, and anti-smoking campaigns that equate cigarettes with fear and disgust (see Figure 13.1). Similarly, the recently failed New York City campaign to ban large-size, sugar-sweetened soft drinks connected the drinks with obesity through vivid images of liquid fat; see for example, You Tube video: Man Drinking Fat. NYC Anti-Soda Ad. Are You Pouring on the Pounds? (retrieved August 18, 2014 from www.youtube.com/watch?v=-F4t8zLGF0c). When people are unsure about risk, probabilities are influenced by the ease or precision with which a probability can be mapped onto an affective impression or emotion (18). Providing these affective associations can influence people's assessment of probabilities, or the chance that something will happen, and having emotions surrounding a situation will also influence people's assessments. These influences extend to feelings of all types, even somewhat distant from the basic emotions of fear or happiness: people are more willing to make decisions that are consistent with existing or recent commitments probably because they feel emotionally more at ease with consistent decisions. This phenomenon has been used to increased compliance with lifestyle modifying interventions, such as by encouraging patients to send a postcard to themselves or a friend stating explicitly what they will change to form a mental commitment that is then consistently followed or not. Emotions are rampant in clinical decision making, so this heuristic is commonplace in health-care choices. As a foundational heuristic, affect also interplays with the other short-cuts described here: it can add a measure of influence to another heuristic at work or can moderate an effect.

13.5.5 Heuristics summary

Heuristics come into play in decision making alone and in combination, and with different importance placed on each. What is important to understand is that these mental short-cuts, these rules of thumb, are used routinely by all of us to deal with uncertainty and time constraints. They can be minimized through structured and systematic thinking, but can rarely be avoided entirely. Most important is to remember that heuristics are omnipresent and should be considered when conducting or guiding decisions, as an analyst or as a clinician.

13.6 Alternatives to 'rational' decision making

Knowing that people are influenced or swayed by various forces that guide their decisions gives us a better understanding of how and why people oftentimes do not behave as the 'rational actors' that we assume they would want to be in decision analysis. Instead, they use heuristics to process information, integrate emotional considerations into choices, and consider other issues (such as equity) in evaluating alternatives – all of which are at least in part antithetical to utility theory, the cornerstone of decision analysis. It is important to remember that decision theory says how people *should* make choices under certain assumptions, not how they *do* behave in actuality. Other theories offer insight into the reality of people's choices and decision making, and the psychology underlying choice. This section of the chapter provides an understanding of the empiric basis of choice.

13.6.1 Prospect theory

When Kahneman and Tversky were describing their observations of how people use heuristics in making judgments, they also proposed Prospect theory to provide a theoretical platform to explain the effect of these and other mechanisms on choices (2). Prospect theory has been debated, adapted, and modified since this time, but it remains the primary alternative to Expected Utility theory to describe decision making under uncertainty. At its core, Prospect theory has three main tenets: (a) for anticipated changes of similar size, 'losses' loom larger to people than do 'gains'; (b) people are 'risk averse' for gains (to preserve benefits) and 'risk seeking' for losses (to avoid harms); and (c) people prefer certain outcomes to those that involve chance. These tenets describe how people react to information about things: how they perceive and process information about outcomes, whether they see them as positive or negative, how they 'feel' about them, and how they interpret (or misinterpret) information about the chance of them occurring. Essentially, this theory describes how the presentation or receipt of a set of outcomes or events influences people's choices. We already know that heuristics guide how people process information, and now we are considering a theory that explains how that information processing determines choices in predictable ways.

13.6.1.1 Framing effects

Framing refers to how a situation is presented to a person, or how a question is phrased. It's the 'frame' that is put around a particular choice.

EXAMPLE 3	**Alternative therapies for lung cancer – part 1(19)**

Think about the following situation:

Surgery for lung cancer involves an operation on the lungs. Most patients are in the hospital for two or three weeks and have some pain around their incisions; they spend a month or so recuperating at home. After that, they generally feel fine.

Radiation therapy for lung cancer involves the use of radiation to kill the tumor and requires coming to the hospital about four times a week for six weeks. Each treatment takes a few minutes and during the treatment, patients lie on a table as if they were having an x-ray. During the course of treatment, some patients develop nausea and vomiting, but by the end of the six weeks they also generally feel fine.

Thus, after the initial six weeks or so, patients treated with either surgery or radiation therapy feel about the same.

Of 100 people having surgery, ten will die during treatment, 32 will have died by one year, and 66 will have died by five years. Of 100 people having radiation therapy, none will die during treatment, 23 will die by one year, and 78 will die by five years.

Which treatment would you prefer?

EXAMPLE 4   **Alternative therapies for lung cancer – part 2(19)**

Think about the same situation:

Surgery for lung cancer involves an operation on the lungs. Most patients are in the hospital for two or three weeks and have some pain around their incisions; they spend a month or so recuperating at home. After that, they generally feel fine.

Radiation therapy for lung cancer involves the use of radiation to kill the tumor and requires coming to the hospital about four times a week for six weeks. Each treatment takes a few minutes and during the treatment, patients lie on a table as if they were having an x-ray. During the course of treatment, some patients develop nausea and vomiting, but by the end of the six weeks they also generally feel fine.

Thus, after the initial six weeks or so, patients treated with either surgery or radiation therapy feel about the same.

Of 100 people having surgery, 90 will survive the surgery, 68 will be alive at one year, and 34 will be alive at five years. Of 100 people having radiation therapy, all will survive the treatment, 77 will be alive at one year, and 22 will be alive at five years.

Which treatment would you prefer?

Consider Examples 3 and 4 that were published in seminal research on framing effects by McNeil and colleagues in the early 1980s (19). Was your preference for surgery or radiation the same in each? As you will notice, surgery has a higher risk of post-treatment death compared to radiation, but has a higher five-year survival probability. The outcome data are the same in both examples but in Example 3 they are presented in terms of the probability of death (i.e., mortality) and in Example 4 they are presented in terms of the probability of living (i.e., survival). The only difference is the *framing* of the outcomes, how they are described. If you were like most people in the original experiment, you found surgery more attractive when the outcomes were presented in terms of survival rather than death: surgery looks better when it's described in terms of how many people survive post-operatively than when it's described in terms of how many people die on the table or immediately thereafter. There's no doubt that long-term survival is better with surgery than radiation, but surgery's post-operative outcome seems to 'loom larger' when it is described in terms of a 10% chance of death than a 90%

chance of survival. This is a classic example of framing affecting preferences: people tend to avoid losses, such as mortality, so when a similar outcome is presented as a loss they shy away from it compared to the same outcome being presented as a gain (i.e., survival). The investigators found this framing effect irrespective of whether respondents were patients, students, or physicians, so it is relatively omnipresent.

Since decisions and options can be described in a multitude of ways, the idea that how something is framed can affect choice implies that people are vulnerable, if you will, to simple details about the presentation of options. Kahneman and Tversky originally presented the hypothesis and supporting data that showed that people are subject to framing effects, and this has been confirmed by many others. It is important to be cognizant of this fact when presenting information to people and when evaluating decisions.

13.6.1.2 Losses versus gains

Prospect theory holds that people think about outcomes relative to some 'reference point,' meaning some point of comparison. People's reference point is usually their current situation: how much money they currently have, or their current health. Someone's reference point can sometimes be what they would *like* their current situation to be, their 'aspired' situation. But more commonly, if someone is offered a $1 million prize they view that money relative to how much money they have right now. You can imagine that the $1 million would be perceived differently by you than by Bill Gates or Warren Buffett.[2]

Equally sized changes that are considered 'gains' are viewed differently than those that are considered 'losses.' According to Prospect theory, 'losses loom larger than gains.' This aversion to losses is generally called just that: 'loss aversion.' It has also been described as an 'endowment effect' or a 'status quo bias.' It means that one places higher value on things one currently has and is contemplating losing, compared with things one does not now have but might have in the future (20). The general idea throughout is that people are particularly averse to making themselves worse off, and will go to what might seem like disproportionate lengths to keep themselves from getting worse compared with what they will do to improve their situation. Think about the lung cancer treatment examples (3,4): death is undoubtedly a loss compared to being alive, while survival is essentially a continuation of the status quo. Hence presented with an outcome framed in terms of a clear loss, people are generally averse toward that scenario compared to the exact same outcome framed in terms of a continuation of the status quo.

---

[2] Bill Gates and Warren Buffett are ranked #2 and #3 respectively on *The World's Billionaires* list published by Forbes.com (as of May 2012).

This behavior is demonstrated throughout domains of life. Kahneman conducted experiments with inconsequential items, like coffee mugs, to demonstrate that people place value on things that they possess regardless of intrinsic value (21). Imagine there are two groups of people: the people in one group are each given a nice ceramic coffee mug from their alma mater. The other group is shown these nice ceramic mugs from their alma maters. The people in the group given the mugs are asked how much they would sell theirs for. The people in the group who have seen pictures of the mugs are asked how much they would pay to buy one for themselves. Which group do you think values the mug higher? If you were in the second group contemplating buying one of these mugs, how much would you pay for it: $5? $7? $10? Now think if you were in the first group and already had one of these mugs. Would you sell it for $5? For $7? $10? In general, people require *more* money to part with their mug than they would pay to buy one. So the *loss* of a mug they already have is worth more than the *gain* of a new mug. Alternately stated, the mug they possess is worth more than the mug they could buy.

Now think of how this applies to health decisions in general. If each individual person has a reference point, a status quo, or their current 'endowment' of health, they may be more reluctant to part with any health, to become worse off, than they would be willing to invest to improve their health. People will generally endure uncomfortable and invasive treatments to avoid a condition worsening but they are generally reluctant to engage in health promoting activities. Think of the lung transplant patient who refuses to stop smoking.

13.6.1.3 Risk aversion and risk seeking

Framing can also be thought of as how people think about risk: their risk 'posture.' As described in Chapter 4, people feel differently about different types of risks. This is in addition to how they perceive information about hazards, as described earlier in this chapter in the section on heuristics. Prospect theory holds that people are 'risk averse' for gains and 'risk seeking' (or 'risk loving') for losses. That means that people do not like to take risks when they involve gains, and are eager to take risks when they involve (i.e., avoid) losses. In a practical example this becomes clearer:

EXAMPLE 5A   **Disease outbreak (1)**

Imagine that the US is preparing for the outbreak of an unusual Asian disease, which is expected to kill 600 people. Two alternative programs to combat the disease have been proposed. Assume that the exact scientific estimate of the consequences of the programs are as follows:

If Program A is adopted, 200 people will be saved.

If Program B is adopted, there is 1/3 probability that 600 people will be saved, and 2/3 probability that no people will be saved.

Which of the two programs would you favor?

EXAMPLE 5B   **Disease outbreak**

Now imagine two different programs have been proposed. Assume that the exact scientific estimate of the consequences of the programs are as follows:

If Program C is adopted 400 people will die.

If Program D is adopted there is 1/3 probability that nobody will die, and 2/3 probability that 600 people will die.

Which of these two programs would you favor?

Looking closely at the examples, you will notice that all the programs have the same expected value: of the 600 people that the outbreak is expected to kill, all four programs result in 200 living and 400 dying. The differences are in framing: Programs A and C offer certain outcomes, while B and D offer uncertain ones, where there is a chance of two outcomes. In addition, A and B are presented in terms of people being saved, while C and D are presented in terms of people dying. Apart from the wording, options A and C are in fact identical and options B and D are identical. But again, all four offer the same outcome. Which did you prefer?

When tested experimentally, Kahneman and Tversky found that most people offered the choice between programs A and B (Example 5a) preferred saving 200 people for sure over taking a chance of saving 600 or none (72% in fact [1]). When presented the options framed in terms of people dying (Example 5b), most people (78%) preferred the 2/3 chance of 600 people dying or 1/3 chance of none, rather than the sure deaths of 400. When the choice was framed as a gain as in Example 5a, that is, saving people, subjects were *averse* to taking a risk; they preferred the certain outcome of Program A. Conversely, when the choice was framed as a *loss* as in 5b, that is, people dying, subjects *sought* a risk; they preferred the chance outcome of Program D. In both cases the expected values of the sure and chance outcomes were the same, but people were more willing to take a risk if the outcome represented a loss and were less willing to take a risk if the outcome represented a gain.

Despite clear differences in how people react to, understand, and perceive messages framed in different ways (19), we still do not have clear evidence to support any single, consistent approach to effect behavior change. The cigarette warning labels in Figure 13.1 are three examples of many that were developed to address message receptivity by different subsets of the population (22, 23). You will notice that these examples all use a negative emotional frame (harm children, cause cancer, risks to health), but the right-most one includes the outcome framed as a gain (reduces serious risks). Thus, most important is understanding the elements of framing that may affect the different elements of communication (perception, understanding, persuasion) and to be intentional in their inclusion or exclusion in messages.

13.6.1.4 Certainty effect

The final piece of Prospect theory for discussion is the certainty effect. The certainty effect describes how people's preferences lean toward things that are certain over things that have an element of chance. This holds true even if the certain outcome is itself less desirable. For example, most people would prefer a guaranteed one week vacation to a nearby beach over a 50% chance of a two-week vacation to a tropical island. This is somewhat different than our discussion of heuristics above, which explained how people interpret and understand probabilities. The certainty effect applies once people have settled upon their understanding of a probability. After probability information has been integrated and understood in people's minds, they show a preference for the probabilities that are 100% or 0%, the certain probabilities, over all the rest. This observation can be extended to see that people view differences between probabilities depending upon where that difference falls on the probability continuum: the difference between a 1% risk of death and a 0% risk of death is more meaningful to people than the difference between a 3% risk of death and a 2% risk of death. Even though both differences in absolute terms are equivalent, arriving at certainty that death will not occur, at the 0% risk, holds added importance for people compared with reducing risk from a very small chance to a slightly lower very small chance, as is in the 3% to 2% difference.

The certainty effect was first described by Maurice Allais and is known as the Allais paradox (24). Kahneman and Tversky demonstrated the paradox with monetary choices, and observed that people's behavior could be considered 'irrational' since the certain outcomes that people tended to prefer had lower expected value than the ones that involved chance. Consider the following experiment they performed (2):

Choice A offers an 80% chance of winning $4000 or a 20% chance of winning nothing.

Choice B offers a 100% chance of winning $3000.

If offered to choose one of these, which would you take?

As you can see, Choice A has an expected value of 0.8*$4000 = $3200, which exceeds Choice B's value of $3000 (1.0*$3,000). Yet 80% of respondents in Kahneman and Tversky's experiment chose B, the $3000 for sure, over choice A that involved an element of chance but a higher expected value of $3200. The certainty effect has been confirmed with other monetary choices, different probabilities, and different outcomes. The implications for medical decision making are substantial: in a field where little is actually certain, people's strong desire for sure outcomes must be remembered during the decision making process. If people come to believe that an outcome is certain, either in actuality or through their perception of probability information, we know that they will place added meaning on that certainty, beyond what is expected from a 'rational' perspective.

13.6.2 Regret theory

Although Prospect theory has gained prominence as an alternative to Expected Utility theory, other alternatives have been explored as well. One that is particularly relevant to medical decision making is Regret theory (25). Developed by Loomes and Sugden, Regret theory holds that an important consideration in people's decision among choices is the 'what might have been' aspect of the alternative not chosen. The possible 'regret' that accompanies making a choice that turns out badly, or the 'rejoicing' that accompanies a choice that turns out well, are significant considerations in decision making under this framework. Regret theory holds that the incorporation of these components into decisions explains some of the apparent irrationality of decisions and makes them instead appear to be rational. Loomes and Sugden provide an example of comparing the loss of £100 due to a tax increase with the loss of the same amount bet on a horse race. The betting loss would likely be experienced more painful because it would inspire more regret of what might otherwise have been done with the money, than the compulsory nature of the tax increase which also eliminates alternative uses of the money. Conversely, the theorists propose that one would rejoice more from a £100 gain from a bet than from a £100 gain from a tax reduction.

Applied to health decisions, Regret theory holds intuitive appeal. People may be worried about making the 'wrong' decision, particularly when making a medical decision for a loved one, and this anticipated regret may weigh heavily on their choice. If Regret theory holds true, this anticipation has a value for people and as such is a reasonable and rational factor to include in decision making. So a choice between surgery and 'watchful waiting' for prostate cancer, for example, may reasonably include consideration of the regret one might feel if the cancer progresses and the surgery were not chosen.

A tangible example of Regret theory is how people make choices about cellular telephone service plans. Many companies in the USA offer a set number of 'minutes' that a customer can use in a particular month for a flat fee, and any usage over this amount is charged at a very high rate per minute. People generally purchase plans with more minutes than they need because of the fear of exceeding the flat amount and incurring the high per-minute penalty charges. In a sense, they anticipate regret at making the wrong choice, and over-purchase minutes to avoid this experience. People generally do not calculate the expected value of the cost of the plan with more minutes compared with the probability of exceeding the usage quota times the cost/minute of the extra calls. Regret theory explains that people make decisions incorporating this consideration of what *might have been* rather than purely optimizing the expected value of different outcomes. In this way, similar outcomes have different utility to people, or they are experienced and valued differently, based on expectations of regret or rejoicing.

Regret theory offers an alternative explanation to Prospect theory for people's choices when faced with decisions that include uncertainty. Both offer insight into how psychological forces influence decision making and add complementarity to the psychology of choice.

13.6.3 Intuitive decision making

Many physicians and patients rely on their intuition to make important health-care decisions. As we have seen, our intuition may be misled by heuristics and biases. At the same time, our intuition also has strengths. Although decision analysis is generally considered a rational analytical approach to decision making, the underlying philosophy is to *integrate* the rational analytical aspects of a decision problem, i.e., the evidence, with the psychological subjective aspects, i.e., our values. Integrating the evidence and values may be done qualitatively based on an intuitive balance sheet or quantitatively by calculating the expected value of each option.

Even though decision analysis advocates rational decision making, the final decision is generally not based on one hard number from the analysis. The process itself is probably more important than the final result and the insight gained during the process usually has more effect than the numbers that are calculated. Having taken into account all the information you have found during the process and after looking at the problem from various different viewpoints in multiple ways, you finally need to use your judgment and *intuition* to decide whether the analysis sufficiently reflects reality, whether the intangibles have been sufficiently considered, which evidence and values apply to the situation at hand, whether the crucial information is available, and finally whether your decision should be based on the results. In this sense, decision making attempts consciously to reconcile rationality and intuition, that is, what is going on in our head with that which is going on in our heart.

An integrated decision approach might proceed as follows: first, the rational components: get a good overview of all objective aspects of the problem and attempt to identify subjective ones. Second, the intuitive process: sleep on it, move onto something else, let the unconscious mind process the information. Third, integrate heart and head: allow both rational and intuitive aspects a say in the final decision, fully aware of the strengths and limitations of each. Finally: evaluate the outcome of the decision in a rational way accounting for hindsight bias and regret, to assess need for reconsideration and to inform future decisions.

The intuitive nature of decision making is well known and acknowledged, yet hard to measure and integrate into an analysis. The psychological aspects are numerous and far reaching. This chapter has skimmed the surface of decision psychology to raise awareness of this intuitive component rather than trying to be exhaustive about the subject. Awareness of our humanness, and the integral element of our psyches in all decisions at all levels, is the first step toward improving the decision process and outcomes.

13.7 Summary

This chapter has served to enrich the information provided in this book, to understand the reality of people's decision making side-by-side with the optimal ways of analyzing choice. Having an understanding and appreciation of the psychology of judgment and choice helps us to better interpret and predict people's decisions in clinical encounters. It also helps us as analysts to know how our own psychology may be influencing our work, to ensure that we incorporate these forces intentionally (if so desired) rather than by default. Though decision analysis adds a systematic and objective layer to the process of choice, we must always remember that people are not machines and the optimal choice may not on the surface appear to be a rational one. People generally optimize their own utility, or in other words, make decisions that are in their own best interest, and decision analysis can provide information and guidance about how this goal is best achieved. The psychology of choice helps us understand what that best interest may be to each person, and how we can provide the best assistance in the decision process for individuals and for society as a whole. At the end of the day, the goal of decision analysis is to assist with decision making, not to prescribe choices. This chapter on the psychology of choice provides a lens through which we can see how people may diverge from what we may think is the 'best' choice, and it reminds us that despite our rigorous analytic techniques, optimal choice is often in the eye of the beholder and must be respected as such.

REFERENCES

1. Tversky A, Kahneman D. The framing of decisions and the psychology of choice. *Science.* 1981;211:453–58.
2. Kahneman D, Tversky A. Prospect theory: an analysis of decision under risk. *Econometrica.* 1979;47(2):263–91.
3. Kahneman D, Slovic P, Tversky A, eds. Judgment under Uncertainty: Heuristics and Biases. New York: Cambridge University Press; 1982.
4. Kahneman D. *Thinking, Fast and Slow.* New York: Farrar, Straus and Giroux; 2011.
5. McFadden D. Rationality for economists? *J Risk Uncertainty.* 1999;19(1–3):73–105.
6. Slovic P, Fischhoff B, Lichtenstein S. Characterizing perceived risk. In: Kates R, Hohenemser C, Kasperson R, eds. Perilous Progress: Managing the Hazards of Technology. Boulder, CO: Westview; 1985.
7. Ariely D. *Predictably Irrational.* New York: HarperCollins Publishers; 2008.
8. Katapodi MC, Lee KA, Facione NC, Dodd MJ. Predictors of perceived breast cancer risk and the relation between perceived risk and breast cancer screening: a meta-analytic review. *Prev Med.* 2004;38(4):388–402.
9. Tversky A, Kahneman D. Judgment under uncertainty: heuristics and biases. *Science.* 1974;185:1124–31.
10. Avis NE, Smith KW, McKinlay JB. Accuracy of perceptions of heart attack risk: what influences perceptions and can they be changed? *Am J Public Health.* 1989; 79(12):1608–12.
11. Cull A, Anderson ED, Campbell S, et al. The impact of genetic counselling about breast cancer risk on women's risk perceptions and levels of distress. *Br J Cancer.* 1999;79(3–4):501–8.
12. Gurmankin AD, Domchek S, Stopfer J, Fels C, Armstrong K. Patients' resistance to risk information in genetic counseling for BRCA1/2. *Arch Intern Med.* 2005; 165(5):523–9.
13. Kassirer J, Wong J, Kopelman R. Learning Clinical Reasoning. 2nd edn. Philadelphia, PA: Lippincott, Williams and Wilkins; 2010.
14. Brewer NT, Chapman GB, Schwartz JA, Bergus GR. The influence of irrelevant anchors on the judgments and choices of doctors and patients. *Med Decis Making.* 2007;27(2):203–11.
15. Earle CC, Landrum MB, Souza JM, et al. Aggressiveness of cancer care near the end of life: is it a quality-of-care issue? *J Clin Oncol.* 2008;26(23):3860–6.
16. Holmboe ES, Concato J. Treatment decisions for localized prostate cancer: asking men what's important. *J Gen Intern Med.* 2000;15(10):694–701.

17. Xu J, Dailey RK, Eggly S, Neale AV, Schwartz KL. Men's perspectives on selecting their prostate cancer treatment. *J Natl Med Assoc.* 2011;103(6):468–78.

18. Bateman I, Dent S, Peters E, Slovic P, Starmer C. The affect heuristic and the attractiveness of simple gambles. *J Behav Decis Making.* 2007;20(4):365–80.

19. McNeil B, Pauker S, Sox H, Tversky A. On the elicitation of preferences for alternative therapies. *N Engl J Med.* 1982;306:1259–62.

20. Kahneman D, Knetsch J, Thaler R. The endowment effect, loss aversion, and status quo bias. *J Econ Perspect.* 1991;5(1):193–206.

21. Kahneman D, Knetsch J, Thaler R. Experimental tests of the endowment effect and the Coase theorem. *J Polit Econ.* 1990;98(6):1325–48.

22. Bansal-Travers M, Hammond D, Smith P, Cummings KM. The impact of cigarette pack design, descriptors, and warning labels on risk perception in the U.S. *Am J Prev Med.* 2011;40(6):674–82.

23. Nonnemaker J, Farrelly M, Kamyab K, Busey A, Ann N. *Experimental Study of Graphic Cigarette Warning Labels.* Research Triangle Park, NC: RTI International; 2010.

24. Allais M. Le comportement de l'homme rationnel devant le risque: critique des postulats et axiomes de l'école Américaine. *Econometrica.* 1953;21(4):503–46.

25. Loomes G, Sugden R. Regret theory: An alternative theory of rational choice under uncertainty. *Econ J.* 1982;92(4):805–24.

Index